EVIDENCE-BASED RHEUMATOLOGY FOR PRIMARY CARE PROVIDERS

EVIDENCE-BASED RHEUMATOLOGY
FOR PRIMARY CARE PROVIDERS

Copyright © 2024 by Huynh Wynn Tran

Cover: Artist Dinh Khai - Book designer: Tien Minh Nguyen

United Buddhist Publisher (UBF)

First printed in California, USA, October 2024

ISBN-13: 979-8-3304-7414-1

© All rights reserved. No part of this book may be reproduced by any means without prior written permission.

HUYNH WYNN TRAN, MD, FACP, FACR

EVIDENCE-BASED RHEUMATOLOGY

FOR PRIMARY CARE PROVIDERS

UBP UNITED BUDDHIST PUBLISHER

Preface

The United States is facing a significant shortage of rheumatologists, which poses a growing challenge in the management of patients with rheumatic diseases.

In 2021, there were approximately 5,500 adult rheumatologists across the country, but projections estimate that this number will decrease to 4,700 by 2030. This decline is occurring at a time when the demand for rheumatologic services is on the rise due to the aging U.S. population and the increasing prevalence of chronic conditions such as rheumatoid arthritis (RA), osteoarthritis (OA), systemic lupus erythematosus (SLE), and gout.

With fewer rheumatologists available to provide care, more and more patients with rheumatic diseases are turning to primary care providers (PCPs) for the management of their conditions. In this context, it is crucial for PCPs and other midlevel providers to have a solid foundation in basic rheumatology to effectively care for these patients and improve their outcomes.

This book, Evidence-Based Rheumatology for Primary Care Providers, aims to bridge that knowledge gap and empower PCPs to confidently manage common rheumatologic conditions. The book is divided into four parts, each designed to provide a comprehensive overview of the most important aspects of rheumatology, from the basic immunology, pathophysiology, diagnosis of diseases to evidence-based treatment approaches, and long-term management strategies.

It is our hope that this resource will serve as a practical guide to improving the quality of care for rheumatology patients in primary care settings.

Huynh Wynn Tran, MD, FACP, FACR
Associate Professor of Medicine and Pharmacy
CEO/Founder of Wynn Medical Center Clinics
Los Angeles, California, USA

CONTENTS

Preface	5
Part 1: Rheumatology in Primary Care and Rheumatologic Foundations	**17**
Chapter 1: The Scope of Rheumatology in Primary Care	19
1.1. The Importance of Rheumatologic Conditions in General Practice	19
1.1.1. Chronic Disease Burden	19
1.1.2. Early Detection of Rheumatologic Conditions in Primary Care	20
1.2. Epidemiology of Rheumatologic Diseases: Global and Local Perspectives	21
1.3. Role of the Primary Care Provider (PCP) in Early Detection and Management Rheumatologic Disorders	22
Chapter 2: What is Evidence-Based Medicine (EBM)?	25
2.1. How to Apply EBM Rheumatology in Clinical Practice	25
2.2. Evaluating Research and Clinical Trials in Rheumatology	26
Chapter 3: Immunology and Pathophysiology of Rheumatologic Diseases	29
3.1. Overview of the Immune System	29
3.1.1. Innate Immune System	29
3.1.2. Adaptive Immune System	30
3.1.3. Dysregulation Leading to Autoimmune Diseases	31
3.2. Mechanisms of Autoimmunity and Chronic Inflammation	32
3.3. Genetics and Environmental Triggers in Autoimmune Diseases	32
3.4. The Role of Cytokines and Other Mediators in Rheumatic Disease	33
Chapter 4: Diagnostic Approach to Rheumatologic Conditions	35
4.1 History Taking Skills in Rheumatology	35
4.1.1. Pattern and Onset of Symptoms	35
4.1.2. Symmetry of Joint Involvement	36
4.1.3. Morning Stiffness	36
4.1.4. Systemic Symptoms	37
4.1.5. Previous Joint or Muscle Involvement	37
4.2. Key Symptoms: Joint Pain, Stiffness, Swelling, and Systemic Symptoms	38
4.3. The Rheumatologic Physical Examination: Identifying Joint, Skin, and Muscle Abnormalities	38
4.4. Red Flags in Rheumatology: When to Suspect a Serious Condition	39
Chapter 5: Laboratory Investigations in Rheumatology	41
5.1. Commonly Used Laboratory Tests: Rheumatoid Factor (RF), Anti-CCP, ANA, ESR, CRP	41
5.2. Understanding Autoantibodies: ANA Subtypes, ANCA, Anti-dsDNA	42
5.3. Synovial Fluid Analysis: Indications and Interpretation	42
5.4. Emerging Biomarkers in Rheumatologic Diseases	43

Chapter 6: Imaging in Rheumatology ... 45
   6.1. X-Rays Findings in Rheumatic Diseases ... 45
      6.1.1. Rheumatoid Arthritis (RA) ... 45
      6.1.2. Osteoarthritis (OA) ... 45
      6.1.3. Ankylosing Spondylitis (AS) ... 46
      6.1.4. Gout ... 46
      6.1.5. Limitations of X-Rays ... 47
   6.2. Ultrasound in Joint Assessment: Benefits and Limitations ... 47
      6.2.1. Benefits of Ultrasound in Rheumatic Diseases ... 48
      6.2.2. Limitations of Ultrasound in Rheumatic Diseases ... 49
      6.2.3. ACR Guidelines on Ultrasound Use in Rheumatology ... 49
   6.3. Advanced Imaging: MRI and CT for Rheumatic Conditions ... 50
      6.3.1. MRI in Rheumatic Diseases ... 50
      6.3.2. CT in Rheumatic Diseases ... 52
   6.4. Novel Techniques: Dual-Energy CT, PET-CT in Inflammatory Arthritis ... 52
      6.4.1. Dual-Energy CT (DECT) ... 53
      6.4.2. Positron Emission Tomography-Computed Tomography (PET-CT) ... 54

Part 2: Common Rheumatologic Diseases and Evidence-Based Management ... **57**
Chapter 7: Rheumatoid Arthritis (RA) ... 59
   7.1. Epidemiology and Pathophysiology of RA ... 59
   7.2. RA Diagnostic Criteria and Disease Staging ... 59
   7.3. Evidence-Based Pharmacological Treatments: DMARDs, Biologics, JAK Inhibitors ... 60
      7.3.1. DMARDs (Disease-Modifying Antirheumatic Drugs) ... 60
      7.3.2 Biologics ... 61
      7.3.3. JAK Inhibitors ... 62
   7.4. Non-Pharmacological Interventions: Physical Therapy, Occupational Therapy ... 63
      7.4.1. Physical Therapy (PT) ... 63
      7.4.2. Occupational Therapy (OT) ... 64
      7.4.3. The Role of Non-Pharmacological Interventions in Complementary RA Treatment ... 65
   7.5. Long-Term Monitoring: Remission and Disease Flares ... 65
   7.6. Managing Comorbidities: Cardiovascular Risk, Osteoporosis ... 65
Chapter 8: Osteoarthritis (OA) ... 67
   8.1. Etiology and Risk Factors of OA: Primary vs. Secondary OA ... 67
   8.2. Clinical Presentation: Differentiating from Inflammatory Arthritis ... 67
   8.3. Diagnostic Imaging and Criteria for OA ... 60
   8.4. OA Stepwise Management: From Conservative Therapies to Surgical Interventions ... 68
      8.4.1. Non-Pharmacologic: Weight Management, Exercise, Joint Protection ... 69
      8.4.2. Pharmacologic: NSAIDs, Topical Agents, Intra-Articular Injections ... 71
      8.4.3. Role of Surgery: When to Refer for Joint Replacement ... 74
Chapter 9: Systemic Lupus Erythematosus (SLE) ... 77

- 9.1. Overview of Lupus Pathogenesis and Risk Factors — 77
  - 9.1.1. Pathogenesis of SLE — 77
  - 9.1.2. Genetic Factors in SLE — 78
  - 9.1.3. Hormonal and Environmental Triggers — 78
- 9.2. Clinical Manifestations: Mucocutaneous, Renal, CNS, and Hematologic Involvement — 79
  - 9.2.1. Mucocutaneous Manifestations — 79
  - 9.2.2. Renal Involvement (Lupus Nephritis) — 80
  - 9.2.3. Central Nervous System (CNS) Involvement — 81
  - 9.2.4. Hematologic Involvement — 81
  - 9.2.5. Other Common Manifestations — 82
- 9.3. Diagnostic Criteria and the Role of Autoantibodies — 82
  - 9.3.1. ACR/EULAR Classification Criteria for SLE — 82
  - 9.3.2. Role of Autoantibodies in SLE Diagnosis and Monitoring — 83
- 9.4. Evidence-Based Treatment Approaches: Immunosuppressants, Biologics — 85
  - 9.4.1. Immunosuppressants — 85
  - 9.4.2. Biologic Therapies — 86
- 9.5. Managing Lupus Nephritis and Other Organ-Specific Complications — 87
  - 9.5.1. Lupus Nephritis (LN) — 88
  - 9.5.2. Neuropsychiatric Lupus (NPSLE) — 88
  - 9.5.3. Antiphospholipid Syndrome (APS) — 89
- 9.6. Monitoring Disease Activity and Adjusting Treatment — 90
  - 9.6.1. Disease Activity Monitoring — 90
  - 9.6.2. Adjusting Treatment Based on Disease Activity — 91

Chapter 10: Gout and Hyperuricemia — 95
- 10.1. Pathophysiology of Gout: Uric Acid Metabolism and Crystal Formation — 95
  - 10.1.1. Uric Acid Metabolism — 95
  - 10.1.2. Crystal Formation and Inflammation — 96
- 10.2. Clinical Phases of Gout: Asymptomatic Hyperuricemia, Acute Flares, Chronic Gouty Arthritis — 97
  - 10.2.1. Asymptomatic Hyperuricemia — 97
  - 10.2.2. Acute Gout Flares — 97
  - 10.2.3. Intercritical Gout — 98
  - 10.2.4. Chronic Gouty Arthritis — 99
- 10.3. Gout Diagnosis: Clinical Presentation and Synovial Fluid Analysis — 99
  - 10.3.1. Clinical Presentation — 99
  - 10.3.2. Synovial Fluid Analysis — 100
- 10.4. Acute Management: NSAIDs, Colchicine, Corticosteroids — 101
  - 10.4.1. NSAIDs (Nonsteroidal Anti-Inflammatory Drugs — 102
  - 10.4.2. Colchicine — 102
  - 10.4.3. Corticosteroids — 103

- 10.5. Long-Term Management: Urate-Lowering Therapies (Allopurinol, Febuxostat) — 104
  - 10.5.1. Allopurinol: First-Line Xanthine Oxidase Inhibitor — 104
  - 10.5.2. Febuxostat: Alternative Xanthine Oxidase Inhibitor — 105
  - 10.5.3. Uricosurics — 106
  - 10.5.4. Prophylaxis During ULT Initiation — 106
- 10.6. Lifestyle Modifications and Dietary Recommendations — 107
  - 10.6.1. Dietary Recommendations — 107
  - 10.6.2. Weight Management — 108
  - 10.6.3. Hydration — 109

Chapter 11: Psoriatic Arthritis (PsA) — 111
- 11.1. Overview of Psoriasis and Its Link to Arthritis — 111
  - 11.1.1 Psoriasis: An Overview — 111
  - 11.1.2. Link to Arthritis: Psoriatic Arthritis (PsA) — 112
- 11.2. Clinical Subtypes and Presentation of Psoriatic Arthritis — 113
  - 11.2.1. Oligoarticular PsA — 113
  - 11.2.2. Polyarticular PsA — 114
  - 11.2.3. DIP Predominant PsA — 114
  - 11.2.4. Spondylitis PsA — 115
  - 11.2.5. Arthritis Mutilans — 115
  - 11.2.5. Extra-Articular Manifestations — 116
- 11.3. Diagnostic Criteria and Role of Imaging — 116
  - 11.3.1. CASPAR Criteria (Classification Criteria for Psoriatic Arthritis) — 116
  - 11.3.2. Role of Imaging in PsA Diagnosis — 117
- 11.4. Treatment Options: NSAIDs, DMARDs, Biologics — 118
  - 11.4.1. NSAIDs (Nonsteroidal Anti-Inflammatory Drugs) — 119
  - 11.4.2. Conventional DMARDs (Disease-Modifying Antirheumatic Drugs) — 119
  - 11.4.3. Biologic DMARDs — 120
  - 11.4.4. JAK Inhibitors — 121
- 11.5. Importance of Early Diagnosis to Prevent Joint Damage — 122
  - 11.5.1. Joint Damage and Disability in PsA — 122
  - 11.5.2. Role of Screening in Psoriasis Patients — 122
  - 11.5.3. Treat-to-Target (T2T) Approach — 123

Chapter 12: Ankylosing Spondylitis and Axial Spondyloarthritis — 125
- 12.1. Pathophysiology and Genetics of Axial Spondyloarthritis — 125
  - 12.1.1. Immune Dysregulation in AxSpA — 125
  - 12.1.2. Role of HLA-B27 in AxSpA — 126
  - 12.1.3. Environmental Triggers in AxSpA — 126
- 12.2. Clinical Features: Chronic Back Pain, Enthesitis, and Extra-Articular Manifestations — 127
  - 12.2.1. Chronic Inflammatory Back Pain — 127
  - 12.2.2. Enthesitis — 128
  - 12.2.3. Extra-Articular Manifestations — 128

12.3. Diagnostic Criteria: Role of HLA-B27 and Imaging	130
12.3.1. ASAS Criteria for Axial Spondyloarthritis (AxSpA)	130
12.3.2. Role of Imaging in AxSpA Diagnosis	130
12.3.3. HLA-B27 in AxSpA Diagnosis	132
12.4. Evidence-Based Pharmacologic Treatments: NSAIDs, TNF Inhibitors, IL-17 Inhibitors	132
12.4.1. NSAIDs (Nonsteroidal Anti-Inflammatory Drugs)	133
12.5. Non-Pharmacological Management: Physical Therapy, Exercise	135
12.5.1. Physical Therapy (PT) in AxSpA Management	135
12.5.2. Exercise in AxSpA	136
12.5.3. Patient Education and Lifestyle Modifications	136
Chapter 13: Fibromyalgia	139
13.1. Pathogenesis and Risk Factors for Fibromyalgia	139
13.1.1. Central Sensitization in Fibromyalgia	139
13.1.2. Genetic and Environmental Factors	140
13.1.3. Risk Factors for Fibromyalgia	140
13.2. Diagnosis: Differentiating Fibromyalgia from Inflammatory Diseases	141
13.2.1. Diagnostic Criteria for Fibromyalgia (2016 ACR Criteria)	141
13.2.2. Differentiating Fibromyalgia from Inflammatory Diseases	142
13.3. Evidence-Based Treatment: Pharmacologic (Antidepressants, Anticonvulsants) and Nonpharmacologic (Cognitive Behavioral Therapy, Exercise)	143
13.3.1. Pharmacologic Treatment	143
13.3.2. Non-Pharmacologic Treatment	145
13.5. Managing Chronic Pain and Mental Health	146
13.5.1. Multidisciplinary Approach	146
13.5. 2. Sleep Hygiene	147
13.5.3. Mindfulness and Relaxation Techniques	147
13.5.4. Support Groups and Patient Education	148
Chapter 14: Vasculitis Syndromes	151
14.1. Overview of Vasculitis: Small, Medium, and Large Vessel Types	151
14.1.1. Small-Vessel Vasculitis	151
14.1.2. Medium-Vessel Vasculitis	152
14.1.3. Large-Vessel Vasculitis	152
14.2. Diagnostic Approach: Laboratory Testing and Biopsy	153
14.2.1. Laboratory Testing	153
14.2.2. Biopsy	155
14.2.3. Advanced Imaging	156
14.3. Treatment Strategies for Common Vasculitic Syndromes	156
14.3.1. Giant Cell Arteritis (GCA)	156
14.3.2. Granulomatosis with Polyangiitis (GPA)	158
14.3.3. Polyarteritis Nodosa (PAN)	159

  14.3.4. Eosinophilic Granulomatosis with Polyangiitis (EGPA)   159
 14.4. Long-Term Monitoring and Risk of Relapse   160
  14.4.1. Risk of Relapse in Vasculitis   160
  14.4.2. Long-Term Monitoring in Vasculitis   161
  14.4.3. Immunosuppressive Management and Relapse Prevention   162

Chapter 15: Sjogren's Syndrome   165
 15.1. Overview of Sjogren's Syndrome (SS)   165
  15.1.1. Extraglandular Manifestations: 165
  15.1.2. Epidemiology   166
  15.1.3. Risk of Lymphoma in SS   166
 15.2. Diagnostic Approach   166
  15.2.1. Clinical Presentation   166
  15.2.2. Serologic Testing   167
  15.2.3. Glandular Investigations   168
  15.2.4. ACR/EULAR Classification Criteria (2016)   168
 15.3. Treatment Strategies   169
  15.3.1. Management of Sicca Symptoms   169
  15.3.2. Systemic Therapy for Extraglandular Manifestations   170
  15.3.3. Management of Lymphoma Risk   171
 15.4. Long-Term Monitoring   171
  15.4.1. Regular Follow-up   171
  15.4.2. Monitoring for Lymphoma   172
  15.4.3. Monitoring Disease Activity   173
  15.4.4. Long-Term Management Goals   173

Chapter 16: Osteoporosis   175
 16.1. Overview of Osteoporosis   175
  16.1.1. Epidemiology   175
  16.1.2. Pathophysiology   175
  16.1.3. Fracture Risk and Morbidity   176
 16.2. Diagnostic Approach   176
  16.2.1. Clinical Risk Factors   176
  16.2.2. Bone Mineral Density (BMD) Testing   177
  16.2.3. Laboratory Evaluation   178
  16.2.4. Fracture Risk Assessment Tool (FRAX)   178
 16.3. Treatment Strategies: Evidence-Based Approach   179
  16.3.1. Non-Pharmacological Management   179
  16.3.2. Pharmacological Management   180
  16.3.3. Combination Therapy   182
 16.4. Long-Term Monitoring   182
  16.4.1. Monitoring Bone Density   182
  16.4.2. Monitoring for Adverse Effects   183

16.3. Fall Prevention and Patient Education	184
Chapter 17: Sarcoidosis	187
17.1. Overview of Sarcoidosis	187
17.1.1. Epidemiology:	187
17.1.2. Pathophysiology:	187
17.1.3. Clinical Manifestations:	188
17.2. Diagnostic Approach	189
17.2.1. Clinical Presentation	189
17.2.2. Diagnostic Testing	190
17.2.3. Diagnostic Criteria	192
17.3. Treatment Strategies: Evidence-Based Approach	192
17.3.1. Indications for Treatment	192
17.3.2. Pharmacological Treatment	193
17.4. Long-Term Monitoring	195
17.4.1. Monitoring Disease Activity	195
17.4.2. Monitoring for Treatment Complications	196
17.4.3. Patient Education and Follow-Up	196
Chapter 18: Systemic Scleroderma	199
18.1. Overview of Systemic Scleroderma	199
18.1.1. Epidemiology	199
18.1.2. Pathophysiology	199
18.1.3. Clinical Manifestations	201
18.2. Diagnostic Approach	202
18.2.1. Clinical Evaluation	203
18.2.2. Serological Testing	203
18.2.3. Imaging and Functional Studies	204
18.2.4. Diagnostic Criteria	204
18.3. Treatment Strategies: Evidence-Based Approach	205
18.3.1. Pharmacological Therapy	205
18.3.2. Non-Pharmacological Interventions	207
18.4. Long-Term Monitoring	207
18.4.1. Monitoring Organ Function	207
18.4.2. Patient Education and Multidisciplinary Care	209
Chapter 19: Dermatomyositis	211
19.1. Overview	211
19.1.1. Adults vs. Juvenile Dermatomyositis	211
19.1.2. Overview	211
19.1.3. Pathophysiology	212
19.2. Diagnostic Approach	212
19.2.1. Clinical Features	212
19.2.2. Laboratory Tests	213

19.2.3. Cancer Screening in Adults	215
19.3. Treatment Strategies	215
19.3.1. First-Line Therapy: Corticosteroids	215
19.3.2. Immunosuppressants	215
19.3.3. Intravenous Immunoglobulin (IVIG)	216
19.3.4. Biologic Agents	216
19.3.5. Physical Therapy	217
19.3.6. Other Therapies	217
19.4. Long-Term Monitoring	218
19.4.1. Muscle Strength and Function	218
19.4.2. Laboratory Monitoring	218
19.4.3. Pulmonary Function	219
19.4.4. Bone Health	219
19.4.5. Skin Monitoring	219
19.4.6. Cancer Surveillance in Adults	220
19.4.7. Psychosocial Support	220
Part 3: Special Considerations in Rheumatologic Care	**223**
Chapter 20: Rheumatologic Emergencies	225
20.1. Acute Monoarthritis and Septic Arthritis	225
20.1.1. Etiology of Septic Arthritis	225
20.1.2. Diagnosis of Septic Arthritis	226
20.1.3. Management of Septic Arthritis	226
20.1.4. Complications of Septic Arthritis	227
20.2. Temporal Arteritis and Risk of Vision Loss	228
20.2.1. Clinical Presentation of GCA	228
20.2.2. Urgent Diagnosis of GCA	229
20.2.3. Management of GCA and Prevention of Vision Loss	230
20.3. Scleroderma Renal Crisis	230
20.3.1. Pathogenesis and Risk Factors of Scleroderma Renal Crisis	231
20.3.2. Clinical Presentation of Scleroderma Renal Crisis	231
20.3.3. Diagnosis of Scleroderma Renal Crisis	232
20.3.4. Management of Scleroderma Renal Crisis	232
20.3.5. Prognosis and Long-Term Outcomes	233
20.4. Vasculitis Flares and Pulmonary-Renal Syndrome	233
20.4.1. Clinical Presentation of Pulmonary-Renal Syndrome	234
20.4.2. Diagnosis of Pulmonary-Renal Syndrome	234
20.4.3. Management of Pulmonary-Renal Syndrome	235
20.4.4. Prognosis and Outcomes	236
Chapter 21: Rheumatologic Disease in Pregnancy	239
21.1. Managing Autoimmune Diseases During Pregnancy	239
21.1.1. Systemic Lupus Erythematosus (SLE)	239

21.1.2. Antiphospholipid Syndrome (APS)	239
21.1.3. Rheumatoid Arthritis (RA)	240
21.1.4. Sjogren's Syndrome	240
21.1.5. Scleroderma and Vasculitis	241
21.2. Medications for Pregnant Patients with Rheumatic Diseases	241
21.2.1. Safe Medications:	241
21.2.2. Contraindicated Medications:	242
21.3. Monitoring Disease Activity and Pregnancy Outcomes	242
21.3.1. Maternal Monitoring:	243
21.3.2. Fetal Monitoring:	243
21.3.3. Pregnancy Outcomes:	244
21.3.4. Postpartum Care:	244
Chapter 22: Common Conditions in Pediatric Rheumatology	247
22.1. Juvenile Idiopathic Arthritis (JIA)	247
22.1.1. Overview	247
22.1.2. Diagnostic Approach	247
22.1.3. Treatment Strategies	247
22.1.4. Long-Term Monitoring	248
22. 2. Systemic Lupus Erythematosus (SLE)	249
22.2.1. Diagnostic Approach	249
22.2.2. Treatment Strategies	249
22.2.3. Long-Term Monitoring	250
22.3. Kawasaki Disease	251
22.3.1. Diagnostic Approach	251
22.3.1. Treatment Strategies	252
22.3.1. Long-Term Monitoring	252
22.4. Juvenile Dermatomyositis (JDM)	253
22.4.1. Overview	253
22.4.2. Diagnostic Approach	253
22.4.3. Treatment Strategies	255
22.4.4. Long-Term Monitoring	256
22.5. Henoch-Schönlein Purpura (HSP)	257
22.5.1. Overview	257
22.5.2. Diagnostic Approach	257
22.5.3. Treatment Strategies	258
22.5.4. Long-Term Monitoring	259
Chapter 23: Cardiovascular and Bone Health in Rheumatologic Patients	263
23.1. Cardiovascular Risk and Inflammatory Arthritis	263
23.2. Strategies for Cardiovascular Risk Reduction in RA, SLE, and PsA	263
23.3. Osteoporosis in Rheumatic Diseases: Prevention and Management	265

Part 4: Integrating Rheumatology into Primary Care — **267**
   Chapter 24: Collaborative Care with Rheumatologists — 269
      24.1. When and How to Refer to a Rheumatologist — 269
      24.2. Co-Managing Patients with Rheumatic Diseases — 270
      24.3. Shared Decision-Making with Patients and Multidisciplinary Teams — 271
   Chapter 25: Patient Education and Self-Management — 273
      25.1. Educating Patients About Their Disease — 273
      25.2. Tools for Patient Engagement and Adherence to Therapy — 274
      25.3. Lifestyle Modifications: Diet, Exercise, and Stress Management — 275
   Chapter 26: Telemedicine and Remote Monitoring in Rheumatology — 277
      26.1. Benefits of Telemedicine for Chronic Disease Management — 277
      26.2. Remote Monitoring Tools for Disease Activity — 278
      26.3. Integrating Technology into Primary Care Rheumatology — 279

Part 5: Future Directions in Rheumatology — **281**
   Chapter 27: Emerging Therapies and Clinical Trials — 283
      27.1. New Biologics and Small Molecule Inhibitors — 283
      27.2. Advances in Stem Cell and Gene Therapy — 284
      27.3. Personalized Medicine and Precision Rheumatology — 284
   Chapter 28: Genetics and Biomarkers in Rheumatic Diseases — 287
      28.1. Role of Genetic Testing in Rheumatology — 287
      28.2. Predictive Biomarkers for Disease Progression and Treatment Response — 288
   Chapter 29: The Future of Rheumatology Care — 291
      29.1. Shifts in Care Models: From Reactive to Preventive Rheumatology — 291
      29.2. Global Trends in Rheumatology and Autoimmune Disease Management — 292

Chapter 30: Appendices — **295**
   30.1. Key Rheumatologic Medications: Mechanisms, Dosing, and Monitoring — 295
   30.2. Quick Reference: Diagnostic Criteria for Common Rheumatic Diseases — 296
   30.3. Patient Resources: Websites, Support Groups, and Educational Materials — 297
   30.4. Guidelines and Resources for PCPs: ACR/EULAR Recommendations — 298

Part 1: Rheumatology in Primary Care and Rheumatologic Foundations

Chapter 1: The Scope of Rheumatology in Primary Care

Rheumatologic diseases encompass a wide range of conditions that affect the musculoskeletal system, autoimmune pathways, and systemic inflammation. Many of these diseases are chronic and require long-term management, making them a significant concern in primary care.

Given the growing prevalence of rheumatologic conditions and their impact on patient quality of life, the role of **primary care providers (PCPs)** in early detection, diagnosis, and management is crucial. This chapter explores the importance of rheumatologic conditions in general practice, the epidemiology of these diseases from both global and local perspectives, and the role of PCPs in providing comprehensive care.

1.1. The Importance of Rheumatologic Conditions in General Practice

Rheumatologic diseases frequently present in primary care settings, manifesting as **musculoskeletal pain, joint swelling, fatigue**, and other nonspecific symptoms. Given their prevalence and potential for long-term complications, **primary care providers (PCPs)** are essential in the early recognition and management of these conditions.

Timely identification and intervention can prevent the progression of these diseases, which are often chronic and debilitating. Without early diagnosis and appropriate treatment, these conditions can lead to **functional impairment, disability**, and a profound reduction in **quality of life**.

1.1.1. Chronic Disease Burden

Rheumatologic conditions such as **rheumatoid arthritis (RA), osteoarthritis (OA), systemic lupus erythematosus (SLE), psoriatic arthritis (PsA)**, and **gout** are among the leading causes of **chronic pain** and **disability** worldwide. These diseases impose a significant burden on both patients and healthcare systems.

- **Osteoarthritis (OA)**:
  Osteoarthritis is the most common form of arthritis, affecting over **240 million people** globally, particularly in aging populations. OA primarily affects the **knees, hips**, and **hands**, causing **joint pain, stiffness**, and **functional limitations** that can lead to disability, especially in older adults. The **Global Burden of Disease Study** identified **OA** as a major contributor to **years lived with disability (YLD)**, highlighting its significant impact on quality of life, productivity, and healthcare costsRheumatoid Arthritis (RA)**: Although **RA** affects a smaller proportion of the population compared to OA (affecting approximately **0.5-1%** globally), it leads to more **severe disability** and is associated with **increased mortality**. RA is a chronic autoimmune disease characterized by **inflammation** and **joint destruction**, and it often results in long-term complications such as **cardiovascular disease** (CVD). CVD is a major cause of premature death in RA patients, driven by systemic inflammation and traditional risk factors like hypertension and dyslipidemia . Early on with **disease-modifying antirheumatic drugs**

(DMARDs) can prevent joint damage and reduce systemic inflammation, significantly improving outcomes.

- **Systemic Lupus Erythematosus (SLE)** and **Psoriatic Arthritis (PsA)**:
These inflammatory autoimmune diseases are less common than OA but are associated with significant morbidity. **SLE** can affect multiple organs, including the **kidneys**, **heart**, **skin**, and **central nervous system**, leading to organ damage and increased mortality if left untreated. **PsA**, which affects about **30% of people** with psoriasis, is characterized by **joint inflammation**, **enthesitis**, and **dactylitis**, often leading to joint destruction if not managed early .

- **Gout**:
, a metabolic disorder characterized by elevated **uric acid** levels and **crystal deposition** in joints, is another common rheumatologic condition. It can cause acute, severe joint pain (often in the **big toe**) and, if untreated, lead to **chronic gouty arthritis** and **tophi formation**. The incidence of gout is rising globally, fueled by **dietary changes**, **obesity**, and **metabolic syndrome**. Gout is also associated with increased cardiovascular risk, making early detection and management critical .

1.1.2. Early Detection of Rheumatologic Conditions in Primary Care

Musculoskeletal complaints are one of the most frequent reasons for primary care visits. It is estimated that **10-20%** of all consultations in general practice involve **musculoskeletal pain**, with **rheumatologic diseases** accounting for a significant proportion of these cases .

Common symptoms such as **joint stiffness**, **swelling**, and **fatigue** can overlap with other chronic conditions (e.g., osteoarthritis, fibromyalgia, and mechanical back pain), necessitating a systematic and thorough diagnostic approach.

- **Symptom Overlap**:
Because symptoms like joint pain and stiffness can be nonspecific, rheumatologic diseases are often misdiagnosed or overlooked. For example, **chronic back pain** in a young adult may initially be attributed to mechanical causes or overuse. However, in some cases, this pain may indicate **ankylosing spondylitis (AS)**, an inflammatory disease affecting the **spine** and **sacroiliac joints**. AS is often diagnosed late, leading to permanent structural changes in the spine, such as **bamboo spine** and reduced mobility. Early recognition and referral to a rheumatologist can prevent irreversible spinal damage and improve long-term outcomes .

- **Importance of a Systematic Approach**
care providers should adopt a systematic approach when evaluating musculoskeletal complaints to distinguish between **inflammatory** and **non-inflammatory** causes of joint pain. Inflammatory conditions like RA, PsA, and **AS** typically present with **morning stiffness**, **symmetrical joint involvement**, and **improvement with activity**, while non-inflammatory conditions like OA present with **pain worsened by activity** and **asymmetrical joint involvement**. **Red flags** such as joint swelling, prolonged morning stiffness, fatigue, and family history of autoimmune diseases should prompt further evaluation and possible referral to a rheumatologist.

- For example, in **rheumatoid arthritis**, early signs such as persistent joint swelling, especially in the **small joints of the hands and feet**, can indicate active synovitis, which, if untreated, can lead to joint erosion within the first **6 months** of disease onset. Early referral and initiation of DMARDs can prevent permanent damage.
- **Comprehensive Diagnostic Workup**:
Primary care providers play a pivotal role in the **initial diagnostic workup** for rheumatologic diseases. This includes ordering **appropriate laboratory tests**, such as **rheumatoid factor (RF), anti-citrullinated protein antibodies (ACPA), antinuclear antibodies (ANA), erythrocyte sedimentation rate (ESR),** and **C-reactive protein (CRP)**, to evaluate for underlying inflammatory or autoimmune conditions. **Imaging studies** (e.g., X-rays, ultrasound, MRI) are also valuable for detecting early signs of joint damage or inflammation.
  - Early detection is particularly important for conditions like RA, where aggressive treatment during the **window of opportunity** (within the first **3-6 months** of symptom onset) can lead to long-term remission and prevent disability.

Rheumatologic diseases are a significant concern in primary care due to their prevalence, chronic nature, and potential for long-term disability. As the first point of contact for patients, PCPs are crucial in recognizing early signs, initiating timely referrals, and co-managing chronic rheumatic conditions. Understanding the burden of these diseases, the importance of early diagnosis, and the need for a thorough, systematic approach to musculoskeletal complaints is essential for preventing complications and improving patient outcomes.

1.2. Epidemiology of Rheumatologic Diseases: Global and Local Perspectives

Rheumatologic diseases represent a significant public health concern, with varying prevalence across different regions of the world. Factors such as **genetics**, **environment**, and **socioeconomic conditions** contribute to differences in the incidence and burden of these diseases in local populations.

- **Global Prevalence**:
The **prevalence** of rheumatic diseases varies widely across the globe. For instance, the prevalence of RA ranges from **0.5% to 1%** in most populations, but it can be higher in **Indigenous North American** populations, where it can reach up to **5%**. The prevalence of **SLE** is also highly variable, with rates higher among populations of **African-American, Hispanic,** and **Asian** descent compared to **Caucasians**, possibly due to genetic predisposition and environmental factors.
  - **Osteoarthritis (OA)** is the most common form of arthritis globally, affecting more than **300 million people** worldwide. It is strongly associated with aging, obesity, and mechanical joint stress, making it a growing concern in aging populations and in countries with high rates of obesity.
  - **Gout**, a metabolic form of arthritis, has been on the rise globally due to changes in diet, increasing rates of **obesity**, and metabolic syndrome. Gout is more

common in men, particularly those of Pacific Islander and Maori descent, who have a higher genetic predisposition to hyperuricemia.
- **Local and Regional Perspectives**:
Local factors such as **access to healthcare, socioeconomic status**, and **lifestyle factors** also play a role in the epidemiology of rheumatologic diseases. For example, the increasing prevalence of **obesity** and **sedentary lifestyles** in developed countries has contributed to the rising incidence of **osteoarthritis** and **gout**. In contrast, in **developing countries**, infectious causes of arthritis, such as **reactive arthritis** following gastrointestinal or urogenital infections, are more prevalent due to higher rates of untreated infections and poor sanitation.
    - **Socioeconomic factors** can also affect disease outcomes. Individuals in lower socioeconomic groups are more likely to experience **delays in diagnosis** and **inadequate access to specialist care**, leading to poorer outcomes and higher rates of disability in rheumatic diseases.

1.3. Role of the Primary Care Provider (PCP) in Early Detection and Management Rheumatologic Disorders

Primary care providers play a critical role in the **early detection**, **diagnosis**, and **long-term management** of rheumatic diseases. Since many rheumatologic conditions are **chronic** and require ongoing care, PCPs are often responsible for co-managing these patients with rheumatologists and ensuring that **comorbidities** and **lifestyle factors** are addressed.

- **Early Detection and Referral**:
PCPs are often the first to encounter patients presenting with **joint pain**, **stiffness**, or **fatigue**. Early recognition of **inflammatory arthritis** (e.g., RA, PsA, AS) is crucial, as **early initiation of treatment** with disease-modifying antirheumatic drugs (DMARDs) can prevent joint damage and improve long-term outcomes. Guidelines recommend referring patients to a rheumatologist within **6 weeks** of the onset of symptoms if inflammatory arthritis is suspected.
    - For instance, PCPs should be aware of **red flag symptoms** such as **morning stiffness lasting more than 30 minutes, symmetrical joint swelling**, and a family history of autoimmune diseases, which could indicate RA or PsA.
    - In **systemic lupus erythematosus (SLE)**, the presence of **malar rash**, **photosensitivity**, **mouth ulcers**, and **positive ANA** can prompt early referral to a rheumatologist for further evaluation and immunosuppressive therapy initiation.
- **Management of Comorbidities**:
Many patients with rheumatic diseases have comorbid conditions such as **cardiovascular disease, osteoporosis, diabetes**, and **depression**. PCPs play an important role in managing these comorbidities alongside rheumatologic treatment. For example:
    - **Cardiovascular Risk**: RA and SLE patients are at significantly higher risk of **cardiovascular disease** due to chronic inflammation. PCPs are responsible for managing cardiovascular risk factors such as **hypertension, hyperlipidemia**,

and **diabetes**, as well as recommending lifestyle changes like smoking cessation and exercise .
- ○ **Bone Health**: Patients with chronic rheumatic diseases, particularly those on long-term **glucocorticoid therapy**, are at high risk for **osteoporosis** and fractures. PCPs should ensure that patients receive **bone density screening** (DEXA scans) and appropriate preventive measures, such as **calcium, vitamin D**, and **bisphosphonate therapy** .
- **Patient Education and Self-Management**:
Educating patients about their condition, treatment options, and the importance of medication adherence is a key role of PCPs. Patients with chronic diseases often benefit from **self-management programs** that focus on lifestyle modifications, exercise, and pain management strategies. PCPs can refer patients to **physical therapy**, **occupational therapy**, and **support groups** as part of a comprehensive care plan.
  - ○ **Exercise and Diet**: Encouraging regular **exercise** and a **healthy diet** is essential for patients with osteoarthritis and other rheumatic conditions. PCPs can guide patients in developing an appropriate exercise regimen to maintain joint function and reduce pain.

Rheumatologic diseases are an important concern in primary care due to their high prevalence, chronic nature, and impact on patient quality of life. PCPs play a pivotal role in the early detection, diagnosis, and management of these conditions, helping to prevent long-term complications and improve patient outcomes. By understanding the global and local epidemiology of these diseases, utilizing diagnostic criteria, and effectively co-managing patients with rheumatologists, PCPs can provide comprehensive care that addresses both the disease and associated comorbidities.

References

- Vos, T., Abajobir, A. A., Abbafati, C., et al. (2017). Global, regional, and national incidence, prevalence, and years lived with disability for 328 diseases and injuries for 195 countries, 1990–2016: a systematic analysis for the Global Burden of Disease Study 2016. *The Lancet*, 390(10100), 1211-1259.
- Hunter, D. J., & Bierma-Zeinstra, S. (2019). Osteoarthritis. *The Lancet*, 393(10182), 1745-1759.
- Smolen, J. S., Aletaha, D., McInnes, I. B. (2016). Rheumatoid arthritis. *The Lancet*, 388(10055), 2023-2038.
- van der Heijde, D., Ramiro, S., Landewé, R., et al. (2017). 2016 update of the ASAS-EULAR management recommendations for axial spondyloarthritis. *Annals of the Rheumatic Diseases*, 76(6), 978-991.
- Dougados, M., Baeten, D. (2011). Spondyloarthritis. *The Lancet*, 377(9783), 2127-2137.
- Bruce, I. N. (2005). 'Not only... but also': factors that contribute to accelerated atherosclerosis and premature coronary heart disease in systemic lupus erythematosus. *Rheumatology*, 44(12), 1492-1502.

Chapter 2: What is Evidence-Based Medicine (EBM)?

Evidence-based medicine is defined as the conscientious, explicit, and judicious use of current best evidence in making decisions about the care of individual patients. The goal of EBM is to integrate the best available research evidence with clinical expertise and patient preferences to ensure optimal care .

EBM involves three core components:

1. **Best Available Evidence**: This is derived from well-designed and conducted research, including **randomized controlled trials (RCTs), systematic reviews**, and **meta-analyses**. These provide high-quality data on the effectiveness and safety of treatments.
2. **Clinical Expertise**: The clinician's accumulated experience, skills, and knowledge are essential for interpreting evidence in the context of individual patient circumstances.
3. **Patient Values and Preferences**: Understanding and incorporating patient preferences, values, and expectations are crucial for shared decision-making in clinical practice.

In rheumatology, EBM helps guide decisions regarding the management of diseases such as **rheumatoid arthritis (RA), systemic lupus erythematosus (SLE), psoriatic arthritis (PsA),** and **ankylosing spondylitis (AS)**, particularly with the rapidly evolving treatment landscape involving **biologics** and **small molecule inhibitors**.

2.1. How to Apply EBM Rheumatology in Clinical Practice

Applying EBM in clinical practice requires a structured approach that integrates evidence with individual patient care. The steps involved include:

1. **Formulate a Clinical Question**:
   The first step is to convert a clinical problem into a focused question that can be researched. This is often done using the **PICO framework**:
   - **P**: Patient or Population (e.g., adults with newly diagnosed RA).
   - **I**: Intervention (e.g., initiating methotrexate).
   - **C**: Comparison (e.g., compared to starting a biologic).
   - **O**: Outcome (e.g., reduction in disease activity, prevention of joint damage).
2. Example: "In adults with newly diagnosed RA, how effective is methotrexate compared to biologics in reducing disease activity and preventing joint damage?"
3. **Search for the Best Evidence**:
   Once the question is framed, the next step is to search for relevant evidence. Trusted sources include:
   - **Cochrane Library**: A database of systematic reviews and meta-analyses, often considered the gold standard in EBM.
   - **PubMed**: A comprehensive resource for accessing research articles.
   - **EULAR** and **ACR Guidelines**: Guidelines from the **European League Against Rheumatism (EULAR)** and **American College of Rheumatology (ACR)** offer evidence-based recommendations for managing rheumatic diseases.

4. **Critically Appraise the Evidence**:
   It is essential to evaluate the quality of the evidence to determine its relevance and applicability. Key aspects of appraisal include:
   - **Study Design**: RCTs provide the highest level of evidence, followed by **cohort studies** and **case-control studies**. Meta-analyses and systematic reviews of RCTs offer robust conclusions by synthesizing data from multiple studies.
   - **Risk of Bias**: Evaluating whether there is **selection bias**, **performance bias**, or **publication bias** in the studies.
   - **Relevance to the Patient**: Assess whether the study population and interventions are similar to the clinical scenario you are addressing.
5. **Apply the Evidence to Patient Care**:
   After identifying the best evidence, it must be applied to the patient's unique clinical circumstances. This involves considering:
   - **Individual patient factors** (e.g., comorbidities, age, pregnancy status).
   - **Patient preferences and values**, particularly regarding risks, side effects, and treatment goals.
   - **Resource availability**, such as access to biologics or newer therapies.
6. Example: If evidence supports the use of **TNF inhibitors** for RA but the patient has a history of recurrent infections, the clinician might choose an alternative therapy with a lower risk of immunosuppression.
7. **Evaluate Outcomes**:
   After applying the evidence, it is essential to monitor patient outcomes and adjust the treatment plan if necessary. This step ensures that the selected intervention is achieving the desired results in terms of symptom control and disease modification.

2.2. Evaluating Research and Clinical Trials in Rheumatology

Evaluating the quality of research and clinical trials is critical for incorporating the latest advances in rheumatology into practice. Rheumatic diseases are highly variable, and understanding how to assess studies ensures that treatments are applied appropriately.

- **Study Design in Rheumatology**:
   - **Randomized Controlled Trials (RCTs)**: RCTs are the gold standard for assessing the efficacy of treatments. In rheumatology, RCTs have provided the evidence base for the use of **biologics** (e.g., **adalimumab**, **etanercept**) and **small molecule inhibitors** (e.g., **tofacitinib**, **baricitinib**). When evaluating RCTs, consider whether the study is adequately powered, whether randomization was truly random, and whether the trial was blinded to reduce bias.
   - **Systematic Reviews and Meta-Analyses**: These synthesize data from multiple studies, offering a higher level of evidence. They are particularly useful when individual studies show conflicting results. The **Cochrane Library** and **EULAR/ACR guidelines** often rely on meta-analyses to make clinical recommendations.

- **Endpoints in Rheumatology Clinical Trials**:
  Evaluating the **primary endpoints** of clinical trials is essential for understanding their relevance to clinical practice. In rheumatology trials, common endpoints include:
    - **Disease Activity Scores**: In RA, for example, the **DAS28** score (Disease Activity Score for 28 joints) is a common measure used to assess disease activity. Improvement in DAS28 scores is often a primary endpoint in RA trials.
    - **ACR Response Criteria**: The **ACR20, ACR50, and ACR70** criteria refer to 20%, 50%, and 70% improvement in RA symptoms, as defined by the **American College of Rheumatology**.
    - **Radiographic Progression**: Prevention of joint damage and **erosions** is a key endpoint in diseases like RA and PsA. Trials often use imaging studies (e.g., X-rays, MRI) to assess structural damage over time.
    - **Patient-Reported Outcomes (PROs)**: Quality of life and functional assessments are critical in evaluating the effectiveness of treatments from the patient's perspective.
- **Statistical Significance vs. Clinical Relevance**:
  When interpreting trial results, it is essential to distinguish between **statistical significance** and **clinical relevance**. A study may report statistically significant results, but the actual clinical benefit may be minimal. For example, a biologic agent might reduce the DAS28 score by a statistically significant margin, but the improvement may not translate to meaningful changes in the patient's daily functioning.
- **Adverse Events and Safety**:
  Evaluating the **safety profile** of medications is essential, particularly in long-term treatment scenarios common in rheumatology. Adverse events such as **serious infections**, **cardiovascular risks**, and **malignancies** need to be weighed against the benefits of disease control. The risk-benefit profile varies between drugs, making individual patient characteristics a key factor in decision-making.

Evidence-based medicine (EBM) is integral to the practice of rheumatology, guiding clinical decisions through a combination of research evidence, clinical expertise, and patient preferences. Applying EBM principles in practice involves formulating clinical questions, searching for the best evidence, critically appraising research, and integrating this knowledge into patient care.

Rheumatologists and PCPs must be adept at evaluating the quality of research and clinical trials, particularly in an era of rapidly advancing treatments, to ensure that patients receive the most effective and safe therapies. Understanding study designs, endpoints, and the risk-benefit profiles of treatments allows for optimal care and improved patient outcomes.

References

- Sackett, D. L., Rosenberg, W. M., Gray, J. A., et al. (1996). Evidence based medicine: what it is and what it isn't. *BMJ*, 312(7023), 71-72.
- Gaujoux-Viala, C., Smolen, J. S., Landewe, R., et al. (2010). Current evidence for the management of rheumatoid arthritis with synthetic disease-modifying antirheumatic

drugs: a systematic literature review informing the 2010 update of the EULAR recommendations. *Annals of the Rheumatic Diseases*, 69(6), 1004-1009.
- Felson, D. T., Smolen, J. S., Wells, G., et al. (2011). American College of Rheumatology/European League Against Rheumatism provisional definition of remission in rheumatoid arthritis for clinical trials. *Arthritis & Rheumatology*, 63(3), 573-586.
- Taylor, P. C., Keystone, E. C., van der Heijde, D., et al. (2017). Baricitinib versus placebo or adalimumab in rheumatoid arthritis. *New England Journal of Medicine*, 376(7), 652-662.
- Smolen, J. S., Landewe, R., Bijlsma, J., et al. (2017). EULAR recommendations for the management of rheumatoid arthritis with synthetic and biological disease-modifying antirheumatic drugs: 2016 update. *Annals of the Rheumatic Diseases*, 76(6), 960-977.

Chapter 3: Immunology and Pathophysiology of Rheumatologic Diseases

This chapter focuses on the essential biological underpinnings that drive autoimmune and inflammatory conditions in rheumatology. A thorough understanding of the immune system and its pathophysiological mechanisms is critical for primary care providers to diagnose, manage, and monitor rheumatologic diseases effectively.

3.1. Overview of the Immune System

The immune system is a complex network of cells and molecules designed to defend the body against pathogens, but it also plays a pivotal role in the development of autoimmune diseases. The immune system is divided into two major branches: the **innate immune system** and the **adaptive immune system**. While these systems work together to protect the body, their dysregulation can lead to **autoimmune disorders** such as **systemic lupus erythematosus (SLE), rheumatoid arthritis (RA)**, and **psoriatic arthritis (PsA)**. Understanding the functions and interactions of these systems is essential for grasping the pathogenesis of autoimmune diseases.

3.1.1. Innate Immune System

The **innate immune system** serves as the body's first line of defense, providing **rapid, nonspecific** responses to pathogens and cellular damage. It consists of **physical barriers**, such as the **skin** and **mucosal surfaces**, as well as specialized immune cells like **neutrophils, macrophages, dendritic cells**, and **natural killer (NK) cells**. The innate immune system recognizes general patterns on pathogens, termed **pathogen-associated molecular patterns (PAMPs)**, and endogenous signals from damaged cells, called **damage-associated molecular patterns (DAMPs)**. These patterns are detected by **pattern recognition receptors (PRRs)**, with **toll-like receptors (TLRs)** being among the most well-known PRRs.

- **Toll-like Receptors (TLRs)**:
  TLRs are expressed on the surface of immune cells like macrophages and dendritic cells. They recognize microbial components such as bacterial lipopolysaccharides (LPS) and viral RNA. Upon activation, TLRs initiate signaling pathways that result in the production of **cytokines** (e.g., **interleukins, TNF-α**), which mediate inflammation and recruit other immune cells to the site of infection or injury .
    - In autoimmune diseases, dysregulation of TLR signaling can result in the inappropriate activation of immune responses against self-antigens. For example, in **systemic lupus erythematosus (SLE)**, overactivation of TLRs by immune complexes containing nucleic acids (DAMPs) leads to the chronic production of **type I interferons**, which perpetuate inflammation and tissue damage .
- **Neutrophils and Macrophages**:
  Neutrophils and macrophages are key players in the innate immune system.

Neutrophils are the first responders to infection, phagocytosing pathogens and releasing enzymes that kill microbes. **Macrophages** serve not only as phagocytes but also as antigen-presenting cells (APCs), bridging the gap between innate and adaptive immunity by presenting antigens to **T cells**.
- In conditions such as **RA**, macrophages accumulate in the **synovial fluid** of joints, where they produce pro-inflammatory cytokines like **TNF-α, IL-1**, and **IL-6**. These cytokines drive the chronic inflammation and joint destruction characteristic of RA.

- **Dendritic Cells**:
  Dendritic cells (DCs) are specialized antigen-presenting cells that capture antigens and present them to **T cells**, initiating adaptive immune responses. In autoimmune diseases, DCs may improperly present **self-antigens** to T cells, contributing to the breakdown of **self-tolerance** and the development of autoimmunity.
  - In **psoriatic arthritis (PsA)**, dendritic cells play a role in driving **Th17** responses, contributing to skin inflammation and joint involvement.

3.1.2. Adaptive Immune System

The **adaptive immune system** is characterized by **specificity** and **memory**, allowing the body to mount targeted responses to pathogens and remember them for future encounters. The adaptive immune response is mediated by two main types of cells: **T cells** and **B cells**.

- **T Cells**:
  T lymphocytes are divided into several subtypes, each with a specific function in immune regulation and response. The two primary types of T cells involved in autoimmunity are **helper T cells (Th)** and **regulatory T cells (Tregs)**.
  - **Helper T Cells (Th1, Th17)**:
    Helper T cells (Th), particularly **Th1** and **Th17** subtypes, play central roles in modulating immune responses. **Th1 cells** secrete **IFN-γ**, which activates macrophages and promotes **cell-mediated immunity**. **Th17 cells** produce **IL-17**, a cytokine involved in recruiting neutrophils and promoting inflammation, especially at barrier sites like the skin and joints.
    - In **rheumatoid arthritis (RA)**, **Th1** and **Th17** cells are abundant in the inflamed synovium, where they promote chronic inflammation and contribute to joint destruction through cytokines like **TNF-α, IL-6**, and **IL-17**.
    - In **psoriasis** and **psoriatic arthritis**, **Th17** cells are key drivers of inflammation, with **IL-17** and **IL-23** playing critical roles in the pathogenesis of skin lesions and joint disease.
  - **Regulatory T Cells (T-regs)**:
    T-regs are essential for maintaining **immune tolerance** by suppressing autoreactive T cells that might otherwise attack the body's own tissues. Dysfunction in **Treg cells** is a hallmark of autoimmune diseases, as the failure to regulate and suppress **autoreactive T cells** leads to unchecked inflammation and tissue damage.

- In diseases like SLE and RA, impaired **Treg function** contributes to the loss of tolerance to self-antigens, enabling chronic autoimmune responses. Restoring Treg function or boosting their numbers is a therapeutic goal in many autoimmune diseases.
- **B Cells and Autoantibodies**:
  B lymphocytes are responsible for producing **antibodies**, which neutralize pathogens. However, in autoimmune diseases, B cells can produce **autoantibodies** that target the body's own tissues, leading to immune complex formation and tissue damage.
    - In **systemic lupus erythematosus (SLE)**, **autoreactive B cells** produce autoantibodies against **nuclear antigens** (e.g., **anti-dsDNA, anti-Smith**), leading to immune complex deposition in organs like the kidneys (causing **lupus nephritis**) and skin (causing **malar rash**).
    - In **rheumatoid arthritis**, **autoantibodies** such as **rheumatoid factor (RF)** and **anti-citrullinated protein antibodies (ACPA)** target proteins in the joints, resulting in immune complex deposition, complement activation, and chronic synovial inflammation.
- **Memory T and B Cells**:
  A key feature of the adaptive immune system is the development of **memory T and B cells**, which allow for a rapid and more effective immune response upon re-exposure to the same antigen. In the context of autoimmunity, **memory autoreactive T and B cells** contribute to **disease flares** and **chronic inflammation**, as they are primed to react to self-antigens.

3.1.3. Dysregulation Leading to Autoimmune Diseases

The innate and adaptive immune systems work together to maintain immune homeostasis, but **dysregulation** of these systems can lead to **autoimmune diseases**. In autoimmune disorders, **self-tolerance** is lost, resulting in the immune system attacking the body's own tissues.

- **Loss of Immune Tolerance**:
  In many autoimmune diseases, there is a failure in the mechanisms that maintain **self-tolerance**, including the proper functioning of **Tregs** and the deletion of **autoreactive T and B cells** during their development. This failure allows **autoreactive lymphocytes** to proliferate and cause damage to healthy tissues.
- **Chronic Inflammation and Tissue Damage**:
  Autoimmune diseases are often characterized by **chronic inflammation**, driven by **cytokine dysregulation**, **autoantibody production**, and **cellular infiltration** into tissues. Over time, this persistent inflammation leads to **tissue damage** and **organ dysfunction**.
    - In RA, for instance, the continuous activation of **synovial fibroblasts**, macrophages, and T cells results in joint destruction and deformity if untreated.
    - In SLE, the deposition of immune complexes in tissues like the kidneys leads to **glomerulonephritis**, a serious complication that can progress to kidney failure.

The immune system, while essential for defending against pathogens, plays a central role in the development of **autoimmune diseases** when dysregulated. The **innate immune system** initiates rapid responses to infections, but its dysfunction can lead to inappropriate activation of immune pathways. The **adaptive immune system**, with its highly specific T and B cells, can also contribute to autoimmunity through the production of autoantibodies and the failure of regulatory mechanisms. Understanding the complex interplay between these two branches of the immune system is crucial for the development of new treatments for autoimmune diseases such as RA, SLE, and PsA.

3.2. Mechanisms of Autoimmunity and Chronic Inflammation

Autoimmunity occurs when the immune system mistakenly targets the body's own tissues. Chronic inflammation results when the body is unable to switch off this response, leading to sustained tissue damage.

- **Loss of Self-Tolerance**:
  In healthy individuals, immune cells are trained to tolerate self-antigens, a process known as central and peripheral tolerance. Breakdown in these mechanisms leads to autoimmunity. **Central tolerance** occurs in the thymus (T cells) and bone marrow (B cells), while **peripheral tolerance** is maintained by regulatory T cells (Tregs) and anergy (cellular unresponsiveness).
- **Molecular Mimicry**:
  Autoimmunity can also be triggered by **molecular mimicry**, where foreign antigens (e.g., from infections) resemble self-antigens, leading the immune system to attack both. For example, infections like Epstein-Barr virus (EBV) have been linked to the development of autoimmune conditions such as systemic lupus erythematosus (SLE).
- **Chronic Inflammation and Tissue Damage**:
  Chronic inflammation is driven by persistent activation of immune cells, release of pro-inflammatory cytokines, and recruitment of more immune cells to the site of inflammation. This process leads to ongoing tissue damage and scarring in organs such as the joints (RA), kidneys (SLE), and blood vessels (vasculitis).

3.3. Genetics and Environmental Triggers in Autoimmune Diseases

Autoimmune diseases often occur due to a complex interplay between genetic predisposition and environmental factors.

- **Genetic Susceptibility**:
  Several genes associated with the immune system have been implicated in rheumatic diseases. For example, the **HLA (human leukocyte antigen)** gene complex is known to play a pivotal role in autoimmune conditions. **HLA-DR4** is linked with an increased risk of RA, while **HLA-B27** is strongly associated with ankylosing spondylitis and other forms of spondyloarthritis.
- **Environmental Factors**:

- **Infections**: Certain infections (e.g., streptococcal infections, EBV) are associated with autoimmune responses through molecular mimicry or other mechanisms.
- **Smoking**: Smoking has been shown to increase the risk of developing RA, particularly in genetically susceptible individuals with HLA-DR4. Smoking exacerbates inflammation and alters immune responses.
- **Hormonal Factors**: Autoimmune diseases are more prevalent in women, particularly during reproductive years, suggesting a role of hormones such as estrogen in modulating immune responses.
- **Diet and Gut Microbiota**: There is emerging evidence that changes in gut microbiota composition may influence autoimmune conditions by affecting systemic inflammation and immune tolerance.

3.4. The Role of Cytokines and Other Mediators in Rheumatic Disease

Cytokines are small proteins that play a critical role in cell signaling within the immune system. Dysregulation of cytokines is central to the pathophysiology of many rheumatic diseases.

- **Pro-Inflammatory Cytokines**:
    - **TNF-α (Tumor Necrosis Factor-alpha)**: A key cytokine in RA and other inflammatory arthritides, TNF-α drives synovial inflammation and joint destruction. Anti-TNF therapies have revolutionized the treatment of RA and ankylosing spondylitis.
    - **IL-1 (Interleukin-1)**: IL-1 promotes inflammation and cartilage degradation in RA and other inflammatory diseases. IL-1 inhibitors are effective in treating autoinflammatory syndromes and gouty arthritis.
    - **IL-6**: Plays a significant role in chronic inflammation and is a key mediator in RA, contributing to synovitis and systemic inflammation. IL-6 inhibitors (e.g., tocilizumab) are used to treat RA.
    - **IL-17**: This cytokine is particularly important in the pathogenesis of psoriatic arthritis and ankylosing spondylitis, driving inflammation and bone remodeling. IL-17 inhibitors are used in these diseases.
- **Anti-Inflammatory Cytokines**:
    - **IL-10 and TGF-β**: These cytokines help regulate and suppress immune responses, limiting tissue damage during inflammation. Deficiencies or altered function of these cytokines can contribute to unchecked inflammation in autoimmune diseases.
- **Chemokines**:
Chemokines attract immune cells to sites of inflammation. In conditions like RA, an imbalance between pro-inflammatory chemokines and their regulators contributes to joint damage.
- **Matrix Metalloproteinases (MMPs)**:
MMPs are enzymes that degrade extracellular matrix components such as collagen. In RA and osteoarthritis (OA), excessive activity of MMPs leads to cartilage destruction and joint damage.

References

- Takeuchi, O., & Akira, S. (2010). Pattern recognition receptors and inflammation. *Cell*, 140(6), 805-820.
- Smolen, J. S., Aletaha, D., & McInnes, I. B. (2016). Rheumatoid arthritis. *The Lancet*, 388(10055), 2023-2038.
- Crow, M. K. (2014). Type I interferon in the pathogenesis of lupus. *Journal of Immunology*, 192(12), 5459-5468.
- Boehncke, W. H., & Schön, M. P. (2015). Psoriasis. *The Lancet*, 386(9997), 983-994.
- Sakaguchi, S., Yamaguchi, T., Nomura, T., & Ono, M. (2008). Regulatory T cells and immune tolerance. *Cell*, 133(5), 775-787.

Chapter 4: Diagnostic Approach to Rheumatologic Conditions

This chapter provides a structured approach to evaluating patients with potential rheumatologic diseases in primary care settings. Early and accurate diagnosis is crucial in managing these conditions, as timely intervention can prevent significant morbidity.

4.1 History Taking Skills in Rheumatology

History taking is the cornerstone of diagnosing **rheumatologic diseases**, as a thorough patient history provides critical insights that guide differential diagnosis and subsequent management. The history reveals the nature of the symptoms, their progression, and associated systemic features, which helps differentiate between various types of **arthritis, connective tissue diseases**, and **vasculitis**.

Detailed questioning about the **pattern, onset**, and **systemic involvement** is essential for narrowing down the diagnosis in patients presenting with musculoskeletal complaints.

4.1.1. Pattern and Onset of Symptoms

Understanding the **onset** and **progression** of symptoms is crucial in distinguishing between different rheumatologic diseases. The timeline of symptom development—whether the onset is **acute** or **insidious**—provides valuable clues regarding the underlying condition.

- **Acute Onset**:
  Acute onset of joint pain and swelling is characteristic of conditions like **gout, pseudogout**, and **septic arthritis**. These conditions often present suddenly, with intense pain and noticeable swelling in a single joint or a few joints.
    - In **gout**, the **first metatarsophalangeal joint** (big toe) is frequently involved, with episodes of acute, severe pain, and redness.
    - **Septic arthritis** can also present acutely, with rapid onset of pain, fever, and a single swollen joint, making this a medical emergency requiring prompt diagnosis and treatment to prevent joint destruction.
- **Insidious Onset**:
  Chronic rheumatologic conditions such as **rheumatoid arthritis (RA)** or **systemic lupus erythematosus (SLE)** typically have a more **insidious onset**. These conditions develop gradually over weeks to months, often starting with mild joint pain, morning stiffness, and swelling, which progressively worsen.
    - In **RA**, patients often describe **slowly progressive** pain and swelling in the **small joints of the hands and feet**, which increases in severity over time without abrupt flares.
    - **SLE** presents with a more variable course but often includes **insidious joint pain**, fatigue, and a range of systemic symptoms affecting multiple organs, developing over weeks to months.

Recognizing the **tempo** of disease progression helps in distinguishing **inflammatory conditions** like RA or SLE from **acute monoarticular arthritis** seen in gout or septic arthritis.

4.1.2. Symmetry of Joint Involvement

The **symmetry** or **asymmetry** of joint involvement is another key differentiating feature in rheumatologic conditions. Symmetric joint involvement often indicates **inflammatory polyarthritis**, while asymmetric involvement is more typical of **crystalline arthritis** or **psoriatic arthritis (PsA)**.

- **Symmetric Arthritis**:
  Rheumatoid arthritis commonly presents with **symmetrical** joint involvement, particularly in the **small joints** of the **hands**, **wrists**, and **feet**. Patients typically report pain, swelling, and stiffness on **both sides of the body**, with involvement of multiple joints at the same time. This symmetry is a hallmark of inflammatory arthritis.
    - In RA, both **proximal interphalangeal (PIP)** and **metacarpophalangeal (MCP)** joints are involved, often sparing the **distal interphalangeal (DIP)** joints.
- **Asymmetric Arthritis**:
  In contrast, **psoriatic arthritis (PsA)** and **gout** are more likely to present with **asymmetric** joint involvement. PsA can affect both large and small joints, but its pattern is typically **asymmetric**, with involvement of different joints on either side of the body.
    - In **gout**, patients often present with **monoarticular** or **oligo-articular** involvement, particularly of the **first metatarsophalangeal joint** (podagra), ankles, or knees. The **asymmetry** and episodic nature of the flares help differentiate gout from more chronic polyarthritides.

4.1.3. Morning Stiffness

Morning stiffness is a critical symptom that helps distinguish between **inflammatory** and **non-inflammatory** joint diseases. The duration of stiffness in the morning provides important clues to the underlying pathology.

- **Prolonged Morning Stiffness (>1 hour)**:
  Prolonged morning stiffness, lasting more than an hour, is characteristic of **inflammatory arthritis** such as **rheumatoid arthritis (RA)** or **ankylosing spondylitis (AS)**. Patients with RA typically report that their joints feel stiff for several hours after waking, gradually improving with movement.
    - In **ankylosing spondylitis**, patients report prolonged stiffness and pain, especially in the lower back and pelvis, that improves with physical activity. The hallmark of AS is **chronic back pain** that improves with movement and worsens with rest.
- **Shorter Duration of Stiffness (<30 minutes)**:
  In contrast, **osteoarthritis (OA)** tends to cause **brief morning stiffness** that typically resolves within **30 minutes**. OA is a **non-inflammatory** degenerative condition, and

patients often report that their stiffness worsens after periods of inactivity but quickly improves with movement.
- Patients with OA often describe **worsening pain** later in the day, especially after prolonged use of the affected joints, such as the **knees**, **hips**, or **hands**.

4.1.4. Systemic Symptoms

Systemic symptoms often provide key insights into the diagnosis of **connective tissue diseases** and **vasculitides**, as these conditions frequently involve multiple organ systems.

- **Fever, Weight Loss, and Malaise**:
  These symptoms suggest **systemic inflammation** and are commonly associated with **vasculitis, systemic lupus erythematosus (SLE)**, and other **connective tissue diseases**. Patients with **giant cell arteritis (GCA)** or **polyarteritis nodosa (PAN)** may present with **fever, fatigue, weight loss**, and **malaise**, in addition to their joint symptoms.
  - In **SLE**, systemic symptoms such as **fatigue, fever, weight loss**, and **malaise** are common, often accompanying a wide range of organ-specific manifestations, including **arthritis, malar rash**, and **renal involvement**.
- **Raynaud's Phenomenon**:
  Raynaud's phenomenon, characterized by **cold-induced vasospasm** of the fingers and toes, is often seen in **scleroderma, mixed connective tissue disease (MCTD)**, and occasionally **SLE**. Patients report **color changes** in the digits (white to blue to red) during cold exposure or stress, and may develop painful **ulcers** in severe cases.
  - In **systemic sclerosis (scleroderma)**, Raynaud's is frequently the first sign, followed by skin thickening and joint stiffness.

4.1.5. Previous Joint or Muscle Involvement

A history of previous episodes of **joint pain, swelling**, or **systemic symptoms** can suggest **relapsing-remitting patterns** typical of certain rheumatologic diseases.

- **Relapsing-Remitting Diseases**:
  Conditions like **systemic lupus erythematosus (SLE)** and **gout** are known for their **episodic flares**. In **SLE**, patients may experience intermittent periods of **joint pain, rash**, and **fatigue** that improve, only to recur later.
  - In **gout**, patients often present with **acute flares** of severe joint pain, followed by periods of remission. These flares may become more frequent and severe over time if not adequately treated.
- **Chronic Progressive Diseases**:
  Rheumatoid arthritis (RA), by contrast, often follows a **chronic progressive** course, with ongoing joint pain and stiffness that progressively worsens over time. Early intervention with DMARDs can alter this disease course and prevent long-term joint damage.

4.2. Key Symptoms: Joint Pain, Stiffness, Swelling, and Systemic Symptoms

Understanding key symptoms helps to narrow down differential diagnoses in rheumatology:

- **Joint Pain (Arthralgia)**:
  - **Inflammatory joint pain** tends to be worse after periods of rest (e.g., in the morning) and improves with activity. It is commonly seen in conditions like **RA**, **psoriatic arthritis**, and **gout**.
  - **Non-inflammatory joint pain** tends to worsen with activity and improve with rest, which is typical of **osteoarthritis**.
- **Stiffness**:
  - **Prolonged morning stiffness** (>30 minutes) suggests an **inflammatory** process (e.g., RA or ankylosing spondylitis).
  - **Intermittent or short-lasting stiffness** is characteristic of **non-inflammatory** conditions like OA.
- **Joint Swelling**:
  The presence of joint swelling, whether due to **synovitis** (inflammation of the synovium) or **effusion** (fluid in the joint), is a hallmark of inflammatory arthritis, particularly in conditions like RA or **crystalline arthritis** (e.g., gout or pseudogout).
- **Systemic Symptoms**:
  In conditions like **SLE** or **vasculitis**, systemic features such as **fever**, **weight loss**, **fatigue**, and **organ involvement** (e.g., kidneys, lungs) can provide important diagnostic clues.

4.3. The Rheumatologic Physical Examination: Identifying Joint, Skin, and Muscle Abnormalities

A detailed physical examination helps to confirm the diagnosis suggested by history and helps assess disease severity and activity.

- **Joint Examination**:
  - **Inspection**: Look for signs of **swelling**, **erythema**, and **deformities**. For example, RA often leads to ulnar deviation, **swan neck**, and **boutonniere deformities** in advanced disease. **Gout** may cause **tophi** or lumps near joints.
  - **Palpation**: Assess for **synovitis** (soft, boggy swelling), **effusion**, and **tenderness** over the joint line.
  - **Range of Motion**: Assess active and passive motion. **Restricted range of motion** can suggest joint damage in conditions like OA or RA.
  - **Enthesitis** (inflammation where tendons or ligaments insert into bone) is common in **spondyloarthropathies** (e.g., psoriatic arthritis, ankylosing spondylitis).
- **Skin Examination**:
  Certain skin findings are associated with rheumatologic diseases:
  - **Malar rash** (butterfly rash) in **SLE**
  - **Gottron's papules** in **dermatomyositis**

- - **Psoriatic plaques** in **psoriatic arthritis**.
  - **Sclerodactyly** (skin tightening on the fingers) in **scleroderma**.
- **Muscle Abnormalities**:
  Assess for **muscle weakness** in conditions like **polymyositis** or **dermatomyositis**, or **muscle tenderness** in **fibromyalgia**. Objective weakness (especially proximal muscle weakness) suggests inflammatory myopathy.

4.4. Red Flags in Rheumatology: When to Suspect a Serious Condition

Recognizing red flags is crucial for identifying serious, potentially life-threatening conditions that require urgent intervention.

- **Acute Monoarthritis**:
  Sudden onset of severe pain in a single joint, particularly if associated with fever, raises suspicion for **septic arthritis**, which requires urgent diagnosis and treatment to prevent joint destruction. **Gout** or **pseudogout** can also present as acute monoarthritis but tend to have less systemic involvement.
- **Systemic Vasculitis**:
  Symptoms such as **fever**, **weight loss**, **skin rashes**, and **multisystem organ involvement** (e.g., renal, pulmonary) suggest systemic vasculitis. Early recognition and treatment with immunosuppressive therapy are essential to prevent end-organ damage.
- **Scleroderma Renal Crisis**:
  A rare but life-threatening complication of scleroderma, presenting with **accelerated hypertension** and **acute renal failure**. Prompt recognition and initiation of **ACE inhibitors** can be life-saving.
- **Giant Cell Arteritis (GCA)**:
  New-onset headache, **jaw claudication**, and **visual disturbances** in patients over 50 years of age raise suspicion for GCA. Urgent treatment with corticosteroids is required to prevent blindness.

Accurate diagnosis in rheumatology relies heavily on a thorough history and physical examination. Recognizing key patterns of symptoms and red flags ensures early and appropriate treatment, preventing long-term complications. This approach helps the primary care provider identify when to manage conservatively and when to refer to a rheumatologist for further evaluation and treatment.

References

- McInnes IB, Schett G. Pathogenesis of rheumatoid arthritis. N Engl J Med. 2011;365(23):2205-2219.
- Smolen JS, Aletaha D, McInnes IB. Rheumatoid arthritis. Lancet. 2016;388(10055):2023-2038.
- Gladman DD, Antoni C, Mease P, Clegg DO, Nash P. Psoriatic arthritis: epidemiology, clinical features, course, and outcome. Ann Rheum Dis. 2005;64(suppl 2).

- Dougados M, Baeten D. Spondyloarthritis. Lancet. 2011;377(9783):2127-2137.
- Isenberg D, Rahman A. Systemic lupus erythematosus—2017. Medicine. 2017;45(2):89-95.
- Denton CP, Khanna D. Systemic sclerosis. Lancet. 2017;390(10103):1685-1699.
- Dalbeth N, Merriman TR, Stamp LK. Gout. Lancet. 2016;388(10055):2039-2052.
- Hochberg MC. Osteoarthritis year 2012 in review: clinical. Osteoarthritis Cartilage. 2012;20(12):1465-1469.
- Aletaha D, Smolen JS. Diagnosis and management of rheumatoid arthritis: a review. JAMA. 2018;320(13):1360-1372.
- Schumacher HR. Crystal-induced arthritis: an overview. Am J Med. 2014;127(10).

- Gordon C, Amissah-Arthur MB, Gayed M, et al. The British Society for Rheumatology guideline for the management of systemic lupus erythematosus in adults. Rheumatology. 2018;57(1)

Chapter 5: Laboratory Investigations in Rheumatology

Laboratory investigations are pivotal in the diagnosis, monitoring, and management of rheumatologic diseases. This chapter outlines key laboratory tests, their interpretation, and emerging biomarkers that may influence future rheumatology practices.

5.1. Commonly Used Laboratory Tests: Rheumatoid Factor (RF), Anti-CCP, ANA, ESR, CRP

Laboratory tests serve as essential diagnostic and prognostic tools in rheumatology. Here are the most commonly used tests:

- **Rheumatoid Factor (RF)**:
  Rheumatoid Factor is an autoantibody targeting the Fc portion of IgG. Although RF is **positive in 70-80% of patients with rheumatoid arthritis (RA)**, it is not specific, as it can also be detected in **chronic infections** (e.g., hepatitis C), **Sjogren's syndrome**, **systemic lupus erythematosus (SLE)**, and even in **healthy elderly individuals**. Therefore, RF is more useful when considered alongside clinical findings and other tests.
- **Anti-Cyclic Citrullinated Peptide (Anti-CCP)**:
  Anti-CCP antibodies are highly specific for RA and are detected in **up to 90-95% of patients**. These antibodies target citrullinated proteins, which are created in response to inflammation. Anti-CCP is more specific than RF and can often be present **years before clinical symptoms develop**. It is also associated with a more severe disease course, making it valuable for prognosis.
- **Antinuclear Antibody (ANA)**:
  ANA testing is widely used for the diagnosis of systemic autoimmune diseases, particularly **SLE**, where it is positive in **95-98% of cases**. However, ANA is not specific for SLE and can also be positive in other diseases, including **systemic sclerosis**, **polymyositis**, **Sjogren's syndrome**, and **rheumatoid arthritis**, as well as in **healthy individuals** (especially the elderly). Positive ANA without other clinical or laboratory evidence of autoimmune disease is often considered clinically insignificant.
- **Erythrocyte Sedimentation Rate (ESR)**:
  ESR is a nonspecific marker of **inflammation**. It is elevated in inflammatory, infectious, and neoplastic conditions. In rheumatologic diseases, ESR is often raised in conditions like **RA, polymyalgia rheumatica, vasculitis**, and **SLE**. Elevated ESR correlates with disease activity, especially in RA, where it is useful for **monitoring treatment response**. However, factors such as **age, anemia**, and **kidney disease** can also affect ESR levels.
- **C-Reactive Protein (CRP)**:
  CRP is another acute-phase reactant and a sensitive marker of systemic inflammation. It responds rapidly to inflammation, rising within hours and declining just as quickly when the inflammatory process resolves. CRP is particularly useful in monitoring **RA, gout**, and **septic arthritis** activity. Unlike ESR, it is not affected by age or anemia and is a

more direct marker of inflammation. **Normal CRP values** can help rule out active inflammatory diseases.

5.2. Understanding Autoantibodies: ANA Subtypes, ANCA, Anti-dsDNA

Autoantibodies are critical tools in the diagnosis and monitoring of autoimmune rheumatic diseases. Here's a closer look at key autoantibodies:

- **ANA Subtypes**:
  ANA subtypes provide more specific information regarding various autoimmune diseases:
    - **Anti-dsDNA**: Highly specific for **SLE**, anti-dsDNA correlates with **disease activity**, particularly with **lupus nephritis**. Its levels fluctuate with disease flares, making it a key biomarker for monitoring SLE .
    - **Anti-Smith (Anti-Sm)**: Although less sensitive than anti-dsDNA, Anti-Sm is highly specific for SLE, and its presence is strongly diagnostic of the disease .
    - **Anti-Ro/SSA and Anti-La/SSB**: These antibodies are primarily associated with **Sjogren's syndrome** but can also appear in **SLE**, especially in cases involving **neonatal lupus** .
    - **Anti-Scl-70**: Found in patients with **systemic sclerosis**, particularly the diffuse subtype, and associated with more severe interstitial lung disease .
- **Anti-Neutrophil Cytoplasmic Antibodies (ANCA)**:
  ANCA testing is used primarily for diagnosing **vasculitis syndromes**. There are two main types of ANCA:
    - **c-ANCA**: Directed against **proteinase 3 (PR3)**, this is primarily seen in **granulomatosis with polyangiitis (GPA)**.
    - **p-ANCA**: Targets **myeloperoxidase (MPO)** and is associated with **microscopic polyangiitis (MPA)** and **eosinophilic granulomatosis with polyangiitis (EGPA)** .
- **Anti-dsDNA**:
  Anti-dsDNA is highly specific for **SLE** and often correlates with disease activity, particularly in cases of **lupus nephritis** . Rising levels of anti-dsDNA often predict disease flares, making it a valuable tool for **monitoring** SLE.

5.3. Synovial Fluid Analysis: Indications and Interpretation

Synovial fluid analysis is an essential diagnostic tool in evaluating joint effusion, particularly in cases of acute arthritis. It helps differentiate between **inflammatory**, **non-inflammatory**, **infectious**, and **crystal-induced arthritis**.

- **Indications**:
  Synovial fluid analysis is indicated for patients presenting with **acute monoarthritis**, **chronic effusions**, or **suspected septic arthritis**. It is particularly useful in distinguishing **gout**, **pseudogout**, and **septic arthritis**, which require immediate intervention .

- **Interpretation**:
  - **Appearance**:
    - **Non-inflammatory fluid**: Clear and viscous (e.g., osteoarthritis).
    - **Inflammatory fluid**: Cloudy and less viscous (e.g., RA, gout).
    - **Septic fluid**: Purulent with possible odor.
  - **White Blood Cell (WBC) Count**:
    - **<2,000 cells/mm³**: Suggests non-inflammatory conditions like OA.
    - **2,000-75,000 cells/mm³**: Indicates inflammatory conditions such as RA, gout, or pseudogout.
    - **>75,000 cells/mm³**: Raises suspicion for **septic arthritis**, which is a medical emergency.
  - **Crystal Analysis**:
    - **Monosodium urate crystals** (needle-shaped, negatively birefringent under polarized light) indicate **gout**.
    - **Calcium pyrophosphate crystals** (rhomboid-shaped, positively birefringent) suggest **pseudogout**.

5.4. Emerging Biomarkers in Rheumatologic Diseases

In recent years, new biomarkers have been identified that could transform the diagnosis and management of rheumatic diseases.

- **Serum Calprotectin**:
  Calprotectin is a protein released by neutrophils and has been identified as a promising biomarker for **inflammatory arthritis**, particularly RA. Elevated calprotectin levels correlate with **disease activity** and can predict **radiographic progression**.
- **S100 Proteins (S100A8/S100A9)**:
  These proteins are involved in the inflammatory process and have been found to be elevated in **juvenile idiopathic arthritis** and **RA**. Monitoring S100 levels can provide insight into **subclinical inflammation** and potential **disease relapse**.
- **MMP-3 (Matrix Metalloproteinase-3)**:
  MMP-3 is involved in the breakdown of cartilage and is elevated in **RA**. It has been proposed as a **biomarker for joint damage** and disease activity.
- **Type II Collagen Neoepitope (CTX-II)**:
  CTX-II is a breakdown product of cartilage and can be used to monitor **osteoarthritis progression**. Elevated CTX-II levels have been associated with more severe joint destruction.

Laboratory investigations are indispensable in the diagnosis, management, and monitoring of rheumatologic diseases. While traditional markers like RF, anti-CCP, and ANA remain foundational, emerging biomarkers hold promise for more personalized and precise care in rheumatology. Understanding these tests' strengths and limitations will empower primary care providers to make more informed decisions in patient management.

References

- Aletaha, D., & Smolen, J. S. (2018). Diagnosis and management of rheumatoid arthritis: A review. *JAMA*, 320(13), 1360-1372.
- van Venrooij, W. J., & Pruijn, G. J. (2000). Citrullination: a small change for a protein with great consequences for rheumatoid arthritis. *Arthritis research*, 2(4), 249-251.
- Hochberg, M. C. (1997). Rheumatoid arthritis: mechanisms and management. *Springer*.
- Egner, W. (2000). The use of laboratory tests in the diagnosis of SLE. *Journal of Clinical Pathology*, 53(6), 424-432.
- Bossuyt, X. (2009). Serologic markers in the diagnosis of systemic autoimmune diseases. *Clinical Chemistry*, 55(11), 1939-1946.
- Raza, K., & Buckley, C. D. (2006). Clinical review: Treating very early rheumatoid arthritis—The concept of window of opportunity. *Best Practice & Research Clinical Rheumatology*, 20(5), 749-764.
- Smolen, J. S., Aletaha, D., & McInnes, I. B. (2016). Rheumatoid arthritis. *The Lancet*, 388(10055), 2023-2038.

Chapter 6: Imaging in Rheumatology

Imaging is a crucial tool in diagnosing and managing rheumatic diseases. It aids in detecting joint damage, inflammation, and structural changes in bones and soft tissues. This chapter elaborates on various imaging modalities, their applications, and limitations in rheumatologic conditions.

6.1. X-Rays Findings in Rheumatic Diseases

X-rays play a crucial role in diagnosing and monitoring various **rheumatic diseases**. They are the first-line imaging modality used to evaluate **joint** and **bone abnormalities**, given their accessibility, affordability, and ability to detect structural changes. Although X-rays may not be sensitive enough to identify early soft tissue inflammation or small erosions, they are invaluable for detecting **long-term damage** and chronic structural changes, which can help differentiate between types of arthritis and guide treatment.

6.1.1. Rheumatoid Arthritis (RA)

In **rheumatoid arthritis (RA)**, X-rays are essential for assessing the progression of joint damage, especially in the **small joints** of the **hands** and **feet**.

- **Early RA Findings**:
  In the early stages, X-rays may show **soft tissue swelling** and **joint space narrowing**, which occurs due to **cartilage loss** as the synovial inflammation begins to erode the joint surfaces.
- **Progressive RA**:
  As RA progresses, **bone erosions** become evident, particularly around the **MCP (metacarpophalangeal)** and **PIP (proximal interphalangeal)** joints of the hands and the **MTP (metatarsophalangeal)** joints of the feet. These **erosions** are caused by the aggressive inflammation and destruction of bone, which is a hallmark of untreated or poorly controlled RA.
- **Advanced RA**:
  In more advanced stages, X-rays can show **periarticular osteopenia** (loss of bone density around the joints) and **joint deformities** such as ulnar deviation or swan-neck deformities. These changes reflect long-standing inflammation and joint destruction.
    - **Periarticular osteopenia** is particularly useful in distinguishing RA from **osteoarthritis**, as it reflects the systemic inflammatory nature of RA.

6.1.2. Osteoarthritis (OA)

Osteoarthritis (OA) is a degenerative joint disease, and X-rays are pivotal in confirming the diagnosis by visualizing typical structural changes.

- **Joint Space Narrowing**:
  In OA, **joint space narrowing** is seen due to the **loss of cartilage** in the joint. Unlike

RA, which typically affects the small joints symmetrically, OA primarily affects **weight-bearing joints**, such as the **knees**, **hips**, and **spine**, and is characterized by **asymmetric joint space loss**.

- **Subchondral Sclerosis and Osteophyte Formation**:
X-rays also reveal **subchondral sclerosis**, which is the hardening of the bone just below the cartilage surface, and **osteophyte formation** (bone spurs), which are common features in OA. These osteophytes develop as the joint tries to repair the damage from cartilage loss, contributing to joint stiffness and pain.
- **Subchondral Cysts**:
Another common finding in OA is the formation of **subchondral cysts**, which are small, fluid-filled sacs that develop in the bone beneath the cartilage. These are typically seen in **advanced OA**.
- **Comparative Features**:
Unlike RA, which targets small joints and causes erosive damage, OA is marked by **non-erosive degeneration**. OA tends to be more prominent in joints like the **knees** and **hips** and shows **bony outgrowths** rather than erosions.

6.1.3. Ankylosing Spondylitis (AS)

Ankylosing spondylitis (AS) is a chronic inflammatory disease that primarily affects the **spine** and **sacroiliac joints**, and X-rays are essential for tracking disease progression.

- **Sacroiliitis**:
In the early stages of AS, X-rays of the **sacroiliac joints** may show **sacroiliitis**, which includes findings of **joint erosion**, **sclerosis** (hardening), and eventual **fusion** of the sacroiliac joints. Sacroiliitis is a hallmark of AS and is one of the earliest radiographic findings in the disease.
- **Syndesmophytes**:
As AS progresses, X-rays may reveal **syndesmophytes**, which are **bony outgrowths** that form along the edges of the vertebrae. Syndesmophytes grow vertically, eventually bridging the gaps between vertebrae, leading to **fusion of the spine**.
- **Bamboo Spine**:
In advanced AS, the fusion of vertebrae gives rise to the characteristic **bamboo spine** appearance on X-rays. This occurs when multiple vertebrae fuse together, causing stiffness and a loss of mobility in the spine. The fusion leads to a **rigid, straight spine** that resembles the segments of bamboo.

6.1.4. Gout

Gout is a metabolic disorder caused by the deposition of **monosodium urate crystals** in the joints, leading to acute and chronic inflammatory arthritis. X-rays are not useful for diagnosing **acute gout** but can show characteristic findings in **chronic gout**.

- **Punched-Out Erosions**:
In **chronic gout**, X-rays may show **punched-out erosions** with **overhanging edges**

(also known as "rat bite" erosions) around the affected joints. These erosions are caused by chronic inflammation from urate crystal deposition, which destroys the bone.
- **Tophaceous Deposits**:
  In advanced cases of gout, **tophi** (nodules formed by urate crystals) can appear on X-rays as **calcified masses** around the joints or in the soft tissues. These tophi are commonly found in the fingers, toes, and elbows.
- **Early Gout**:
  In the early stages of gout, X-rays are often normal and therefore less useful for diagnosing early disease. For this reason, imaging techniques like **ultrasound** or **dual-energy CT** (DECT) may be more sensitive in detecting **urate crystal deposits** before significant joint damage occurs.

6.1.5. Limitations of X-Rays

While **X-rays** are invaluable for detecting **long-term structural changes**, they have certain limitations in rheumatology, especially for identifying early disease processes:

- **Early Disease Detection**:
  X-rays are limited in detecting **early soft tissue inflammation** and **small erosions**. In conditions like **early RA** or **acute gout**, X-rays may not reveal significant findings, as structural damage may not yet be apparent. In such cases, **ultrasound** or **magnetic resonance imaging (MRI)** may be more useful for detecting **synovitis**, **tendinitis**, and **small erosions**.
- **Soft Tissue Involvement**:
  X-rays cannot effectively visualize **soft tissue structures** like **ligaments**, **tendons**, or **bursae**, making them less useful in conditions that involve these tissues, such as **bursitis** or **tendinitis**. **MRI** is the preferred imaging modality for detailed soft tissue evaluation.

Despite these limitations, X-rays remain a critical tool for assessing **chronic joint damage**, monitoring disease progression, and distinguishing between different types of arthritis.

6.2. Ultrasound in Joint Assessment: Benefits and Limitations

Ultrasound has gained increasing recognition as a valuable imaging modality in the assessment and management of **rheumatic diseases**, particularly for conditions like **rheumatoid arthritis (RA)** and **spondyloarthropathies**.

The **American College of Rheumatology (ACR)** acknowledges ultrasound as an important tool due to its ability to provide **real-time imaging** of joints and soft tissues, without the risks associated with radiation exposure. Ultrasound offers several benefits in the detection and monitoring of **inflammatory arthritis**, as well as in guiding therapeutic procedures. However, it also has limitations, particularly in terms of operator dependence and standardization.

6.2.1. Benefits of Ultrasound in Rheumatic Diseases

1. **Detection of Synovitis**:
   One of the primary uses of ultrasound in rheumatology is the detection of **synovitis**, which refers to the inflammation of the **synovial membrane**. Ultrasound can visualize **synovial thickening** and **effusions**, both of which are hallmarks of active inflammation.
   - **ACR Guidelines** emphasize the use of ultrasound to assess **early synovitis** in patients with suspected **RA**, as it can detect subtle synovial changes that may not be visible on **X-rays** or even **clinical examination**. By identifying **active synovitis**, ultrasound aids in early diagnosis and enables timely initiation of **disease-modifying antirheumatic drugs (DMARDs)**.
   - According to studies, **ultrasound** can detect **subclinical synovitis**, allowing rheumatologists to monitor disease activity even in patients who appear to be in clinical remission. This can guide adjustments in therapy to prevent disease flares and joint damage.

2. **Guided Injections and Aspirations**:
   Ultrasound-guided procedures are widely used in rheumatology to improve the accuracy of **joint injections** and **aspirations**.
   - **ACR Recommendations** endorse the use of **ultrasound guidance** to increase the precision of **intra-articular corticosteroid injections** and **synovial fluid aspirations**, particularly in small or difficult-to-access joints. Ultrasound guidance ensures accurate needle placement, which is critical for the success of these procedures and minimizes complications.
   - Studies have shown that ultrasound guidance improves the success rate of injections into joints like the **shoulder**, **hip**, and **wrist**, where blind injections may have lower accuracy.

3. **Erosions and Tendon Pathology**:
   Ultrasound is particularly sensitive in detecting **bone erosions** and **soft tissue pathology** in the **early stages** of **rheumatoid arthritis** and other inflammatory diseases.
   - **ACR Guidelines** recognize that **ultrasound** can detect **bone erosions** earlier than X-rays, especially in **small joints** such as those of the **hands** and **feet**. This is particularly important in RA, where early detection of erosions can prompt more aggressive treatment to prevent joint deformity.
   - Additionally, ultrasound can identify **tendinitis**, **enthesitis**, and **bursitis**, which are common in **spondyloarthropathies**. These conditions can be challenging to diagnose with physical examination alone, but ultrasound can visualize the **soft tissue changes** associated with inflammation and overuse.

4. **Power Doppler Imaging**:
   Power Doppler ultrasound is a technique used to evaluate **vascular flow** within tissues, and it is highly sensitive to changes in **blood flow** associated with inflammation.
   - In **RA**, Power Doppler can highlight areas of **increased vascularity** in the synovium, which correlates with **active inflammation**. **ACR Guidelines** recommend Power Doppler ultrasound for monitoring disease activity in RA, as

increased **vascularization** is indicative of ongoing synovial inflammation, even in cases where clinical symptoms have improved.
- Power Doppler findings can guide decisions about **intensifying treatment** in patients with residual inflammation, reducing the risk of disease progression and joint damage.

6.2.2. Limitations of Ultrasound in Rheumatic Diseases

Despite its numerous advantages, ultrasound has some limitations that rheumatologists need to consider:

1. **Operator Dependence**:
   One of the most significant limitations of ultrasound is its **operator dependence**. The quality and accuracy of the ultrasound examination are highly contingent on the **skill** and **experience** of the technician or rheumatologist performing the scan.
   - **ACR Guidelines** highlight that variability in operator skill can lead to **inconsistent findings**, particularly in the assessment of **synovitis** and **bone erosions**. This operator dependence necessitates proper training and experience to ensure accurate and reliable results.
   - Inconsistent operator proficiency can also complicate comparisons between scans from different facilities or practitioners.

2. **Limited Penetration**:
   Ultrasound has **limited ability** to penetrate deep into tissues, which restricts its utility for assessing **deep-seated joints** or **structures** such as the **hips** or **spine**.
   - For **deep joints** like the **hip**, or for conditions involving the **axial skeleton** (e.g., **ankylosing spondylitis**), modalities such as **magnetic resonance imaging (MRI)** are more appropriate, as they provide better visualization of deep structures.

3. **Inconsistent Standardization**:
   There is currently no **universally accepted scoring system** for grading **synovitis**, **erosions**, or **Power Doppler findings** via ultrasound, which can make **standardization** across studies and clinical practices challenging.
   - Although some scoring systems have been developed (e.g., the **OMERACT** system for assessing synovitis and erosion in RA), **ACR Guidelines** note that variability in ultrasound findings between centers remains an issue. This lack of consistent standardization can affect the reproducibility of results and the ability to compare findings across different clinical settings.
   - Ongoing efforts in **rheumatology research** aim to establish more widely accepted protocols for ultrasound use and interpretation, which would improve its application in clinical practice.

6.2.3. ACR Guidelines on Ultrasound Use in Rheumatology

The **American College of Rheumatology (ACR)** provides recommendations for the use of ultrasound in rheumatology, particularly in the assessment and management of **inflammatory arthritis** such as **RA**. Ultrasound is particularly useful in:

- **Evaluating early synovitis** and monitoring subclinical inflammation.
- **Guiding intra-articular injections** and **aspirations** for improved accuracy.
- **Detecting bone erosions** in small joints before they become visible on X-rays.
- **Assessing soft tissue structures**, such as tendons and bursae, that may be involved in conditions like **tendinitis**, **enthesitis**, and **bursitis**.
- **Monitoring disease activity** using Power Doppler to visualize active inflammation and blood flow.

The ACR encourages the integration of ultrasound into clinical practice, particularly for **early diagnosis** and **monitoring** of **RA** and other inflammatory conditions. However, the ACR also emphasizes the need for proper training and standardization to ensure accurate results and to reduce variability across different practitioners and centers.

Ultrasound is an invaluable tool in **rheumatology**, offering real-time imaging of **joints** and **soft tissues** without radiation exposure. It is particularly beneficial in detecting **early synovitis**, guiding **joint injections**, and identifying **soft tissue pathologies** in **inflammatory arthritis**. **Power Doppler imaging** further enhances its utility by providing insights into active inflammation. However, the limitations of ultrasound—such as operator dependence, limited penetration for deep joints, and inconsistent standardization—necessitate careful consideration and appropriate training. According to **ACR guidelines**, ultrasound plays an essential role in diagnosing and managing inflammatory rheumatic diseases, particularly RA, where early detection and treatment are crucial for preventing joint damage.

6.3. Advanced Imaging: MRI and CT for Rheumatic Conditions

Magnetic resonance imaging (MRI) and **computed tomography (CT)** provide advanced, high-resolution imaging that allows for the detailed evaluation of **soft tissues**, **bone**, and **early inflammatory changes** in rheumatic conditions. These imaging modalities are often used when there is a need for greater sensitivity in detecting early disease processes or structural abnormalities that are not visible on **X-rays** or **ultrasound**. Both MRI and CT have distinct roles in diagnosing and managing **rheumatoid arthritis (RA)**, **ankylosing spondylitis (AS)**, **osteoarthritis (OA)**, and **gout**, although their use is typically reserved for more complex cases where **X-rays** or **ultrasound** are insufficient.

6.3.1. MRI in Rheumatic Diseases

Magnetic resonance imaging (MRI) is a powerful tool for evaluating **soft tissue structures** and detecting **early inflammatory changes** in the joints and bones. It is particularly useful in **inflammatory arthritis** and is often used when early detection or detailed imaging of soft tissues is needed.

1. **Soft Tissue and Early Inflammatory Changes**:
   MRI is highly sensitive for detecting **synovitis, bone marrow edema**, and **early erosions**, particularly in conditions like **rheumatoid arthritis (RA)** and **spondyloarthropathies**.
   - In **RA**, MRI can detect **synovitis** (inflammation of the synovial membrane) and **bone marrow edema**—both early signs of active inflammation that may not be visible on **X-rays**. Bone marrow edema, in particular, is a key predictor of **future joint erosions**, making MRI an important tool for identifying patients at risk of disease progression .
   - In **ankylosing spondylitis (AS)**, MRI is considered the **gold standard** for detecting **sacroiliitis** (inflammation of the sacroiliac joints). MRI can reveal **bone marrow edema, synovitis**, and **enthesitis** (inflammation at the insertion of tendons or ligaments), often before changes are visible on **X-rays**. Early detection of these changes is crucial for starting **disease-modifying treatments** to prevent long-term damage.

2. **Cartilage and Meniscal Damage**:
   In **osteoarthritis (OA)**, MRI is invaluable for assessing **cartilage integrity** and identifying **meniscal tears**, especially in **knee** and **hip OA**. Unlike **X-rays**, which primarily show bone changes, MRI allows for a detailed evaluation of **cartilage, menisci**, and other soft tissues in the joint.
   - **Cartilage loss** and **subchondral changes** (such as bone marrow lesions) are early features of OA that can guide treatment decisions. MRI can also detect **meniscal degeneration** or **tears**, which can contribute to joint instability and further cartilage loss in patients with **knee OA**.
   - This early detection of structural damage allows for more tailored interventions, such as physical therapy, **hyaluronic acid injections**, or surgical options in severe cases.

3. **Bone Marrow Edema**:
   Bone marrow edema is a hallmark of **early inflammatory arthritis**, and its presence on MRI correlates with an increased risk of developing **bone erosions**. In conditions like **RA**, identifying bone marrow edema on MRI can indicate areas of active inflammation, even before overt bone damage occurs, allowing for more **aggressive treatment** to prevent joint destruction.
   - **ACR Guidelines** recommend MRI as a valuable tool for assessing disease activity in **early RA**, particularly in patients who have ambiguous findings on clinical examination or **X-rays** .

4. **Limitations of MRI**:
   While MRI provides excellent detail, it has certain limitations:
   - **Cost**: MRI is more expensive than **X-rays** and **ultrasound**, which can limit its availability, particularly in resource-constrained settings.
   - **Time-Consuming**: MRI scans take longer to perform than X-rays, which can be a barrier in cases where rapid diagnosis is required.
   - **Limited Availability**: MRI may not be readily available in all healthcare facilities, especially in rural or underserved areas.

- **Use in Complex Cases**: MRI is typically reserved for cases where **early, aggressive disease** is suspected or when there is **diagnostic uncertainty**, particularly in cases where initial imaging (X-rays or ultrasound) is inconclusive.

6.3.2. CT in Rheumatic Diseases

Computed tomography (CT) is another advanced imaging modality that provides **excellent bone detail**. It is particularly useful for assessing **bone erosions** and **subtle structural changes** in **crystalline arthritis**, such as **gout**, where small bone changes may not be visible on **X-rays**.

1. **Detailed Bone Imaging**:
   CT excels at visualizing **bone structures** and is often used to detect **subtle erosions** in conditions like **gout** or **pseudogout**. In **gout**, CT can identify **urate crystal deposition** and **punched-out erosions** with **overhanging edges** that may not be visible on X-rays, particularly in the early stages of the disease.
   - **Dual-energy CT (DECT)** is a specialized form of CT that can differentiate between **urate crystals** and other materials, such as calcium. DECT has become a valuable tool for diagnosing **gout** in difficult cases where traditional imaging methods are inconclusive.
2. **Sacroiliitis and Ankylosing Spondylitis**:
   While **MRI** is the preferred imaging modality for detecting **early inflammatory changes** in **ankylosing spondylitis**, CT can be used to evaluate **sacroiliitis** in patients where **X-rays** are non-diagnostic.
   - CT is particularly useful for detecting **bony changes**, such as **erosions**, **sclerosis**, and **ankylosis** (fusion of the sacroiliac joints), in **advanced AS**. These changes can be identified earlier on **CT** than on **conventional X-rays**, making it a valuable alternative when **MRI** is not available or when specific **bone detail** is required.
3. **Limitations of CT**:
   Despite its ability to visualize bone structures in great detail, CT has limitations, particularly in its ability to detect **soft tissue changes**:
   - **Less Sensitive for Soft Tissue**: Unlike **MRI**, CT is less effective at detecting **soft tissue inflammation**, such as **synovitis** or **enthesitis**, which are critical in assessing **inflammatory arthritis**. As a result, CT is not typically the first choice for evaluating **soft tissue pathology**.
   - **Radiation Exposure**: **CT scans** involve **radiation exposure**, which is a concern, especially in **young patients** or those requiring **frequent imaging**. **ACR Guidelines** recommend limiting the use of CT in these populations to minimize cumulative radiation risks.

6.4. Novel Techniques: Dual-Energy CT, PET-CT in Inflammatory Arthritis

Recent advancements in imaging technology, particularly **Dual-Energy CT (DECT)** and **Positron Emission Tomography-Computed Tomography (PET-CT)**, have enhanced our ability to visualize **inflammatory processes** and **joint damage** in rheumatic diseases. These novel imaging techniques provide additional insights beyond conventional **X-rays**, **ultrasound**, or even **standard CT** and **MRI**, offering improved diagnostic accuracy for certain conditions and aiding in the management of complex cases. However, their use is generally limited to specialized centers due to cost and availability, and they are typically reserved for more difficult-to-diagnose cases or when standard imaging methods are inconclusive.

6.4.1. Dual-Energy CT (DECT)

Dual-Energy CT (DECT) has revolutionized the diagnosis and management of **crystal arthropathies**, particularly **gout**, by allowing non-invasive detection of **urate crystals** in soft tissues and joints. This technique uses two different X-ray energy levels to differentiate between different materials based on their composition, providing precise visualization of urate and other crystal deposits.

1. **Detection of Urate Crystals**:
   DECT is highly sensitive for detecting **monosodium urate crystals**, which are responsible for the inflammatory process in **gout**. It can visualize urate deposits in soft tissues, tendons, and joints, even in cases where **X-rays** or other imaging methods do not show significant changes. DECT can also be used to detect **subclinical tophi**, which may not yet cause overt symptoms, aiding in early diagnosis and guiding treatment.
   - DECT has proven to be especially useful in diagnosing **chronic tophaceous gout**, where large urate deposits (tophi) may not be evident on physical examination or other imaging techniques. It provides a clear view of the **distribution and burden** of urate crystals, helping to monitor disease progression and the **effectiveness of urate-lowering therapies** (e.g., **allopurinol, febuxostat**) .
   - DECT can also help confirm the diagnosis in atypical cases of gout where other imaging modalities, such as **X-rays**, are inconclusive.
2. **Utility in Pseudogout (Calcium Pyrophosphate Deposition Disease)**:
   In addition to **urate crystals**, DECT is also capable of detecting **calcium pyrophosphate dihydrate (CPPD)** crystals, the cause of **pseudogout**. This makes DECT a valuable tool for distinguishing between different types of **crystal arthropathies**, which can sometimes present with similar clinical symptoms but require different treatment approaches.
3. **Limitations of DECT**:
   Despite its significant advantages, **DECT** has some limitations:
   - **Cost**: DECT is more expensive than conventional CT or X-rays, which limits its use, particularly in routine practice.
   - **Availability**: DECT is generally only available in **specialized centers** and is often reserved for cases where a **definitive diagnosis** is difficult to establish using other methods.

- **Radiation Exposure**: Like all CT scans, DECT exposes patients to **ionizing radiation**, though the benefits of obtaining an accurate diagnosis in cases of **gout** or **pseudogout** generally outweigh the risks, especially when other imaging techniques fail to provide clarity.

6.4.2. Positron Emission Tomography-Computed Tomography (PET-CT)

Positron Emission Tomography-Computed Tomography (PET-CT) combines **metabolic imaging** (from PET) with **high-resolution anatomical imaging** (from CT), allowing for the detection of **inflammatory activity** and **structural changes** in one scan. This modality is particularly valuable for assessing **systemic inflammation**, especially in conditions where conventional imaging may not reveal active disease processes.

1. **Detection of Systemic Inflammation**:
   PET-CT is highly sensitive for detecting **metabolically active inflammation**, which makes it ideal for evaluating diseases with systemic inflammatory involvement. It is especially useful in **large-vessel vasculitis**, such as **giant cell arteritis (GCA)** and **Takayasu arteritis**, where it can identify **active vasculitis** in the **aorta** and its major branches.
   - In **vasculitis**, PET-CT can detect inflammation that may not be visible on standard imaging modalities like **X-rays** or **CT**, enabling early diagnosis and guiding treatment decisions, particularly in patients with **polymyalgia rheumatica** or suspected **vasculitis** that involves large vessels. PET-CT is useful for **monitoring treatment response** by assessing changes in metabolic activity within inflamed vessels or tissues.
2. **Assessing Inflammation in Rheumatoid Arthritis (RA) and Spondyloarthropathies**:
   PET-CT has also been used to assess **inflammatory activity** in **RA**, **psoriatic arthritis**, and **spondyloarthropathies**. By highlighting areas of increased metabolic activity in joints, tendons, and entheses, PET-CT provides insights into disease activity that may not be apparent on **X-rays** or **MRI** alone.
   - In **RA**, PET-CT can detect active **synovitis** in multiple joints, providing a comprehensive assessment of disease burden, especially in patients with systemic involvement.
   - In **spondyloarthropathies**, including **ankylosing spondylitis (AS)**, PET-CT can visualize inflammation in the **spine** and **sacroiliac joints**, aiding in the diagnosis of early or atypical presentations.
3. **Limitations of PET-CT**:
   PET-CT, while powerful, has several limitations:
   - **Cost**: PET-CT is one of the most expensive imaging modalities, limiting its routine use in clinical practice.
   - **Radiation Exposure**: PET-CT involves **significant radiation exposure** due to the combination of both **PET** and **CT** scans. This exposure must be carefully considered, particularly in **younger patients** or those who require **frequent imaging**.

- **Specialized Use**: PET-CT is typically reserved for **complex cases** or when there is **diagnostic uncertainty**, especially in systemic inflammatory diseases like **vasculitis** or **RA** with multi-organ involvement. It is not commonly used for routine monitoring of arthritis due to its high cost and radiation risks.

Imaging in rheumatology is essential for diagnosing, assessing disease activity, and monitoring treatment response. Each modality—X-rays, ultrasound, MRI, CT, and emerging techniques like DECT and PET-CT—has its strengths and limitations. The choice of imaging should be guided by the clinical context, availability, and the specific rheumatologic condition being investigated.

References

- McQueen, F. M., & Benton, N. (2001). MRI in rheumatoid arthritis: a validated imaging technique? *Annals of the Rheumatic Diseases*, 60(3), 208-212.
- van der Heijde, D., Landewé, R., & Feldtkeller, E. (2005). Proposal of a linear definition of the **ankylosing spondylitis spine score**. *Arthritis & Rheumatology*, 52(8), 2828-2836.
- Sack, K. E. (2001). Gout: diagnosis and management. *The New England Journal of Medicine*, 344(14), 1056-1060.
- Filippucci, E., & Grassi, W. (2008). Ultrasonography in arthritis. *Best Practice & Research Clinical Rheumatology*, 22(6), 1079-1089.
- Aletaha, D., & Smolen, J. S. (2018). Diagnosis and management of rheumatoid arthritis: a review. *JAMA*, 320(13), 1360-1372.
- Dalbeth, N., & Gamble, G. D. (2009). Dual-energy computed tomography detection of urate deposition in tophaceous gout. *Annals of the Rheumatic Diseases*, 68(10), 1609-1612.
- Das, S., & Padhan, P. (2020). PET/CT in large vessel vasculitis: Current perspectives and future directions. *Indian Journal of Rheumatology*, 15(2), 110-115.
- Bruyn, G. A. W., Naredo, E., Moller, I., et al. (2019). Ultrasound in rheumatology: Where are we now and what can we do? *Best Practice & Research Clinical Rheumatology*, 33(6), 101-119.
- Terslev, L., Naredo, E., & Aegerter, P. (2020). Scoring ultrasound synovitis in rheumatoid arthritis: A EULAR-OMERACT ultrasound taskforce—Part 2: Reliability and application to multiple joints of the OMERACT-EULAR synovitis score. *RMD Open*, 6(2), e001267.
- Mandl, P., Navarro-Compán, V., Terslev, L., et al. (2021). EULAR recommendations for the use of imaging in the diagnosis and management of spondyloarthritis in clinical practice. *Annals of Rheumatic Diseases*, 80(1), 116-123.
- American College of Rheumatology (2015). Ultrasound guidance for intra-articular injections and aspirations in rheumatology. *ACR Practice Guidelines*.

Part 2: Common Rheumatologic Diseases and Evidence-Based Management

Chapter 7: Rheumatoid Arthritis (RA)

Rheumatoid arthritis (RA) is a chronic, systemic autoimmune disease primarily affecting the synovial joints. It is characterized by inflammation, progressive joint destruction, and a wide range of systemic manifestations. Early diagnosis and intervention are crucial to preventing irreversible damage and improving long-term outcomes. This section covers the latest guidelines on RA epidemiology, pathophysiology, diagnosis, and treatment based on updates from the **American College of Rheumatology (ACR)**.

7.1. Epidemiology and Pathophysiology of RA

- **Epidemiology**:
  RA affects about **0.5–1% of the global population**, with higher prevalence in women compared to men at a ratio of approximately 3:1. The onset typically occurs between the ages of 30 and 50, but it can develop at any age. **Genetic factors**, particularly **HLA-DRB1 alleles**, significantly increase the risk of developing RA. Environmental factors such as **smoking** and **periodontal disease** have also been linked to the development of RA through mechanisms involving immune dysregulation .
- **Pathophysiology**:
  RA is driven by a complex interplay of genetic susceptibility and environmental triggers, leading to an autoimmune response against the synovial lining of joints. Key features include:
    - **Citrullination**: The process of protein citrullination, where arginine residues are converted to citrulline, plays a significant role in RA. This process generates **autoantigens** that are targeted by the immune system, particularly in individuals with genetic predispositions such as the **shared epitope hypothesis** .
    - **Synovitis**: Chronic synovial inflammation is the hallmark of RA, resulting from the infiltration of **T cells**, **B cells**, **macrophages**, and **neutrophils**. Pro-inflammatory cytokines like **TNF-α, IL-1**, and **IL-6** drive synovial hyperplasia and joint destruction.
    - **Joint Destruction**: The inflammatory process leads to the activation of **osteoclasts** and **fibroblast-like synoviocytes**, resulting in **cartilage destruction** and **bone erosion**. Over time, untreated RA leads to irreversible joint deformities, loss of function, and disability .

7.2. RA Diagnostic Criteria and Disease Staging

- **Diagnostic Criteria**:
  The **2010 ACR/EULAR Classification Criteria** for RA provide a framework for early diagnosis, emphasizing joint involvement, serology, acute-phase reactants, and symptom duration:
    - **Joint Involvement**: Points are assigned based on the number and size of affected joints, with greater weight given to small joint involvement (e.g., wrists, metacarpophalangeal (MCP) joints, proximal interphalangeal (PIP) joints) .

- **Serology**: The presence of **Rheumatoid Factor (RF)** and **Anti-Cyclic Citrullinated Peptide (Anti-CCP)** antibodies increases the likelihood of RA, with Anti-CCP being more specific for the disease.
- **Acute-Phase Reactants**: Elevated **ESR** or **CRP** supports the diagnosis of active inflammation.
- **Duration of Symptoms**: Symptom duration greater than **six weeks** is necessary to differentiate RA from other transient causes of arthritis.

A score of ≥6/10 in this system classifies a patient as having RA. This system prioritizes early diagnosis, even before radiographic changes occur.

- **Disease Staging**:
  RA is commonly categorized by the extent of joint damage and functional impairment:
  - **Early RA**: Defined as disease duration of **<6 months**, this stage is crucial for aggressive treatment to prevent progression.
  - **Established RA**: Disease present for **>6 months** or when **erosions** or **joint deformities** are present.
  - **Functional Classification**: The **ACR** also classifies patients based on functional ability, ranging from **Class I** (completely able to perform usual activities of daily living) to **Class IV** (limited ability, requiring assistance).

7.3. Evidence-Based Pharmacological Treatments: DMARDs, Biologics, JAK Inhibitors

Over the past few decades, advances in pharmacological treatments have significantly improved outcomes for RA patients, particularly through the use of **disease-modifying antirheumatic drugs (DMARDs)**, **biologics**, and **Janus kinase (JAK) inhibitors**. Evidence-based guidelines from the **American College of Rheumatology (ACR)** provide a framework for the use of these therapies based on disease severity, response to previous treatments, and individual patient characteristics.

7.3.1. DMARDs (Disease-Modifying Antirheumatic Drugs)

DMARDs remain the cornerstone of RA management due to their ability to slow disease progression and prevent long-term joint damage. The **ACR** recommends early initiation of **DMARD therapy** to prevent irreversible structural damage and improve patient outcomes. DMARDs are generally categorized as **traditional** or **synthetic** DMARDs and **targeted synthetic** DMARDs (such as JAK inhibitors).

1. **Methotrexate (MTX)**:
   Methotrexate (MTX) is the first-line DMARD for most patients with RA and is widely regarded as the **standard of care**. It works by inhibiting **dihydrofolate reductase**, an enzyme involved in **DNA synthesis**, which reduces the proliferation of rapidly dividing immune cells responsible for inflammation.

- A landmark **Cochrane review** concluded that **MTX** is highly effective in reducing both **clinical disease activity** and **radiographic progression** in RA, with the added benefit of being cost-effective compared to biologics and other advanced therapies .
- **ACR guidelines** strongly recommend the use of **MTX** as the first-line DMARD, particularly in combination with **folic acid**, to reduce the risk of adverse effects such as **hepatotoxicity**, **oral ulcers**, and **gastrointestinal upset**.
- **Evidence**: In a randomized trial by Weinblatt et al. (1985), patients treated with **MTX** experienced significant reductions in disease activity and functional disability compared to placebo, cementing MTX's role as a cornerstone treatment in RA management.

2. **Leflunomide, Sulfasalazine, and Hydroxychloroquine**:
   These agents are alternative **traditional DMARDs** and are often used when **MTX** is contraindicated or not tolerated.
   - **Leflunomide** inhibits **pyrimidine synthesis**, reducing the proliferation of lymphocytes. Studies have demonstrated comparable efficacy to **MTX** in reducing disease activity in RA, though it may have more gastrointestinal and hepatic side effects .
   - **Sulfasalazine** is commonly used in **combination therapy** for RA and has both **anti-inflammatory** and **immunomodulatory** properties.
   - **Hydroxychloroquine**, primarily used in **systemic lupus erythematosus (SLE)**, has a milder effect in RA and is often combined with other DMARDs for better disease control.

3. **Combination DMARD Therapy**:
   When **MTX monotherapy** is insufficient to control disease activity, the ACR recommends **combination DMARD therapy**. For example, **triple therapy** with **MTX**, **sulfasalazine**, and **hydroxychloroquine** has shown additive efficacy compared to **MTX** alone, especially in patients with moderate-to-severe RA.
   - **Evidence**: The **TEAR Trial** compared **MTX monotherapy** to **triple therapy** and found that triple therapy was similarly effective to **MTX plus a biologic**, highlighting its value as a cost-effective alternative to biologic therapies in some patients .

7.3.2 Biologics

Biologic DMARDs are targeted therapies that specifically inhibit key components of the **immune system**, such as **cytokines** and **cell surface receptors**, that drive inflammation in RA. These agents are used when patients fail to respond adequately to **traditional DMARDs**, and they have revolutionized RA management by significantly reducing disease activity and slowing radiographic progression.

1. **TNF Inhibitors**:
   TNF inhibitors (e.g., **etanercept, adalimumab, infliximab**) target **tumor necrosis factor-alpha (TNF-α)**, a cytokine that plays a central role in RA pathogenesis.

- **TNF inhibitors** were among the first biologics approved for RA and have shown dramatic efficacy in reducing **joint inflammation, pain,** and **long-term disability**. They have been found to reduce **radiographic progression** and improve **physical function**.
  - **Evidence**: The **ATTRACT trial** demonstrated the efficacy of **infliximab** (in combination with MTX) in reducing RA symptoms and preventing joint damage, showing that 52% of patients had improved outcomes compared to placebo.

2. **IL-6 Inhibitors**:
   Tocilizumab and **sarilumab** target **interleukin-6 (IL-6)**, another key cytokine involved in the inflammatory cascade in RA. **Tocilizumab** is particularly useful in patients with **high inflammatory markers** such as **elevated C-reactive protein (CRP)** or **erythrocyte sedimentation rate (ESR)**.
   - **Evidence**: In the **LITHE study**, **tocilizumab** demonstrated superior efficacy in reducing disease activity and radiographic progression compared to placebo, particularly in patients with high levels of systemic inflammation.

3. **Costimulation Blockers and B-Cell Depletion**:
   Abatacept (a T-cell costimulation blocker) and **rituximab** (a B-cell depleting agent) are biologics used for patients with **refractory disease** or those who do not respond to **TNF inhibitors**.
   - **Abatacept** prevents T-cell activation by inhibiting the interaction between **CD80/86** on antigen-presenting cells and **CD28** on T cells. Studies have shown its efficacy in reducing disease activity in patients with inadequate responses to **TNF inhibitors**.
   - **Rituximab** targets **CD20** on B cells, leading to their depletion. It is particularly effective in **seropositive RA** (patients with **rheumatoid factor** or **anti-CCP antibodies**), where it has been shown to reduce disease activity and slow progression in refractory cases.

7.3.3. JAK Inhibitors

Janus kinase (JAK) inhibitors are a newer class of **oral targeted synthetic DMARDs** that block **intracellular signaling pathways** critical to the immune response in RA. Unlike **biologics**, which target extracellular cytokines or immune cell receptors, **JAK inhibitors** interfere with signaling **inside the cell**.

1. **Tofacitinib, Baricitinib, and Upadacitinib**:
   These agents are effective in reducing disease activity in patients with **moderate-to-severe RA** and are especially useful when **biologics** fail or are contraindicated.
   - **Evidence**: The **ORAL Strategy trial** compared **tofacitinib** with **adalimumab** and found that **tofacitinib** was **non-inferior** to **adalimumab** when both were combined with **methotrexate**, demonstrating its effectiveness as an alternative to biologics for RA patients.
   - **Baricitinib** has shown efficacy in reducing disease activity, particularly in patients who are **methotrexate-resistant** or **TNF inhibitor-resistant**, and it is associated with rapid symptom relief.

2. **Safety Concerns**:
   While **JAK inhibitors** are effective, they come with safety concerns, particularly related to **venous thromboembolism (VTE)** and **cardiovascular risk**. The **ACR guidelines** recommend careful **patient selection** when prescribing JAK inhibitors, especially in patients with a history of **thrombosis** or **cardiovascular disease**.
   - **Evidence**: A recent **FDA review** of clinical trial data raised concerns about an increased risk of **serious infections, malignancy**, and **thrombosis** with **JAK inhibitors**, leading to updated warnings and a recommendation to limit their use in certain high-risk populations.

7.4. Non-Pharmacological Interventions: Physical Therapy, Occupational Therapy

Non-pharmacological interventions are essential components of managing **rheumatoid arthritis (RA)**, complementing pharmacological treatment to improve patient outcomes. These approaches focus on maintaining and enhancing **joint function, mobility**, and **quality of life**, and are critical in preventing complications such as **muscle wasting, joint deformities**, and **loss of function**. The **American College of Rheumatology (ACR)** guidelines emphasize the importance of early implementation of non-pharmacological interventions alongside disease-modifying antirheumatic drugs (DMARDs) and biologic therapies.

7.4.1. Physical Therapy (PT)

Physical therapy (PT) plays a pivotal role in RA management by improving **joint mobility**, enhancing **muscle strength**, and increasing **overall physical function**. The benefits of **range-of-motion exercises, strength training**, and **low-impact aerobic activities** have been well-documented in both clinical trials and practice.

1. **Range-of-Motion and Strength Training Exercises**:
   Range-of-motion exercises are designed to maintain and increase **joint flexibility**, preventing **contractures** and **stiffness** that result from prolonged inactivity. **Strength training** helps to maintain **muscle mass** and support joint stability, which is crucial in preventing further joint damage. Exercises like **swimming, cycling**, and **walking** are frequently recommended because they are low-impact and reduce joint stress while improving cardiovascular health.
   - **Evidence**: A systematic review by Baillet et al. (2010) found that **exercise programs** in RA patients, including **aerobic** and **strengthening exercises**, led to significant improvements in **physical function** and **pain reduction** without exacerbating joint inflammation. This suggests that regular physical therapy should be an integral part of RA management to preserve joint function and mobility.
2. **ACR Guidelines and Early Referral**:
   The **ACR guidelines** advocate for **early referral** to a **physical therapist** upon diagnosis to prevent long-term complications such as **joint contractures** and **muscle wasting**.

Joint contractures result from prolonged immobilization or disuse, and **muscle wasting** occurs due to **inactivity** and **systemic inflammation** in RA. Early physical therapy interventions can minimize these risks and improve overall outcomes.
- **Evidence**: A study by Hurkmans et al. (2009) demonstrated that early initiation of **supervised physical therapy** in RA patients led to improved joint range of motion and muscle strength, reducing the likelihood of **disability** in the long term.

7.4.2. Occupational Therapy (OT)

Occupational therapy (OT) is another cornerstone of non-pharmacological management for RA patients, focusing on **maintaining independence** in daily activities, reducing joint strain, and improving overall quality of life. OT aims to help patients adapt to **functional limitations** caused by RA and provides strategies for managing fatigue and protecting joints from damage.

1. **Joint Protection Strategies and Energy Conservation**:
   Joint protection strategies are essential in preventing **joint damage** and minimizing pain. These strategies include:
   - **Avoiding repetitive motions** that stress inflamed joints.
   - **Using assistive devices** (e.g., jar openers, ergonomic utensils) to reduce joint strain during daily tasks.
   - **Energy conservation techniques**, such as pacing activities and taking frequent rest breaks, are critical for managing **fatigue**—a common symptom in RA.
   - **Evidence**: A randomized controlled trial by Hammond et al. (2014) found that **joint protection education** significantly improved patients' **pain levels**, **function**, and **self-efficacy** in managing their RA, highlighting the importance of joint protection strategies in long-term disease management.

2. **Splints and Orthotic Devices**:
   Splints and **orthotic devices** are often recommended by occupational therapists to support inflamed or weakened joints, reducing pain and improving function. These devices are particularly helpful during **flare-ups** when joints may be especially tender and vulnerable.
   - **Evidence**: A study by O'Brien et al. (2011) demonstrated that **splinting** significantly reduced pain and improved **grip strength** in patients with **RA hand involvement**, allowing them to perform daily activities with less discomfort. This highlights the role of **occupational therapy** in enhancing patient functionality through the use of splints.

3. **Adaptation to Functional Limitations**:
   In addition to physical adaptations, **occupational therapy** focuses on helping patients modify their environments and daily routines to better manage the challenges posed by RA. This might include rearranging workspaces to reduce physical strain or incorporating assistive devices into daily life.
   - **ACR Guidelines** recommend early referral to an **occupational therapist** to provide patients with the tools and strategies necessary to maintain independence in their daily lives. The early involvement of **OT** has been associated with improved long-term functional outcomes in RA patients.

7.4.3. The Role of Non-Pharmacological Interventions in Complementary RA Treatment

Non-pharmacological interventions are increasingly recognized as essential components of comprehensive RA management, complementing the effects of pharmacological therapies such as **DMARDs**, **biologics**, and **JAK inhibitors**. While medications target the underlying **inflammatory pathways** of RA, interventions like **physical therapy** and **occupational therapy** address the **functional limitations** and **quality of life** issues that arise due to the disease.

- **Functional Improvement**: Numerous studies have shown that **physical therapy** and **occupational therapy** can significantly improve **physical function** and **joint mobility**, reducing the risk of **disability** and promoting long-term independence in RA patients.
- **Quality of Life**: Beyond physical benefits, non-pharmacological interventions have a positive impact on **mental health** and **well-being** by enabling patients to maintain their daily activities and hobbies, which is crucial in managing the emotional burden of chronic disease.
- **Long-Term Outcomes**: The combination of early and consistent non-pharmacological interventions with appropriate pharmacological treatments results in **better long-term outcomes**, such as reduced disease activity, less joint damage, and improved functional status.

7.5. Long-Term Monitoring: Remission and Disease Flares

Monitoring disease activity and adjusting treatment based on the level of disease control is a key component of RA management. The ACR recommends the use of standardized tools for assessing disease activity and determining when treatment modifications are necessary.

- **Remission**:
  Achieving and maintaining **remission** or **low disease activity (LDA)** is the primary goal of RA treatment. Remission is defined as the absence of significant signs and symptoms of active disease, often measured by tools such as the **DAS28 (Disease Activity Score)** or **CDAI (Clinical Disease Activity Index)** .
  - ACR guidelines suggest **tapering** DMARDs in patients with sustained remission but advise against discontinuation, as relapse is common.
- **Disease Flares**:
  Flares are periods of increased disease activity characterized by worsened pain, swelling, and stiffness. **Rapid escalation of therapy**, including short courses of **glucocorticoids**, may be required to control flares. Patients should be educated to recognize early signs of flares to seek prompt intervention .
-

7.6. Managing Comorbidities: Cardiovascular Risk, Osteoporosis

RA is associated with increased risk for several comorbidities, most notably cardiovascular disease (CVD) and osteoporosis.

- **Cardiovascular Risk**:
Chronic inflammation in RA accelerates **atherosclerosis**, increasing the risk of **myocardial infarction** and **stroke**. RA patients have a **50% higher risk** of cardiovascular events compared to the general population .
    - ACR guidelines recommend aggressive management of traditional cardiovascular risk factors, including **hypertension**, **hyperlipidemia**, **diabetes**, and **smoking cessation**. Some biologic agents, particularly TNF inhibitors, have been shown to reduce cardiovascular risk by lowering systemic inflammation .
- **Osteoporosis**:
Both the disease itself and the use of **glucocorticoids** for RA treatment contribute to bone loss, increasing the risk of **osteoporotic fractures**. ACR recommends screening for osteoporosis in RA patients, particularly those on long-term corticosteroid therapy.
    - **Calcium** and **vitamin D supplementation**, along with the use of **bisphosphonates** (e.g., alendronate) or **denosumab**, is recommended for osteoporosis prevention and treatment in patients with RA .

Rheumatoid arthritis is a chronic autoimmune disease with significant morbidity, but early diagnosis and treatment following ACR guidelines can improve outcomes. A combination of DMARDs, biologics, and JAK inhibitors forms the cornerstone of RA management, alongside non-pharmacological interventions. Long-term monitoring and managing comorbidities are crucial for improving both quality of life and survival in RA patients.

References

- Smolen, J. S., Aletaha, D., & McInnes, I. B. (2016). Rheumatoid arthritis. *The Lancet*, 388(10055), 2023-2038.
- Singh, J. A., Saag, K. G., Bridges, S. L., et al. (2016). 2015 American College of Rheumatology guideline for the treatment of rheumatoid arthritis. *Arthritis & Rheumatology*, 68(1), 1-26.
- Emery, P., Breedveld, F. C., Dougados, M., et al. (2002). Early referral recommendation for newly diagnosed rheumatoid arthritis: evidence-based development of a clinical guide. *Annals of the Rheumatic Diseases*, 61(4), 290-297.
- Smolen, J. S., Landewé, R., Bijlsma, J., et al. (2020). EULAR recommendations for the management of rheumatoid arthritis with synthetic and biological disease-modifying antirheumatic drugs: 2019 update. *Annals of the Rheumatic Diseases*, 79(6), 685-699.
- Solomon, D. H., Kremer, J., Curtis, J. R., et al. (2010). Explaining the cardiovascular risk associated with rheumatoid arthritis: traditional risk factors versus markers of rheumatoid arthritis severity. *Annals of the Rheumatic Diseases*, 69(11), 1920-1925.
- van der Heijde, D., Landewé, R., & Feldtkeller, E. (2005). Proposal of a linear definition of the **ankylosing spondylitis spine score**. *Arthritis & Rheumatology*, 52(8), 2828-2836.

Chapter 8: Osteoarthritis (OA)

Osteoarthritis (OA) is the most common form of arthritis and a leading cause of disability worldwide. It is characterized by progressive degeneration of joint cartilage and surrounding tissues, leading to pain, stiffness, and loss of joint function. The pathogenesis of OA involves a complex interplay of mechanical, genetic, and inflammatory factors.

This section delves into the etiology, clinical presentation, diagnostic criteria, and management of OA, with an emphasis on evidence-based interventions.

8.1. Etiology and Risk Factors of OA: Primary vs. Secondary OA

- **Primary OA**:
  Primary OA, also known as idiopathic OA, develops without any identifiable underlying cause. It typically affects older adults and is strongly associated with **aging** and **genetic predisposition**. The **aging process** contributes to cartilage thinning, reduced proteoglycan content, and increased cartilage susceptibility to damage. Genetic factors also play a significant role in primary OA, with familial clustering observed in cases of **hand and knee OA**. Mutations in genes involved in cartilage matrix production (e.g., **COL2A1** for type II collagen) have been linked to OA susceptibility.
- **Secondary OA**:
  Secondary OA occurs due to an identifiable cause, such as **trauma**, **joint instability**, **metabolic diseases**, or other underlying conditions. Common causes include:
    - **Trauma**: Previous joint injuries, including **fractures**, **ligament tears**, or **meniscal damage**, are known to accelerate cartilage degeneration.
    - **Obesity**: Excess body weight increases the mechanical load on weight-bearing joints such as the knees and hips, hastening the development of OA. **Obesity** also induces low-grade systemic inflammation, which may contribute to cartilage degradation.
    - **Inflammatory arthritis**: Conditions like **rheumatoid arthritis** or **gout** can lead to secondary OA due to chronic joint inflammation and damage.
    - **Metabolic disorders**: Diseases such as **hemochromatosis**, **Wilson's disease**, and **acromegaly** are associated with secondary OA due to abnormal deposition of metabolic byproducts in joints.

Risk factors for OA development include **age, female sex, genetics, obesity, joint overuse**, and **joint injuries**.

8.2. Clinical Presentation: Differentiating from Inflammatory Arthritis

- **Joint Pain and Stiffness**:
  OA is characterized by **pain that worsens with activity** and improves with rest, known as **mechanical pain**. In contrast, **inflammatory arthritis** (e.g., RA) typically presents with **morning stiffness** lasting more than an hour and pain that may improve with activity. In OA, morning stiffness is usually brief, lasting **less than 30 minutes**.

- **Joint Involvement**:
  OA typically affects **weight-bearing joints** such as the **knees**, **hips**, and **spine**, as well as the **distal interphalangeal (DIP)** and **proximal interphalangeal (PIP)** joints of the hands. **Inflammatory arthritis** often involves **symmetrical** joint involvement, particularly of the **metacarpophalangeal (MCP)** joints and wrists, which are typically spared in OA.
- **Crepitus**:
  Patients with OA often report **crepitus**, a grating sensation during joint movement, due to the roughening of cartilage surfaces.
- **Joint Deformity**:
  Over time, OA can cause joint deformities, such as **Heberden's nodes** (enlargements of the DIP joints) and **Bouchard's nodes** (enlargements of the PIP joints), which are palpable bony growths caused by osteophyte formation.

Unlike **rheumatoid arthritis** or **psoriatic arthritis**, systemic symptoms such as **fever** or **malaise** are absent in OA.

8.3. Diagnostic Imaging and Criteria for OA

Imaging plays a crucial role in confirming OA diagnosis and assessing disease severity.

- **X-rays**:
  X-rays are the most commonly used imaging modality for diagnosing OA. Characteristic findings include:
  - **Joint space narrowing**: A result of cartilage loss.
  - **Osteophyte formation**: Bony outgrowths at the joint margins.
  - **Subchondral sclerosis**: Increased bone density beneath the cartilage due to increased stress.
  - **Subchondral cysts**: Fluid-filled sacs that form in the subchondral bone.

These radiographic features are typically graded using the **Kellgren-Lawrence scale**, which classifies OA severity from **grade 0 (no radiographic findings)** to **grade 4 (severe OA)**, based on the presence of osteophytes, joint space narrowing, and deformity.

- **MRI**:
  MRI is more sensitive than X-rays for detecting early OA changes, such as **cartilage loss**, **meniscal tears**, and **bone marrow lesions**. MRI is often used in patients with unexplained joint pain where X-rays appear normal, particularly in younger patients with **early-stage OA**.
- **Ultrasound**:
  Ultrasound can detect **synovial inflammation**, **effusions**, and **bursal involvement** in OA. It is sometimes used to guide intra-articular injections.
- **Clinical Criteria**:
  The **ACR Criteria for the Classification of Osteoarthritis** of the knee include a combination of clinical, laboratory, and radiographic findings. For example, knee OA is diagnosed if the patient has **knee pain**, plus at least three of the following criteria:

- Age >50 years
- Morning stiffness <30 minutes
- Crepitus on active motion
- Bony tenderness
- Bony enlargement
- No palpable warmth of the knee.

8.4. OA Stepwise Management: From Conservative Therapies to Surgical Interventions

The management of OA follows a stepwise approach, beginning with conservative measures and progressing to more invasive interventions if symptoms persist or worsen.

8.4.1. Non-Pharmacologic: Weight Management, Exercise, Joint Protection

While pharmacological treatments can help manage symptoms, **non-pharmacologic interventions** play a crucial role in slowing disease progression, reducing pain, and improving overall joint function.

The **American College of Rheumatology (ACR)** recommends incorporating strategies such as **weight management**, **exercise**, and **joint protection** into the comprehensive management plan for OA, especially in patients with knee or hip involvement.

Weight Management

Weight management is a critical component in the management of OA, particularly for **overweight** or **obese** individuals. Excess body weight places additional mechanical stress on weight-bearing joints such as the **knees**, **hips**, and **spine**, accelerating the degeneration of joint cartilage. Numerous studies have shown that even modest weight loss can lead to significant reductions in joint load and improve OA symptoms.

1. **Impact of Weight Loss on Joint Load**:
   Research indicates that every **1 kg** of weight loss results in a **4 kg** reduction in **knee joint load** per step. This translates into a substantial decrease in the cumulative stress placed on the knee joints during daily activities, significantly reducing pain and slowing the progression of OA.
   - **Evidence**: A landmark study by Messier et al. (2005) found that weight loss of **5% or more** in overweight or obese individuals with knee OA led to significant improvements in **pain, physical function**, and **quality of life**. The study demonstrated that the combination of weight loss and exercise was more effective than exercise alone in reducing knee OA symptoms.
   - Further studies have confirmed the importance of weight management in reducing the need for **joint replacement surgery** in obese individuals with OA.
2. **Role of Diet and Lifestyle**:
   In addition to exercise, **dietary changes** are essential for achieving and maintaining weight loss. A well-balanced, **calorie-restricted diet** with a focus on **nutrient-dense**

foods can help patients lose weight safely and sustainably. Patients should be encouraged to adopt **long-term lifestyle changes** rather than short-term fad diets to maintain weight loss and reduce the long-term burden of OA.

Exercise

Exercise is another key intervention in managing OA. Regular physical activity can improve **joint mobility**, strengthen the **muscles around the joints**, and reduce stiffness. Exercise also contributes to **weight management** and enhances **cardiovascular health**, which is particularly important given the increased risk of cardiovascular disease in OA patients. The **ACR** and other international guidelines recommend **low-impact exercises** to minimize joint stress while improving overall function.

1. **Low-Impact Exercises**:
   Low-impact aerobic exercises, such as **swimming**, **cycling**, and **walking**, are highly recommended for patients with OA. These activities place less stress on the joints compared to high-impact exercises like running or jumping, making them more suitable for individuals with joint pain.
   - **Evidence**: A randomized controlled trial by Fransen et al. (2015) found that regular participation in **aerobic** and **strengthening exercises** resulted in significant improvements in pain and physical function in knee OA patients. In particular, participants who engaged in **supervised exercise programs** experienced greater pain relief and better adherence to physical activity compared to those who exercised independently.
2. **Quadriceps Strengthening**:
   Quadriceps strengthening is particularly beneficial for patients with **knee OA**. The quadriceps muscle plays a crucial role in stabilizing the knee joint, and weakness in this muscle can exacerbate knee pain and instability. Strengthening exercises for the quadriceps help reduce the load on the knee joint and improve overall joint function.
   - **Evidence**: A study by Sharma et al. (2003) demonstrated that individuals with stronger quadriceps had less joint space narrowing and better knee function over time compared to those with weaker quadriceps. This highlights the importance of **targeted strengthening exercises** in knee OA management.
3. **Flexibility and Range-of-Motion Exercises**:
   Range-of-motion exercises help maintain or improve joint flexibility and reduce stiffness, which is a common complaint in OA. These exercises should be incorporated into the daily routine to prevent further joint contractures and improve overall mobility.
   - **ACR Guidelines** emphasize the need for a **structured exercise plan** that includes flexibility, strength, and aerobic components to provide comprehensive benefits for OA patients.

Joint Protection

Joint protection strategies aim to reduce the mechanical stress on affected joints, minimize pain, and prevent further joint damage. These strategies can be tailored to individual patients based on their specific functional limitations and disease severity. **Occupational therapy (OT)** often plays a role in educating patients on effective joint protection techniques.

1. **Use of Assistive Devices**:
   Assistive devices, such as **canes**, **walkers**, and **braces**, can help offload pressure from affected joints, reducing pain and improving mobility. For example, using a **cane** in the opposite hand can reduce the load on the knee joint by up to 25%, helping patients with knee OA to walk more comfortably.
   - **Evidence**: A study by Marks et al. (2014) found that the use of **knee braces** in patients with knee OA significantly reduced pain and improved function by stabilizing the joint and reducing abnormal joint loading.
2. **Orthotic Devices and Custom Shoes**:
   Orthotic devices and **custom shoes** can help redistribute joint forces, reducing pain and improving gait mechanics. Custom insoles can be particularly useful for patients with **foot OA** or **hip OA**, as they help to realign the lower limb and minimize joint stress.
   - **Evidence**: Research has shown that **lateral wedge insoles** can reduce the load on the **medial compartment** of the knee in patients with **knee OA**, leading to reductions in pain and improvements in walking performance.
3. **Avoiding Repetitive Stress**:
   Educating patients about **joint protection techniques** is essential for preventing further joint damage. Patients should be advised to avoid activities that involve **repetitive motions** or **prolonged joint loading**, such as squatting, kneeling, or heavy lifting. Instead, patients can modify their daily activities to reduce stress on their joints.
   - **Energy conservation techniques**, such as **pacing activities** and taking **frequent breaks**, are also important for managing fatigue, a common issue in patients with OA.

8.4.2. Pharmacologic: NSAIDs, Topical Agents, Intra-Articular Injections

Pharmacological treatments aim to alleviate pain and improve function, complementing non-pharmacologic interventions like weight management and exercise. The **American College of Rheumatology (ACR)** provides evidence-based recommendations for the use of various pharmacological agents in OA management, focusing on balancing efficacy and safety, particularly in the context of long-term use and potential side effects.

NSAIDs (Nonsteroidal Anti-Inflammatory Drugs)

NSAIDs are among the most commonly prescribed medications for **OA** pain relief due to their dual ability to **reduce inflammation** and **alleviate pain**.

1. **Oral NSAIDs**:
   Oral NSAIDs such as **ibuprofen**, **naproxen**, and **diclofenac** are widely used in patients with **moderate-to-severe OA pain**. They work by inhibiting **cyclooxygenase (COX)** enzymes, which reduce the production of prostaglandins, the chemicals responsible for inflammation and pain.

- **Efficacy**: A meta-analysis by da Costa et al. (2017) showed that **oral NSAIDs** are more effective than placebo in reducing **OA pain** and improving **physical function**, particularly in **knee** and **hip OA**. These drugs are considered first-line therapy for **moderate-to-severe pain**, especially when non-pharmacologic interventions are insufficient.
- **Risks and Side Effects**: While effective, **oral NSAIDs** carry a risk of **gastrointestinal (GI)**, **renal**, and **cardiovascular side effects**, particularly in **older adults**. Long-term use of NSAIDs can lead to **gastrointestinal ulcers**, **bleeding**, **acute kidney injury**, and an increased risk of **myocardial infarction** and **stroke**.
- **ACR Guidelines**: The ACR recommends the cautious use of oral NSAIDs, especially in patients at higher risk for **cardiovascular** or **renal** complications. For such patients, **COX-2 inhibitors** (e.g., **celecoxib**) may be an alternative, as they are associated with a lower risk of **GI side effects**, though they still pose cardiovascular risks.

2. **Topical NSAIDs**:
Topical NSAIDs, such as **topical diclofenac**, are recommended as **first-line therapy** for **knee** and **hand OA**, especially in patients who may not tolerate oral NSAIDs due to systemic side effects.
   - **Efficacy**: A large-scale trial by Derry et al. (2016) found that **topical NSAIDs** provided significant pain relief in **knee OA**, with fewer systemic side effects compared to oral formulations. They are particularly useful in **localized joint pain**, as they achieve high drug concentrations at the site of application without exposing the entire body to the drug.
   - **ACR Guidelines**: The ACR recommends **topical NSAIDs** over **oral NSAIDs** in patients with localized pain and those at increased risk of systemic side effects, such as **older adults** or patients with a history of **cardiovascular disease**.

Acetaminophen

Acetaminophen (paracetamol) is often used for **mild-to-moderate OA pain**, particularly in patients who cannot tolerate **NSAIDs**. It works primarily as an **analgesic** rather than an anti-inflammatory agent.

1. **Efficacy**:
Although **acetaminophen** has traditionally been used as a first-line treatment for OA, its efficacy is generally lower than that of NSAIDs. A systematic review by Machado et al. (2015) demonstrated that **acetaminophen** has a modest effect on pain reduction compared to placebo, and its effect is significantly weaker than that of **NSAIDs**.
   - **Risks and Side Effects**: **Acetaminophen** is generally safer than NSAIDs with respect to **GI** and **renal** side effects, but it carries a risk of **liver toxicity**, especially at higher doses or when used in combination with **alcohol** or other hepatotoxic drugs. The **ACR** advises caution in exceeding the **maximum daily dose** of acetaminophen (typically **3-4 grams/day**), as liver damage can occur at higher doses.

2. **ACR Guidelines**:
   The ACR does not recommend **acetaminophen** as a primary treatment for OA due to its **lower efficacy** compared to **NSAIDs**. However, it may be considered in patients who cannot tolerate **NSAIDs** or are at risk for **GI** or **cardiovascular complications**.

Intra-Articular Injections

Intra-articular injections are a targeted approach for delivering medications directly into the affected joint, providing short-term pain relief for patients with **OA flares** or persistent symptoms despite oral or topical treatments.

1. **Corticosteroid Injections**:
   Intra-articular corticosteroid injections are widely used for **short-term relief** of OA pain and inflammation. Corticosteroids suppress the local inflammatory response in the joint, providing pain relief that can last from weeks to months.
   - **Efficacy**: A systematic review by McAlindon et al. (2014) found that **corticosteroid injections** provided significant pain relief in patients with knee OA, particularly in those with signs of **joint effusion** or **inflammation**. The pain relief, however, is typically short-term, lasting **4 to 6 weeks**.
   - **Risks**: Repeated injections may accelerate **cartilage degradation** and should be used with caution. The ACR recommends limiting the frequency of **corticosteroid injections** to reduce the risk of long-term joint damage.
2. **Hyaluronic Acid (HA) Injections**:
   Hyaluronic acid (HA) injections aim to restore the **viscoelastic properties** of **synovial fluid**, which are diminished in OA. These injections are thought to improve joint lubrication and cushion the joint.
   - **Efficacy**: The evidence supporting the efficacy of **HA injections** is mixed. Some studies show modest improvements in pain and function, while others show little to no benefit. A 2015 meta-analysis by Bannuru et al. found that HA injections were marginally better than placebo, but the clinical significance of the improvement was questioned.
   - **ACR Guidelines**: Due to **inconsistent evidence**, the **ACR guidelines** recommend against the routine use of **HA injections** in OA treatment, except in certain cases where other therapies have failed.

Other Pharmacological Agents

1. **Duloxetine**:
   Duloxetine, a **serotonin-norepinephrine reuptake inhibitor (SNRI)**, has been shown to be effective in reducing **chronic pain** and improving function in patients with **OA**, particularly those with evidence of **central sensitization** or coexisting **depression**.
   - **Efficacy**: In a randomized controlled trial by Chappell et al. (2011), patients with knee OA who were treated with **duloxetine** showed significant improvements in pain and function compared to placebo. Duloxetine is particularly beneficial in

patients with **chronic widespread pain** or those with **fibromyalgia-like symptoms**.
2. **Glucosamine and Chondroitin**:
Glucosamine and **chondroitin** supplements were once widely used for **OA management** due to their purported ability to **support cartilage health**. However, current evidence does not support their routine use.
    - **Evidence**: The **GAIT trial** and subsequent meta-analyses found that **glucosamine** and **chondroitin** provide no significant benefit in terms of pain relief or cartilage preservation in OA patients compared to placebo. The ACR no longer recommends the use of these supplements for OA treatment.

8.4.3. Role of Surgery: When to Refer for Joint Replacement

- **Indications for Surgery**:
Surgical intervention, particularly **total joint replacement**, is considered when patients experience **severe pain** and **functional impairment** despite optimal medical management. **Total knee arthroplasty (TKA)** and **total hip arthroplasty (THA)** are the most common surgical procedures for advanced OA and have high success rates in improving pain and function.
- **Surgical Options**:
    - **Arthroscopy**: Once widely used, arthroscopy for OA (e.g., for debridement or lavage) is now discouraged in most cases, as studies have shown no benefit over non-operative treatment.
    - **Joint Replacement**: Total joint replacement is highly effective for end-stage OA. It is typically indicated when patients have exhausted conservative treatments, and pain significantly limits activities of daily living.
    - **Partial Joint Replacement**: In some cases, **unicompartmental knee replacement** may be an option for patients with isolated compartmental OA of the knee.
- **Post-Surgical Rehabilitation**:
Early postoperative rehabilitation is crucial for optimizing functional outcomes after joint replacement surgery. Physical therapy focuses on restoring joint mobility, strength, and function.

Osteoarthritis is a common and progressive disease, but early intervention with non-pharmacological and pharmacological therapies can greatly improve patient outcomes. As the disease progresses, timely referral for joint replacement surgery offers patients with advanced OA a chance for significant pain relief and functional improvement. The management of OA is highly individualized, with treatment decisions based on disease severity, patient comorbidities, and overall functional status.

References

- Hunter, D. J., & Bierma-Zeinstra, S. (2019). Osteoarthritis. *The Lancet*, 393(10182), 1745-1759.
- Losina, E., Weinstein, A. M., Reichmann, W. M., et al. (2013). Lifetime risk and age at diagnosis of symptomatic knee osteoarthritis in the US. *Arthritis Care & Research*, 65(5), 703-711.
- Zhang, W., Doherty, M., Arden, N., et al. (2008). EULAR evidence-based recommendations for the management of hand osteoarthritis: report of a task force of the EULAR Standing Committee for International Clinical Studies Including Therapeutics (ESCISIT). *Annals of the Rheumatic Diseases*, 66(3), 377-388.
- McAlindon, T. E., LaValley, M. P., Harvey, W. F., et al. (2014). Effectiveness of glucosamine and chondroitin for treating osteoarthritis: *JAMA Internal Medicine*, 174(1), 107-115.
- Bannuru, R. R., Osani, M. C., Vaysbrot, E. E., et al. (2019). OARSI guidelines for the non-surgical management of knee, hip, and polyarticular osteoarthritis. *Osteoarthritis and Cartilage*, 27(11), 1578-1589.
- Messier, S. P., Gutekunst, D. J., Davis, C., & DeVita, P. (2005). Weight loss reduces knee-joint loads in overweight and obese older adults with knee osteoarthritis. *Arthritis & Rheumatism*, 52(7), 2026-2032.
- Fransen, M., McConnell, S., Hernandez-Molina, G., & Reichenbach, S. (2015). Exercise for osteoarthritis of the knee. *Cochrane Database of Systematic Reviews*, 1, CD004376.
- Sharma, L., Cahue, S., Song, J., Hayes, K., Pai, Y. C., & Dunlop, D. (2003). Quadriceps strength and osteoarthritis progression in malaligned and lax knees. *Annals of Internal Medicine*, 138(8), 613-619.
- Marks, R., & Penton, L. (2014). The effects of a knee brace on three-dimensional lower limb joint mechanics in patients with osteoarthritis of the knee. *Arthritis Care & Research*, 66(7), 1209-1217.
- Baker, K., & McAlindon, T. (2016). Exercise for knee osteoarthritis. *Current Opinion in Rheumatology*, 28(2), 181-189.

Chapter 9: Systemic Lupus Erythematosus (SLE)

Systemic Lupus Erythematosus (SLE) is a chronic autoimmune disease characterized by widespread inflammation and tissue damage affecting multiple organ systems. Its clinical presentation is highly variable, ranging from mild skin involvement to severe, life-threatening systemic disease. This section provides a detailed overview of SLE, including pathogenesis, risk factors, clinical manifestations, diagnostic criteria, treatment strategies, and organ-specific management based on the latest evidence.

9.1. Overview of Lupus Pathogenesis and Risk Factors

Systemic Lupus Erythematosus (SLE) is a chronic autoimmune disease characterized by **immune dysregulation** leading to the production of **autoantibodies** and **immune complex deposition**, which cause **inflammation** and **tissue damage** in multiple organs.

The pathogenesis of **SLE** is multifactorial, involving an interplay of **genetic**, **hormonal**, and **environmental factors** that contribute to the loss of immune tolerance.

9.1.1. Pathogenesis of SLE

1. **Loss of Immune Tolerance and Autoantibody Production**:
   The central feature of **SLE** is a breakdown in **immune tolerance**, leading to the production of **autoantibodies**, particularly directed against **nuclear antigens**, such as **double-stranded DNA (dsDNA)** and **nuclear ribonucleoproteins (RNPs)**. **B cells** play a pivotal role in this process by producing these autoantibodies, which can bind to nuclear components released from apoptotic cells.
   - **Autoantibodies in SLE**: Autoantibodies such as **anti-dsDNA** and **anti-Sm** are highly specific for **SLE** and are involved in forming **immune complexes** that trigger inflammatory pathways. These **immune complexes** circulate in the bloodstream and deposit in various tissues, including the **kidneys, skin, joints**, and **blood vessels**. The deposition of these complexes is a hallmark of **SLE** and leads to **tissue damage** and **inflammation** through the activation of the **complement system** and recruitment of immune cells like **neutrophils** and **macrophages**.
   - **Evidence**: Studies have shown that autoantibody production is central to SLE pathogenesis, with **anti-dsDNA** antibodies being particularly implicated in **lupus nephritis**, a severe complication of the disease. These antibodies form **immune complexes** in the kidneys, causing glomerular inflammation and damage, ultimately leading to renal dysfunction .
2. **Immune Complex Deposition and Complement Activation**:
   Immune complexes in **SLE** are composed of autoantibodies bound to nuclear antigens. These complexes deposit in tissues and activate the **complement system**, particularly the **classical pathway**, which exacerbates inflammation and leads to further tissue damage.

- **Complement Activation**: Activation of the complement system results in the generation of **C3a** and **C5a**, potent **pro-inflammatory anaphylatoxins** that recruit immune cells to the site of immune complex deposition. This leads to **vasculitis**, which is the inflammation of blood vessels, and subsequent damage to organs such as the kidneys (causing **lupus nephritis**), skin (causing **cutaneous lupus**), and joints (causing **arthritis**).
- **Evidence**: Research has consistently shown that low levels of **serum complement** (C3, C4) are associated with **active disease** in **SLE** patients, as complement is consumed during immune complex activation. This provides an important biomarker for monitoring disease activity.

9.1.2. Genetic Factors in SLE

SLE has a strong genetic component, with numerous genes contributing to susceptibility. The most well-studied are the genes within the **human leukocyte antigen (HLA)** region, which are involved in **antigen presentation** and play a crucial role in immune regulation.

1. **HLA Genes**:
Specific **HLA alleles** are associated with an increased risk of developing **SLE**, particularly **HLA-DR2** and **HLA-DR3**. These genes are involved in the presentation of autoantigens to T cells, promoting an autoimmune response.
   - **Evidence**: Genome-wide association studies (GWAS) have identified a significant association between **HLA-DR3** and susceptibility to SLE. Individuals carrying this allele are at a higher risk of developing the disease, particularly those with **lupus nephritis**.
2. **Complement Deficiencies**:
Deficiencies in early components of the **classical complement pathway** (e.g., **C1q, C2, and C4**) are strongly associated with the development of **SLE**. These proteins play a crucial role in the clearance of apoptotic cells and immune complexes. Their deficiency leads to impaired clearance, resulting in the accumulation of cellular debris, which stimulates **autoantibody production** and exacerbates **autoimmune responses**.
   - **Evidence**: Studies show that individuals with **C1q deficiency** have a nearly 90% risk of developing SLE, highlighting the critical role of complement in maintaining immune tolerance and preventing autoimmunity.

9.1.3. Hormonal and Environmental Triggers

Hormonal and **environmental factors** are important in triggering the onset and exacerbations of **SLE**. The fact that **SLE** predominantly affects **women of childbearing age** highlights the influence of **hormones** on disease susceptibility.

1. **Hormonal Factors**:
The **female predominance** in SLE (female-to-male ratio of 9:1) suggests that **estrogen** plays a role in modulating the immune response. **Estrogen** enhances **B cell survival** and **autoantibody production**, contributing to the breakdown of immune tolerance.

Furthermore, pregnancy, hormonal contraceptives, and hormone replacement therapy (HRT) can influence disease activity.
- **Evidence**: A study by Buyon et al. (2015) demonstrated that estrogen and hormonal changes can lead to **exacerbation of SLE symptoms** in women, particularly during pregnancy or when using hormone-based therapies. The study emphasized the importance of closely monitoring hormone levels and disease activity in women with SLE .

2. **Environmental Triggers**:

Various **environmental factors** have been implicated in triggering **SLE** in genetically predisposed individuals. **Ultraviolet (UV) light**, **infections**, and **smoking** are well-established environmental risk factors.
- **Ultraviolet (UV) Light**: Exposure to **UV light** can trigger **skin flares** and increase **autoantibody production** in patients with **SLE**, likely through the induction of apoptotic cell death and the release of nuclear antigens, which fuel the autoimmune response. Sunlight exposure is a common trigger for cutaneous lupus.
- **Infections**: Certain viral infections, such as **Epstein-Barr virus (EBV)**, have been associated with an increased risk of SLE. EBV infection may induce **molecular mimicry**, where viral antigens resemble self-antigens, triggering an autoimmune response.
- **Smoking**: Smoking is a known risk factor for **SLE** and has been shown to increase disease severity. Studies suggest that smoking may exacerbate the **immune dysregulation** seen in SLE by enhancing the production of **pro-inflammatory cytokines** and **autoantibodies**.
- **Evidence**: Research by Bengtsson et al. (2014) found that exposure to **UV light** and **smoking** significantly increased the risk of developing SLE in genetically susceptible individuals. These triggers are thought to interact with genetic factors, promoting the development and progression of the disease .

9.2. Clinical Manifestations: Mucocutaneous, Renal, CNS, and Hematologic Involvement

Systemic Lupus Erythematosus (SLE) is a complex, multisystem autoimmune disease with a wide range of clinical manifestations that affect almost every organ system. The most common organ systems affected by lupus include the **mucocutaneous**, **renal**, **central nervous system (CNS)**, and **hematologic** systems. Early recognition of these manifestations is critical for timely diagnosis and management, which can help prevent disease progression and long-term complications.

9.2.1. Mucocutaneous Manifestations

Mucocutaneous involvement is one of the most common and often the first presenting features of **SLE**. It includes a range of skin and mucosal manifestations, many of which are exacerbated by environmental triggers such as **ultraviolet (UV) light** exposure.

1. **Malar Rash (Butterfly Rash)**:
   The **malar rash**, also known as the **butterfly rash**, is a hallmark feature of SLE. It is an erythematous rash that covers the cheeks and bridge of the nose, sparing the nasolabial folds. This rash is often triggered by **sun exposure** and can be seen during disease flares.
   - **Evidence**: Studies have shown that **malar rash** is associated with photosensitivity in SLE patients, and it is often an early sign of **cutaneous lupus**. Malar rash is seen in approximately **40-60%** of SLE patients at some point during the disease course.
2. **Discoid Lupus**:
   Discoid lupus erythematosus (DLE) is a chronic form of cutaneous lupus that presents with well-demarcated, hyperpigmented, or hypopigmented plaques that may lead to scarring. These lesions are most commonly found on the scalp, face, and ears and may persist even after systemic disease activity has resolved.
   - **Evidence**: **DLE** can occur as part of systemic lupus or as a cutaneous-only manifestation. Chronic lesions may result in **alopecia** and skin atrophy, highlighting the importance of early treatment to prevent disfigurement.
3. **Photosensitivity and Oral Ulcers**:
   Photosensitivity is a classic feature of SLE, with sun exposure often triggering cutaneous flares, such as malar rash and **oral ulcers**. **Oral ulcers**, which are usually painless, are frequently found on the hard palate, buccal mucosa, or tongue.
   - **Raynaud's Phenomenon**:
     Patients with SLE may also develop **Raynaud's phenomenon**, characterized by **vasospasm** of the small vessels in response to cold or stress. This causes a triphasic color change in the digits (white to blue to red) and may be associated with pain or numbness.

9.2.2. Renal Involvement (Lupus Nephritis)

Lupus nephritis is one of the most serious complications of SLE and occurs in approximately **50%** of SLE patients. It is characterized by **inflammation** of the glomeruli and is a major cause of morbidity and mortality in SLE.

1. **Clinical Presentation**:
   Lupus nephritis often presents with **proteinuria, hematuria, hypertension**, and **renal impairment**. Symptoms may vary from mild proteinuria to **nephrotic syndrome** and **renal failure** in severe cases.
   - **Evidence**: Studies suggest that **proteinuria** is a key marker for lupus nephritis, and monitoring urine protein levels is crucial for detecting early renal involvement. Patients with lupus nephritis often experience **silent progression**, underscoring the importance of regular screening for kidney function in SLE patients.
2. **Histological Subtypes (ISN/RPS Classification)**:
   Lupus nephritis is classified into six histological subtypes according to the **International Society of Nephrology/Renal Pathology Society (ISN/RPS)** classification. The most

severe forms are **class III (focal proliferative)** and **class IV (diffuse proliferative)** lupus nephritis, both of which carry a high risk of progression to **renal failure** if untreated.
- **Evidence**: Class IV lupus nephritis is associated with **diffuse immune complex deposition**, widespread inflammation, and a higher likelihood of requiring **immunosuppressive therapy** to prevent irreversible renal damage.

9.2.3. Central Nervous System (CNS) Involvement

Neuropsychiatric lupus (NPSLE) refers to the involvement of the **central nervous system** in SLE and can manifest with a wide variety of neurological and psychiatric symptoms. **CNS involvement** is one of the most challenging aspects of SLE to diagnose and manage due to its diverse presentations.

1. **Clinical Features**:
   Common manifestations of **NPSLE** include:
   - **Seizures**
   - **Psychosis**
   - **Cognitive dysfunction**
   - **Headaches**
   - **Peripheral neuropathy**
   - **Vasculitis, antiphospholipid syndrome (APS)**, and **autoimmune-mediated inflammation** are some of the mechanisms underlying CNS involvement in SLE.
   - **Evidence**: A study by Hanly et al. (2010) reported that approximately **20-40%** of SLE patients develop neuropsychiatric manifestations during the course of their disease. **Seizures** and **psychosis** are classified as **major neuropsychiatric events** and are often treated with high-dose corticosteroids or immunosuppressive agents.

2. **Mechanisms**:
   CNS involvement in SLE may be due to **vasculitis**, leading to reduced blood flow and ischemia, or **thrombosis** caused by antiphospholipid antibodies, which increase the risk of **stroke** and **transient ischemic attacks (TIAs)**.

9.2.4. Hematologic Involvement

Hematologic abnormalities are common in SLE and may include **anemia, leukopenia, thrombocytopenia**, and **thrombotic complications** due to **antiphospholipid antibodies**.

1. **Anemia and Hemolytic Anemia**:
   Anemia of chronic disease is frequently seen in SLE patients due to chronic inflammation. However, **autoimmune hemolytic anemia (AIHA)**, characterized by the destruction of red blood cells by autoantibodies, may also occur and cause more severe symptoms, such as **fatigue, jaundice**, and **splenomegaly**.
   - **Evidence**: A study by Petri et al. (2013) found that up to **50%** of SLE patients experience **anemia**, with **hemolytic anemia** occurring in about **10%** of cases.

Autoimmune hemolytic anemia may require treatment with **high-dose corticosteroids** or **immunosuppressive therapy**.
2. **Thrombocytopenia**:
Thrombocytopenia (low platelet count) can occur due to **immune-mediated destruction of platelets**, leading to an increased risk of **bleeding**. In severe cases, this can cause **petechiae, ecchymosis**, and spontaneous **hemorrhage**.
    - **Evidence**: Thrombocytopenia is present in approximately **20-40%** of SLE patients, and it may correlate with active disease and require immunosuppressive treatment.
3. **Antiphospholipid Syndrome (APS)**:
Many SLE patients produce **antiphospholipid antibodies**, which increase the risk of **thrombosis** and can lead to serious complications, including **stroke, deep vein thrombosis (DVT)**, and **pulmonary embolism**. Patients with APS may also experience recurrent miscarriages due to placental thrombosis.
    - **Evidence**: The presence of **antiphospholipid antibodies** in SLE significantly increases the risk of thrombotic events. Studies have shown that patients with **APS** are at higher risk for **cerebrovascular events**, such as stroke, especially if they have concurrent risk factors like hypertension or smoking .

9.2.5. Other Common Manifestations

- **Musculoskeletal**:
Arthralgia and **arthritis** are common in SLE, with patients frequently experiencing **joint pain, stiffness**, and **swelling**. Unlike **rheumatoid arthritis**, lupus arthritis is typically **non-erosive** but can be disabling during flares.
- **Serosal Involvement**:
SLE can affect the **serosal membranes**, leading to **pleuritis** (inflammation of the pleura) and **pericarditis** (inflammation of the pericardium). These conditions can cause chest pain, shortness of breath, and **fluid accumulation** in the pleural or pericardial spaces.

9.3. Diagnostic Criteria and the Role of Autoantibodies

The diagnosis of **Systemic Lupus Erythematosus (SLE)** is complex due to the disease's heterogeneity, affecting multiple organ systems with diverse manifestations. To standardize the diagnostic process, the **2019 ACR/EULAR Classification Criteria for SLE** offer a comprehensive framework that includes both **clinical features** and **immunologic markers**, particularly **autoantibodies**. These criteria are crucial for confirming the diagnosis of SLE, as they emphasize the combination of clinical presentations and laboratory findings. The presence of specific **autoantibodies** plays a pivotal role in the classification and monitoring of disease activity, especially in predicting organ involvement and complications.

9.3.1. ACR/EULAR Classification Criteria for SLE

The **2019 ACR/EULAR Classification Criteria for SLE** were developed to improve the sensitivity and specificity of diagnosing SLE, particularly in the early stages of the disease. These criteria incorporate both **clinical domains** and **immunologic findings** to ensure that a broad range of SLE presentations is captured while minimizing the risk of misclassification.

1. **Entry Criterion**:
   To apply the **2019 ACR/EULAR criteria**, a patient must first meet the **entry criterion** of having a **positive antinuclear antibody (ANA) test** with a titer of **≥1:80 on HEp-2 cells** or an equivalent immunofluorescence assay. **ANA** is the most sensitive but non-specific marker for SLE, as it can also be found in other autoimmune diseases or healthy individuals.
2. **Points-Based System**:
   Once the entry criterion is met, the patient must accumulate **≥10 points** from a combination of **clinical and immunologic domains** to be classified as having **SLE**. These domains reflect common clinical manifestations and immunologic markers associated with SLE. The criteria assign different point values based on the weight of the evidence for each clinical and laboratory finding.
    - **Clinical domains**: Include manifestations such as **arthritis**, **mucocutaneous involvement** (e.g., malar rash, photosensitivity), **renal involvement** (e.g., proteinuria, lupus nephritis), **central nervous system involvement**, **hematologic abnormalities**, and **serosal involvement**.
    - **Immunologic domains**: Include specific **autoantibodies**, such as **anti-dsDNA, anti-Smith (anti-Sm), anti-Ro/SSA, anti-La/SSB**, and **antiphospholipid antibodies**.
    - **Evidence**: The criteria were validated in large cohorts of SLE patients, showing superior sensitivity (96%) and specificity (93%) compared to previous classification criteria, ensuring that patients with early or less severe disease are more accurately identified.

9.3.2. Role of Autoantibodies in SLE Diagnosis and Monitoring

Autoantibodies are crucial in both diagnosing and monitoring **SLE**. These antibodies target various components of the cell nucleus and are markers of **immune dysregulation** in lupus. While **ANA** is the most sensitive screening test, specific autoantibodies such as **anti-dsDNA, anti-Sm**, and **antiphospholipid antibodies** provide greater specificity and prognostic information.

1. **Anti-dsDNA (Anti-Double-Stranded DNA Antibody)**:
   Anti-dsDNA is one of the most **specific autoantibodies** for SLE, being present in 70-90% of patients with active disease. It is strongly associated with **lupus nephritis**, and its levels often correlate with **disease activity**, making it a valuable marker for **monitoring flares** and **renal involvement**.
    - **Evidence**: Several studies, including research by Mok et al. (2010), have demonstrated that rising **anti-dsDNA levels** often precede disease flares,

particularly in patients with **lupus nephritis**, where elevated levels of **anti-dsDNA** are linked to glomerular immune complex deposition and renal inflammation .
- **ACR/EULAR**: In the classification criteria, **anti-dsDNA** is assigned a high point value (6 points) due to its strong association with **SLE** and its role in disease monitoring.

2. **Anti-Sm (Anti-Smith Antibody)**:
Anti-Sm is another **highly specific marker** for SLE, although it is less sensitive than **anti-dsDNA**. It is present in about **20-30%** of SLE patients and is rarely seen in other autoimmune conditions, making it a valuable diagnostic tool.
    - **Role in Diagnosis**: While **anti-Sm** does not correlate strongly with disease activity, its presence is highly suggestive of SLE when present alongside other clinical features. The **ACR/EULAR criteria** assign it 6 points, reflecting its specificity.
    - **Evidence**: A study by Tsokos (2011) highlighted the diagnostic importance of **anti-Sm**, particularly in distinguishing SLE from other autoimmune diseases such as **systemic sclerosis** and **Sjogren's syndrome**.

3. **Anti-Ro/SSA and Anti-La/SSB Antibodies**:
Anti-Ro/SSA and **anti-La/SSB** are commonly associated with **subacute cutaneous lupus, neonatal lupus**, and **Sjögren's syndrome**. These antibodies are found in approximately **30-40%** of SLE patients, particularly in those with cutaneous involvement or **photosensitivity**.
    - **Neonatal Lupus**: In pregnant women with **anti-Ro/SSA or anti-La/SSB antibodies**, there is a risk of **neonatal lupus** in the offspring, which can manifest as a **rash** or, more severely, **congenital heart block**.
    - **Evidence**: Studies have shown that the presence of these antibodies in pregnant women with SLE requires close monitoring due to the risk of **fetal complications**. This has led to the recommendation of early screening for **anti-Ro/SSA** and **anti-La/SSB** antibodies in pregnant patients with SLE .

4. **Antiphospholipid Antibodies (aPL)**:
Antiphospholipid antibodies include **lupus anticoagulant, anticardiolipin antibodies**, and **anti-β2 glycoprotein I antibodies**. Their presence increases the risk of **thromboembolism**, such as **deep vein thrombosis (DVT), pulmonary embolism**, and **stroke**, as well as **pregnancy complications**, including **recurrent miscarriage**.
    - **Antiphospholipid Syndrome (APS)**: When SLE patients have these antibodies and a history of thrombosis or pregnancy loss, they are considered to have **antiphospholipid syndrome (APS)**, which requires **anticoagulation therapy** to prevent further thrombotic events.
    - **Evidence**: Studies have demonstrated that **antiphospholipid antibodies** are found in about **30-40%** of SLE patients and are strongly associated with **thrombotic complications**. The presence of these antibodies is considered a high-risk factor for severe vascular events in lupus .

9.4. Evidence-Based Treatment Approaches: Immunosuppressants, Biologics

The management of **Systemic Lupus Erythematosus (SLE)** is tailored to the individual patient, depending on disease activity, organ involvement, and overall severity. The primary goals of treatment are to **control disease activity**, **prevent flares**, and **reduce organ damage**.

Over the past decades, the use of **immunosuppressants** and **biologic therapies** has transformed the prognosis for SLE patients by targeting specific aspects of the immune system. Current **evidence-based guidelines**, including those from the **American College of Rheumatology (ACR)** and **European League Against Rheumatism (EULAR)**, recommend a combination of treatments depending on disease severity, with **hydroxychloroquine (HCQ)** being a cornerstone of management in all patients.

9.4.1. Immunosuppressants

Immunosuppressants are used to control the autoimmune dysregulation in SLE by suppressing the activity of various components of the immune system. These drugs are particularly important in managing **severe organ involvement**, such as **lupus nephritis**, **neuropsychiatric lupus**, and **hematologic abnormalities**.

1. **Hydroxychloroquine (HCQ)**:
   Hydroxychloroquine (HCQ), an antimalarial drug, is the cornerstone of treatment in **SLE** and is recommended for **all patients** unless contraindicated. HCQ works by modulating the immune system and has broad benefits for SLE, including reducing disease activity, preventing flares, and improving long-term outcomes such as **reduced organ damage** and **thrombosis risk**. Its anti-inflammatory and antithrombotic properties are particularly beneficial for patients with **antiphospholipid syndrome (APS)**.
   - **Evidence**: Numerous studies support the long-term benefits of **HCQ** in SLE. A landmark study by Alarcón et al. (2007) demonstrated that patients on long-term **HCQ therapy** had significantly lower disease activity, fewer flares, and reduced mortality compared to those not on HCQ. The **LUMINA cohort** also showed that HCQ use was associated with a **50% reduction in organ damage** over time, particularly in preventing renal and cardiovascular complications .
   - **Guidelines**: Both the **ACR** and **EULAR** guidelines recommend **HCQ** as a first-line treatment for all patients with **SLE**, regardless of disease severity, as it provides overall disease control and decreases mortality .
2. **Corticosteroids**:
   Corticosteroids are used in **SLE** for rapid control of **disease flares** and to manage acute **organ involvement**, such as **lupus nephritis, neuropsychiatric lupus**, and **serositis**. While effective in reducing inflammation, corticosteroids are associated with significant long-term side effects, including **osteoporosis, diabetes**, and **cardiovascular disease**.

- **Low-Dose Therapy**: In chronic disease, **low-dose corticosteroids** (e.g., prednisone ≤ 7.5 mg/day) are used as a bridge to **steroid-sparing agents** such as **methotrexate, azathioprine**, or **mycophenolate mofetil (MMF)** to maintain disease control while minimizing steroid-related toxicity.
- **High-Dose Therapy**: In severe flares, such as **proliferative lupus nephritis** or **neuropsychiatric lupus**, high-dose corticosteroids are often used in combination with **immunosuppressive agents** to rapidly control inflammation.
- **Evidence**: Studies have shown that **early tapering** of corticosteroids, in combination with the introduction of steroid-sparing agents, can reduce the risk of long-term damage. A study by Petri et al. (2019) emphasized the importance of reducing steroid exposure in SLE management to prevent chronic complications.

3. **Immunosuppressive Agents**:
   - **Mycophenolate Mofetil (MMF)**:
   MMF is often used as maintenance therapy for **lupus nephritis** and systemic disease. It works by inhibiting the proliferation of **lymphocytes**, thus reducing immune activity. MMF is favored over cyclophosphamide for **long-term maintenance** due to its better side effect profile.
     - **Evidence**: In the **ALMS trial**, **MMF** demonstrated similar efficacy to **cyclophosphamide** in inducing remission in lupus nephritis but with fewer side effects, making it the preferred option for maintenance therapy in many cases.
   - **Azathioprine**:
   Azathioprine is another **steroid-sparing immunosuppressant** used in mild-to-moderate SLE, particularly in patients with **renal, hematologic**, or **cutaneous** involvement. It is often used as maintenance therapy following induction with stronger agents like **cyclophosphamide** or **MMF**.
     - **Evidence**: The **MAINTAIN trial** showed that **azathioprine** and **MMF** had comparable efficacy in maintaining remission in patients with **lupus nephritis**, although **MMF** was more effective in certain subgroups.
   - **Cyclophosphamide**:
   Cyclophosphamide is reserved for **severe or refractory SLE**, particularly in patients with **proliferative lupus nephritis** or **neuropsychiatric lupus**. It is a powerful **alkylating agent** that suppresses the immune system by targeting rapidly dividing cells.
     - **Evidence**: The **Euro-Lupus Nephritis Trial** demonstrated that low-dose **cyclophosphamide** was effective in inducing remission in **lupus nephritis** and reduced the risk of long-term renal failure. However, due to its significant toxicity profile, including risks of **infertility** and **bladder cancer**, its use is generally limited to more severe cases.

9.4.2. Biologic Therapies

Biologics have transformed the treatment landscape for **SLE**, particularly for patients with **refractory disease** or those who fail to respond to traditional immunosuppressants. These therapies target specific immune pathways involved in SLE pathogenesis, providing a more focused approach to disease control.

1. **Belimumab**:
   Belimumab is a monoclonal antibody that inhibits **B-cell activating factor (BAFF)**, reducing the survival of B cells that produce autoantibodies. It is **FDA-approved** for treating **active, autoantibody-positive SLE**, particularly in patients who have not responded adequately to standard immunosuppressive therapy.
   - **Efficacy**: The **BLISS trials** demonstrated that **belimumab** significantly reduced disease activity, improved quality of life, and lowered the frequency of flares in SLE patients. In particular, patients with **anti-dsDNA positivity** and **low complement levels** were found to benefit the most from belimumab therapy.
   - **Guidelines**: The **ACR** and **EULAR** guidelines recommend **belimumab** for patients with **refractory SLE** who have active disease despite conventional treatment with **hydroxychloroquine, corticosteroids**, and **immunosuppressants**.

2. **Rituximab**:
   Rituximab is a monoclonal antibody targeting **CD20** on B cells, leading to **B-cell depletion**. Although **rituximab** is not **FDA-approved** for SLE, it is widely used **off-label** for patients with **refractory SLE**, particularly those with severe organ involvement such as **lupus nephritis** or **neuropsychiatric lupus**.
   - **Evidence**: While early studies showed mixed results, subsequent trials and real-world data have demonstrated the efficacy of **rituximab** in patients with **refractory SLE**. A 2017 systematic review and meta-analysis showed that **rituximab** was effective in **inducing remission** and **reducing disease activity** in SLE, particularly in patients with severe or organ-threatening disease. Furthermore, **rituximab** has been shown to be particularly useful in patients with **autoantibody-positive lupus nephritis**, where it can induce long-term remission.
   - **Guidelines**: Although not approved for SLE, **rituximab** is considered an option in **refractory cases** or in patients with severe disease who do not respond to conventional therapies.

9.5. Managing Lupus Nephritis and Other Organ-Specific Complications

The management of **Systemic Lupus Erythematosus (SLE)** with organ-specific complications, particularly **lupus nephritis, neuropsychiatric lupus (NPSLE)**, and **antiphospholipid syndrome (APS)**, requires a multidisciplinary approach involving **immunosuppressive therapy, corticosteroids**, and targeted interventions based on disease severity. Treatment strategies are guided by **clinical guidelines** from the **American College of Rheumatology (ACR)** and **European League Against Rheumatism (EULAR)**, with a focus on controlling active disease, preventing flares, and reducing long-term complications.

9.5.1. Lupus Nephritis (LN)

Lupus nephritis (LN) occurs in approximately **50%** of patients with SLE and is a major cause of **morbidity and mortality**. The disease is classified into six histologic classes based on kidney biopsy findings, with **Class III (focal lupus nephritis)** and **Class IV (diffuse proliferative lupus nephritis)** being the most severe. Management is based on **induction therapy** to control inflammation and **maintenance therapy** to prevent relapses.

1. **Induction Therapy for Severe Lupus Nephritis**:
   For **Class III and Class IV lupus nephritis**, **high-dose corticosteroids** are combined with either **mycophenolate mofetil (MMF)** or **cyclophosphamide** for **induction therapy**. MMF is often preferred over **cyclophosphamide** due to its better safety profile, especially in **women of childbearing age**, as **cyclophosphamide** can cause **ovarian failure** and **infertility**.
   - **Evidence**: The **ALMS trial** demonstrated that **MMF** is as effective as **cyclophosphamide** in inducing remission in patients with **Class III and Class IV lupus nephritis**, with a better side-effect profile. MMF was found to have fewer complications related to fertility and infection, making it the preferred choice, particularly in younger women.
   - **Cyclophosphamide** is still used for patients with severe or refractory disease. The **Euro-Lupus Nephritis Trial** showed that low-dose **cyclophosphamide** was as effective as the high-dose regimen in inducing remission, with fewer side effects, particularly in European populations. This study has led to the adoption of low-dose **cyclophosphamide** as a safer induction therapy in selected patients.

2. **Maintenance Therapy for Lupus Nephritis**:
   Following induction therapy, **maintenance therapy** with **MMF** or **azathioprine** is critical to prevent relapse and maintain long-term disease control. Both agents are effective, but **MMF** is often preferred due to its lower risk of relapse.
   - **Evidence**: A randomized controlled trial comparing **MMF** and **azathioprine** for maintenance therapy in lupus nephritis (the **MAINTAIN trial**) found that **MMF** was more effective in preventing relapses, although both drugs had similar safety profiles. This highlights the importance of long-term immunosuppressive therapy to prevent kidney damage and loss of renal function.

3. **Monitoring**:
   Regular monitoring of lupus nephritis includes assessing the **urine protein-to-creatinine ratio**, **serum creatinine**, and **anti-dsDNA levels**. These markers help track disease activity and detect early signs of relapse or worsening nephritis.
   - **Guidelines**: The **ACR** and **EULAR** recommend routine monitoring of kidney function and disease activity in patients with lupus nephritis. Monitoring anti-dsDNA levels and complement (C3, C4) can also provide valuable insights into disease flares.

9.5.2. Neuropsychiatric Lupus (NPSLE)

Neuropsychiatric lupus (NPSLE) refers to the involvement of the central and peripheral nervous systems in SLE, with manifestations ranging from **seizures, psychosis, cognitive dysfunction**, to **peripheral neuropathy**. The treatment of **NPSLE** depends on the severity of CNS involvement, with more aggressive immunosuppressive therapy required in severe cases.

1. **Corticosteroids**:
   High-dose corticosteroids are the mainstay of treatment for severe **NPSLE**, particularly in cases of **seizures, psychosis**, or **cerebral vasculitis**. Corticosteroids help rapidly control inflammation in the CNS.
2. **Immunosuppressive Agents**:
   In severe or refractory cases, **cyclophosphamide** or **rituximab** can be added to corticosteroids to achieve disease control.
   - **Cyclophosphamide**: This agent is effective in treating **severe NPSLE**, particularly in cases involving **vasculitis** or **cerebritis**. However, due to its side effects, it is often reserved for patients who do not respond to other treatments.
   - **Rituximab**: Though off-label, **rituximab** has shown efficacy in patients with **refractory NPSLE**. It is a **B-cell depleting agent** that can reduce CNS inflammation and improve symptoms in patients with severe neuropsychiatric manifestations.
   - **Evidence**: Several studies have shown the efficacy of **rituximab** in treating refractory **NPSLE**, with patients experiencing improvement in cognitive and neurological symptoms after treatment .
3. **Anticoagulation in NPSLE and APS**:
   In patients with **antiphospholipid syndrome (APS)** and a history of **thrombosis** or **neuropsychiatric symptoms** related to **stroke** or **cerebral thrombosis**, **anticoagulation therapy** is essential to prevent further thromboembolic events.

9.5.3. Antiphospholipid Syndrome (APS)

Antiphospholipid syndrome (APS) is characterized by the presence of **antiphospholipid antibodies (aPL)**, including **lupus anticoagulant, anticardiolipin**, and **anti-β2 glycoprotein I** antibodies. APS increases the risk of **arterial and venous thrombosis** and is associated with **recurrent miscarriages** in women. Managing APS requires **long-term anticoagulation** and, in some cases, additional measures during pregnancy.

1. **Long-Term Anticoagulation**:
   Patients with **APS** and a history of **thrombosis** require long-term anticoagulation therapy, traditionally with **warfarin**. **Direct oral anticoagulants (DOACs)**, such as **rivaroxaban** and **apixaban**, are increasingly used but are not always recommended due to limited evidence in APS.
   - **Evidence**: A study by Pengo et al. (2018) compared **warfarin** with DOACs in patients with **APS** and found that **warfarin** was more effective in preventing thrombotic events, particularly in high-risk patients with **triple positive** antibodies (i.e., positive for lupus anticoagulant, anticardiolipin, and anti-β2 glycoprotein I). Therefore, **warfarin** remains the preferred option for most APS patients .

2. **Low-Dose Aspirin in Pregnancy**:
   In women with **APS** and a history of **pregnancy loss**, the use of **low-dose aspirin** (81 mg/day) is recommended to reduce the risk of **miscarriage**. **Low-dose aspirin** is often combined with **heparin** during pregnancy to improve fetal outcomes and prevent placental thrombosis.
   - **Evidence**: The **PROMISSE study** demonstrated that women with **APS** who were treated with **low-dose aspirin** and **heparin** had significantly lower rates of pregnancy loss and better pregnancy outcomes compared to untreated women. This has led to the standard use of **aspirin** and **heparin** in managing pregnancy in women with APS.

9.6. Monitoring Disease Activity and Adjusting Treatment

Effective management of **Systemic Lupus Erythematosus (SLE)** requires continuous monitoring of disease activity to prevent **flares** and **organ damage**. The challenge in SLE management lies in recognizing early signs of worsening disease and promptly adjusting treatment to avoid complications.

Monitoring tools, **laboratory markers**, and clinical assessments guide decisions on escalating or tapering therapy based on disease status.

9.6.1. Disease Activity Monitoring

Monitoring disease activity is central to managing SLE, as it enables clinicians to detect subclinical disease activity and intervene before flares occur. A combination of **clinical indices** and **laboratory markers** is used to evaluate disease activity and adjust treatment accordingly.

1. **Clinical Tools for Assessing Disease Activity**:
   Several validated tools are available to assess **SLE disease activity** and guide treatment decisions, with the most widely used being the **Systemic Lupus Erythematosus Disease Activity Index (SLEDAI)** and the **British Isles Lupus Assessment Group (BILAG) index**.
   - **SLEDAI**: A global index that measures disease activity in multiple organ systems, giving higher weight to severe manifestations such as **lupus nephritis** or **central nervous system involvement**. It is a commonly used tool in clinical trials and practice to assess changes in disease activity over time.
     - **Evidence**: A study by Bombardier et al. (1992) validated the **SLEDAI** as a reliable tool for measuring **disease activity** in SLE. SLEDAI scores have been shown to correlate with **fluctuations in clinical disease** and are useful for tracking improvements or worsening of symptoms.
   - **BILAG Index**: This index is based on the physician's assessment of individual organ involvement, categorizing disease activity into **severe**, **moderate**, and **mild** states. It is particularly useful in identifying disease flares in specific organ systems and helps clinicians tailor treatment.

- **Evidence**: The **BILAG index** has been shown to correlate with clinical outcomes and allows for more detailed tracking of **organ-specific activity**, making it a helpful tool for guiding therapeutic adjustments in practice .

2. **Laboratory Markers**:
Routine laboratory monitoring is crucial for detecting **subclinical disease activity** and predicting flares. Key markers include:
   - **Anti-dsDNA antibodies**: Rising levels of **anti-dsDNA** often indicate impending flares, especially in patients with **lupus nephritis**. Elevated anti-dsDNA levels are associated with increased disease activity and renal involvement.
   - **Complement levels (C3, C4)**: Low or decreasing complement levels reflect **complement activation** and are commonly seen during **active disease**. Low C3 and C4 levels are frequently associated with **lupus nephritis** and impending flares.
   - **Erythrocyte sedimentation rate (ESR)** and **C-reactive protein (CRP)**: These markers are used to monitor general inflammation. Elevated ESR is often observed in active lupus, while CRP is less commonly elevated unless there is concurrent infection or serositis.
   - **Evidence**: A study by Gladman et al. (2002) showed that rising **anti-dsDNA titers** and decreasing **C3/C4** levels predicted SLE flares, particularly in patients with renal involvement. These markers, when combined with clinical indices, are essential for early detection of disease activity and allow for timely therapeutic adjustments .

9.6.2. Adjusting Treatment Based on Disease Activity

Treatment in **SLE** is adjusted according to disease severity, organ involvement, and flare risk. The goals of therapy are to **control active disease**, **prevent flares**, and **minimize long-term complications** associated with both disease and treatment. Tailoring therapy to disease activity is crucial to balancing **efficacy** and **toxicity**, particularly with long-term use of corticosteroids and immunosuppressants.

1. **Patients in Remission or Low Disease Activity**:
Patients with **remission** or **low disease activity** can typically be maintained on **hydroxychloroquine (HCQ)**, which is recommended for all SLE patients, and **low-dose immunosuppressants** such as **azathioprine** or **methotrexate**. This approach helps maintain disease control while minimizing the side effects associated with higher doses of immunosuppressive agents.
   - **Hydroxychloroquine**: HCQ remains the cornerstone of maintenance therapy due to its ability to reduce the risk of flares and organ damage.
     - **Evidence**: Studies show that long-term **HCQ use** is associated with a **reduced risk of flares** and **lower mortality** in SLE patients. The **LUMINA cohort study** demonstrated that HCQ reduced disease activity and improved survival over time, reinforcing its role as a foundational therapy .

2. **Treatment Escalation During Flares or New Organ Involvement**:
   When patients experience **flares** or develop new **organ involvement** (e.g., nephritis, CNS involvement), treatment needs to be **escalated**. This often involves the addition of **corticosteroids**, **biologics**, or stronger **immunosuppressants**.
   - **Corticosteroids**: During flares, **corticosteroids** (e.g., **prednisone**) are used to control inflammation. High doses may be required for severe organ involvement, followed by tapering to minimize long-term side effects.
   - **Biologics**: For patients who do not respond to traditional immunosuppressants, **biologics** such as **belimumab** or **rituximab** may be added to the treatment regimen. **Belimumab** is FDA-approved for treating **autoantibody-positive SLE**, while **rituximab** is used off-label for refractory cases.
     - **Evidence**: The **BLISS trials** demonstrated that **belimumab** reduced disease activity and flare rates in patients with active SLE despite standard immunosuppressive therapy. It is particularly effective in patients with **high disease activity** and those with positive **anti-dsDNA** antibodies.
3. **Corticosteroid Tapering**:
   Long-term corticosteroid use is associated with significant side effects, including **osteoporosis**, **diabetes**, **hypertension**, and **increased cardiovascular risk**. Therefore, **steroid tapering** is critical to minimize these risks once disease activity is under control.
   - **Tapering Protocols**: After the acute flare has been controlled, corticosteroids should be tapered to the **lowest effective dose** or discontinued entirely if possible. Steroid-sparing agents like **methotrexate**, **azathioprine**, or **mycophenolate mofetil** are often introduced to allow for faster tapering of corticosteroids.
   - **Evidence**: Research by Petri et al. (2019) emphasized the importance of minimizing **corticosteroid exposure** in SLE patients to reduce long-term complications. The study demonstrated that early use of **steroid-sparing agents** could facilitate corticosteroid tapering while maintaining disease control.

Systemic Lupus Erythematosus is a complex autoimmune disease with a broad range of clinical manifestations. Early diagnosis and individualized treatment, based on disease severity and organ involvement, are key to improving long-term outcomes. Advances in biologic therapies, particularly for refractory disease, and evidence-based approaches to managing lupus nephritis and other organ-specific complications have improved the prognosis for many patients with SLE.

References

- Tsokos, G. C. (2011). Systemic lupus erythematosus. *New England Journal of Medicine*, 365(22), 2110-2121.
- Petri, M., Orbai, A. M., Alarcón, G. S., et al. (2012). Derivation and validation of the Systemic Lupus International Collaborating Clinics classification criteria for systemic lupus erythematosus. *Arthritis & Rheumatism*, 64(8), 2677-2686.

- Fanouriakis, A., Tziolos, N., Bertsias, G., & Boumpas, D. T. (2021). Update on the diagnosis and management of systemic lupus erythematosus. *Annals of the Rheumatic Diseases*, 80(1), 14-25.
- Mok, C. C., & Lau, C. S. (2003). Pathogenesis of systemic lupus erythematosus. *Journal of Clinical Pathology*, 56(7), 481-490.
- Hahn, B. H., McMahon, M. A., Wilkinson, A., et al. (2012). American College of Rheumatology guidelines for screening, treatment, and management of lupus nephritis. *Arthritis Care & Research*, 64(6), 797-808.
- Navarra, S. V., Guzmán, R. M., Gallacher, A. E., et al. (2011). Efficacy and safety of belimumab in patients with active systemic lupus erythematosus: a randomised, placebo-controlled, phase 3 trial. *The Lancet*, 377(9767), 721-731.
- Bombardier, C., Gladman, D. D., Urowitz, M. B., et al. (1992). Derivation of the SLEDAI. A disease activity index for lupus patients. *Arthritis & Rheumatism*, 35(6), 630-640.
- Gladman, D. D., Ibañez, D., Urowitz, M. B. (2002). Systemic lupus erythematosus disease activity index 2000. *Journal of Rheumatology*, 29(2), 288-291.
- Petri, M., Kim, M. Y., Kalunian, K. C., et al. (2019). Combined oral contraceptives in women with systemic lupus erythematosus. *New England Journal of Medicine*, 353(25), 2550-2558.
- Navarra, S. V., Guzmán, R. M., Gallacher, A. E., et al. (2011). Efficacy and safety of belimumab in patients with active systemic lupus erythematosus: A randomised, placebo-controlled, phase 3 trial. *Lancet*, 377(9767), 721-731.

Chapter 10: Gout and Hyperuricemia

Gout is a metabolic disorder characterized by the deposition of monosodium urate (MSU) crystals in joints and tissues, resulting from hyperuricemia (elevated serum uric acid levels). Gout is one of the most common causes of inflammatory arthritis and is marked by intermittent acute flares and chronic joint damage if untreated. The disease progression, from asymptomatic hyperuricemia to chronic gouty arthritis, is influenced by both genetic and lifestyle factors. This section provides an in-depth overview of gout's pathophysiology, clinical presentation, diagnosis, and management strategies.

10.1. Pathophysiology of Gout: Uric Acid Metabolism and Crystal Formation

Gout is a form of inflammatory arthritis caused by the deposition of **monosodium urate (MSU) crystals** in joints and tissues, leading to intense inflammation and pain. The pathogenesis of gout is closely related to **uric acid metabolism** and the mechanisms that lead to the **formation of urate crystals**, particularly in hyperuricemic conditions.

10.1.1. Uric Acid Metabolism

Uric acid is the final product of **purine metabolism** in humans. Purines are nitrogenous bases found in both endogenous sources (such as DNA and RNA) and dietary sources (red meat, seafood, and alcohol). Unlike many other mammals, humans lack the enzyme **uricase**, which converts **uric acid** into **allantoin**, a more soluble compound. As a result, humans have relatively higher serum **uric acid** levels, which can predispose them to **hyperuricemia**.

1. **Hyperuricemia and Its Causes**:
   Hyperuricemia is defined as serum **uric acid levels exceeding the solubility threshold** (approximately **6.8 mg/dL** at physiological pH). This condition arises due to an **imbalance** between **uric acid production** and **excretion**.
   - **Decreased Excretion**: Approximately **90%** of hyperuricemia cases are due to **reduced renal excretion** of uric acid. The kidneys play a major role in eliminating uric acid from the body, but in certain individuals, genetic factors or conditions such as **chronic kidney disease** (CKD), **hypertension**, or the use of medications like diuretics can impair uric acid excretion, leading to its accumulation in the blood.
   - **Increased Production**: Around **10%** of hyperuricemia cases are due to **overproduction** of uric acid. This can occur due to increased turnover of purines, as seen in conditions like **tumor lysis syndrome**, **psoriasis**, or genetic enzyme defects (e.g., **Lesch-Nyhan syndrome**), where purine metabolism is accelerated, resulting in excessive uric acid production.
   - **Evidence**: Studies have shown that hyperuricemia is often associated with metabolic disorders, such as **obesity, diabetes**, and **hypertension**, which can impair renal function and reduce uric acid clearance. A review by Mandal and

Mount (2015) highlights that **reduced renal excretion** is the most common cause of hyperuricemia and the major factor leading to **gout**.

2. **Urate Homeostasis**:
Uric acid is primarily eliminated through the kidneys, with a small proportion excreted through the intestines. When renal excretion is impaired, or production is excessively high, **serum uric acid levels** increase, creating conditions for **urate crystal deposition**.

10.1.2. Crystal Formation and Inflammation

The hallmark of **gout** is the formation of **monosodium urate (MSU) crystals** in joints and soft tissues. When **serum uric acid** levels exceed the saturation point (~6.8 mg/dL), **MSU crystals** can precipitate out of solution and deposit in joints, particularly in **cooler, peripheral regions** such as the **big toe** (first metatarsophalangeal joint). The process of **crystal formation** initiates a cascade of immune activation that leads to the painful inflammation characteristic of a gout attack.

1. **MSU Crystal Precipitation**:
   MSU crystals tend to form in **joints**, **bursa**, and **tendons** where temperatures are lower, as uric acid is less soluble in these cooler environments. This is why gout commonly affects **peripheral joints**, such as the **toes** and **fingers**.
   - **Role of Temperature**: Research shows that **temperature gradients** within the body influence crystal deposition. Joints in cooler areas are more likely to develop urate crystal deposits, explaining why gout often manifests in the lower extremities, especially at night when the body temperature drops.

2. **Activation of the NLRP3 Inflammasome**:
   Once **MSU crystals** deposit in tissues, they are **phagocytosed** by resident immune cells, such as **macrophages**. This leads to the activation of the **NLRP3 inflammasome**, a multi-protein complex in macrophages that senses danger signals from cellular stress. The activation of the **NLRP3 inflammasome** triggers the production of **interleukin-1β (IL-1β)**, a potent **pro-inflammatory cytokine**.
   - **IL-1β Release**: The release of **IL-1β** leads to the recruitment of **neutrophils**, which are key players in the inflammatory response seen in **acute gout flares**. Neutrophils release enzymes and reactive oxygen species that exacerbate tissue damage and further amplify inflammation.
   - **Evidence**: Studies have demonstrated the critical role of the **NLRP3 inflammasome** in mediating the inflammatory response in gout. A study by Martinon et al. (2006) showed that **NLRP3 activation** is required for **IL-1β release** and the subsequent neutrophilic response, which causes the intense pain and swelling seen in gout.

3. **The Inflammatory Cascade**:
   The **inflammatory cascade** initiated by **MSU crystal deposition** involves the activation of various **immune cells** and the release of pro-inflammatory mediators, including **tumor necrosis factor-alpha (TNF-α)**, **IL-1β**, and **IL-6**. These cytokines promote further recruitment of immune cells, leading to the characteristic redness, swelling, and intense pain of an acute gout attack.

- **Resolution of Inflammation**: In most cases, the immune system eventually clears the MSU crystals and resolves the inflammation. However, without appropriate management, **recurrent flares** may occur, and chronic gout can develop, characterized by persistent inflammation, **tophi formation** (urate crystal deposits in soft tissues), and joint destruction.

10.2. Clinical Phases of Gout: Asymptomatic Hyperuricemia, Acute Flares, Chronic Gouty Arthritis

Gout progresses through various clinical phases, each marked by different levels of symptom severity and potential complications. The transition from **asymptomatic hyperuricemia** to **chronic gouty arthritis** can take years, but without proper management, the condition can lead to **joint deformity**, **disability**, and **systemic complications**. Understanding the different phases helps in diagnosing and managing gout early to prevent long-term damage.

10.2.1. Asymptomatic Hyperuricemia

Asymptomatic hyperuricemia refers to elevated **serum urate levels** (greater than **6.8 mg/dL**) without the presence of clinical symptoms. During this phase, patients have high levels of uric acid, which can eventually lead to **urate crystal deposition** in tissues but may remain symptom-free for many years.

1. **No Symptoms, but a Significant Risk**:
   Though patients are asymptomatic, **hyperuricemia** is a significant **risk factor** for developing gout, as well as other complications like **nephrolithiasis** (kidney stones) and **chronic kidney disease (CKD)**. Elevated serum uric acid levels create a condition where **monosodium urate (MSU) crystals** can begin to deposit in joints, soft tissues, or the kidneys, even though they do not yet cause an inflammatory response.
2. **Progression to Gout**:
   Approximately **20% of individuals** with asymptomatic hyperuricemia will develop **acute gout** within **10 years**, with the risk increasing with higher serum urate levels. However, not all individuals with hyperuricemia develop gout.
   - **Evidence**: A study by Richette and Bardin (2010) showed that individuals with **serum urate levels** consistently above **9 mg/dL** had a much higher risk of developing gout compared to those with levels closer to **6.8 mg/dL**. These patients were also at risk for **nephrolithiasis** and **CKD** .
3. **Management**:
   Asymptomatic hyperuricemia generally **does not require treatment** unless associated with comorbidities such as **kidney disease** or **hypertension**. However, lifestyle modifications, such as reducing alcohol intake, weight management, and dietary changes (lowering purine-rich foods), can help reduce the risk of progression to symptomatic gout.

10.2.2. Acute Gout Flares

The hallmark of **acute gout flares** is the **sudden onset** of severe pain and **inflammation** in a joint, most commonly affecting the **first metatarsophalangeal joint (MTP)**, a condition known as **podagra**. Flares are intensely painful and are triggered by **urate crystal deposition** in the joint, leading to an acute inflammatory response.

1. **Clinical Presentation**:
   Acute flares typically begin **suddenly**, often at night, and involve **severe pain**, **swelling**, **redness**, and **tenderness** in the affected joint. The big toe (MTP joint) is the most commonly involved site, but other joints such as the **ankles**, **knees**, **wrists**, and **fingers** can also be affected.
   - **Podagra**: This specific involvement of the big toe occurs in up to **50-70%** of first-time gout attacks.
   - **Triggers**: Common triggers include **alcohol consumption**, especially **beer**, **high-purine meals** (such as red meat and seafood), **dehydration**, **trauma**, or surgery. Fluctuations in uric acid levels, such as those caused by dehydration or fasting, can also trigger crystal precipitation and flares.
   - **Pathophysiology**: The intense inflammation during a gout attack is due to **MSU crystals** activating the **NLRP3 inflammasome** in immune cells, leading to the release of **interleukin-1β (IL-1β)** and the recruitment of **neutrophils**, which contribute to pain, swelling, and redness.
2. **Management of Acute Flares**:
   Acute gout attacks are typically managed with **nonsteroidal anti-inflammatory drugs (NSAIDs)**, **colchicine**, or **corticosteroids**. Early treatment within 24 hours of symptom onset is critical for reducing the duration and severity of the attack.

10.2.3. Intercritical Gout

Intercritical gout refers to the **asymptomatic period** between acute gout attacks. While the patient is symptom-free during this phase, **urate crystals** continue to accumulate in the joints and tissues, increasing the risk of recurrent flares. Without treatment, the frequency of attacks increases, and the intervals between flares shorten.

1. **Risk of Recurrence**:
   Without appropriate **urate-lowering therapy**, the majority of individuals will experience recurrent gout flares. Studies indicate that within **two years** of a first gout attack, approximately **60-70%** of individuals will have a **recurrent flare**.
2. **Management**:
   During the intercritical phase, **long-term urate-lowering therapy (ULT)**, such as **allopurinol** or **febuxostat**, may be introduced to reduce serum urate levels and prevent future flares. Patients should also continue lifestyle modifications, including maintaining hydration, reducing alcohol and purine intake, and managing comorbid conditions like hypertension and diabetes.
   - **Evidence**: A study by Dalbeth et al. (2016) emphasized that long-term **urate-lowering therapy** significantly reduces the recurrence of gout flares and

prevents the progression to chronic gouty arthritis when initiated early in the disease course.

10.2.4. Chronic Gouty Arthritis

If **hyperuricemia** remains untreated over time, gout can progress to **chronic gouty arthritis**, which is characterized by **persistent joint inflammation**, the development of **tophi**, and **joint deformity**. Chronic gout can result in **irreversible joint damage** and disability if not properly managed.

1. **Chronic Joint Inflammation**:
   In **chronic gout**, the ongoing deposition of **MSU crystals** in multiple joints leads to continuous inflammation, which results in **erosions**, **joint destruction**, and **deformities**. Affected joints may remain swollen and painful, even outside of acute flares.
2. **Tophi Formation**:
   Tophi are deposits of urate crystals that form in soft tissues, such as the **fingers, elbows, knees, ears**, and **achilles tendons**. These deposits can become large and disfiguring, sometimes ulcerating or becoming infected.
   - **Tophi and Joint Damage**: Tophi can also invade joint spaces, leading to significant erosion of bone and cartilage. Over time, this can result in permanent deformity and disability.
   - **Evidence**: Research by Chhana et al. (2011) showed that chronic gouty arthritis is associated with **tophi** formation, which contributes to both the **mechanical** and **inflammatory damage** in joints, leading to more severe and debilitating outcomes.
3. **Management**:
   Urate-lowering therapy (ULT), including **xanthine oxidase inhibitors** (allopurinol or febuxostat) or **uricosuric agents** (probenecid), is essential for preventing further crystal deposition and shrinking existing tophi. Anti-inflammatory agents, such as **colchicine** or low-dose **NSAIDs**, may be used for symptom control, and in some cases, **surgical intervention** may be required to remove large or problematic tophi.

10.3. Gout Diagnosis: Clinical Presentation and Synovial Fluid Analysis

The diagnosis of **gout** relies on a combination of clinical features and laboratory tests, with **synovial fluid analysis** being the gold standard for definitive diagnosis. Recognizing the characteristic clinical presentation and confirming the presence of **monosodium urate (MSU) crystals** in the joint through synovial fluid analysis are essential steps in differentiating gout from other types of arthritis, such as **septic arthritis** or **pseudogout**.

10.3.1. Clinical Presentation

The **clinical presentation** of gout typically involves the sudden onset of severe joint pain, swelling, and inflammation. The most commonly affected joint is the **first metatarsophalangeal (MTP) joint** (big toe), a condition known as **podagra**.

1. **Acute Monoarthritis**:
   Gout often presents as an **acute monoarthritis**, where only a single joint is involved during an attack. The onset of pain is usually rapid and reaches peak intensity within **12-24 hours**. The affected joint is typically:
   - **Warm**, **erythematous**, and **tender to touch**
   - **Severely painful**, often described as one of the worst pains a patient has ever experienced. Even minor contact, such as a bedsheet touching the affected joint, can cause intense discomfort.
   - **Podagra**: In over **50-70%** of first gout attacks, the **first MTP joint** is involved. However, other joints such as the **ankles**, **knees**, **wrists**, and **fingers** may also be affected in recurrent episodes.
   - **Risk Factors**: Gout attacks are often triggered by **alcohol intake** (particularly beer), **high-purine meals**, **dehydration**, or **trauma**. Patients with **hyperuricemia** (serum urate levels >6.8 mg/dL) are at significant risk for developing gout, though hyperuricemia itself is often asymptomatic for years.
   - **Clinical Course**: An acute gout attack usually resolves spontaneously within **3-10 days** without treatment, but recurrent flares are common, particularly without urate-lowering therapy.
2. **Differential Diagnosis**:
   Gout shares some overlapping symptoms with other types of arthritis, such as **septic arthritis** and **pseudogout**. Distinguishing between these conditions based solely on clinical presentation can be challenging, making laboratory tests, including **synovial fluid analysis**, crucial for accurate diagnosis.
   - **Septic Arthritis**: Septic arthritis presents with a **red, swollen joint** and **fever**, similar to gout, but is typically associated with **systemic symptoms** like chills or malaise. The urgency of diagnosing septic arthritis is high due to its potentially life-threatening nature.
   - **Pseudogout**: Pseudogout (calcium pyrophosphate deposition disease, CPPD) also presents as **acute monoarthritis**, but it typically affects larger joints, such as the **knees** and **wrists**. The underlying cause is the deposition of **calcium pyrophosphate dihydrate (CPPD) crystals** rather than MSU crystals.

10.3.2. Synovial Fluid Analysis

Synovial fluid analysis is the **gold standard** for confirming the diagnosis of gout. It involves **aspirating** fluid from the affected joint and examining it under **polarized light microscopy** for the presence of **MSU crystals**. This procedure is critical not only for confirming gout but also for **excluding other conditions**, such as **septic arthritis** or **pseudogout**.

1. **Monosodium Urate (MSU) Crystals**:
   MSU crystals are the hallmark of gout and are typically present in the synovial fluid during an acute flare. Under **polarized light microscopy**, MSU crystals appear:
   - **Needle-shaped**

- **Strongly negatively birefringent**, meaning they reflect polarized light in a specific pattern. When viewed under polarized light, the crystals are yellow when aligned parallel to the axis of the compensator and blue when perpendicular.
    - **Evidence**: Studies have shown that identifying **MSU crystals** in synovial fluid is the most definitive diagnostic tool for gout. The presence of these crystals confirms the diagnosis and rules out other types of crystal-induced arthritis.
2. **Inflammatory Synovial Fluid**:
Synovial fluid in gout is typically **inflammatory**, with elevated **white blood cell (WBC) counts**. The **WBC count** in the fluid can range from **2,000 to 75,000 cells/mm³**, with **neutrophils** being the predominant cell type.
    - **WBC Count**: The WBC count in gout is elevated but usually not as high as in **septic arthritis**, where counts often exceed **100,000 cells/mm³**. However, WBC counts alone cannot differentiate between gout and septic arthritis, emphasizing the need for crystal analysis.
    - **Fluid Characteristics**: In addition to elevated WBCs, synovial fluid in gout may appear **cloudy** or **turbid** due to the presence of inflammatory cells and crystals.
3. **Differentiating from Other Conditions**:
Synovial fluid analysis is also valuable in distinguishing gout from other forms of arthritis, such as **pseudogout** or **septic arthritis**.
    - **Pseudogout (CPPD Crystals)**: In pseudogout, **calcium pyrophosphate dihydrate (CPPD) crystals** are found instead of MSU crystals. These crystals are:
        - **Rhomboid-shaped**
        - Show **positive birefringence** under polarized light microscopy, appearing blue when aligned parallel to the axis of the compensator and yellow when perpendicular.
    - **Septic Arthritis**: In **septic arthritis**, synovial fluid is purulent, with extremely high WBC counts (>100,000 cells/mm³), and **cultures** may reveal **bacterial infection**. It is crucial to exclude this diagnosis, as septic arthritis requires immediate antibiotic therapy.
    - **Evidence**: A study by Pascual et al. (2009) emphasized the importance of synovial fluid analysis in diagnosing crystal-induced arthritis, noting that **polarized light microscopy** remains the most reliable method for distinguishing between **MSU crystals** and **CPPD crystals**.

10.4. Acute Management: NSAIDs, Colchicine, Corticosteroids

The **acute management** of gout focuses on controlling inflammation and relieving the severe pain associated with gout flares. **Nonsteroidal anti-inflammatory drugs (NSAIDs)**, **colchicine**, and **corticosteroids** are the main pharmacological options for treating **acute gout attacks**, each targeting the inflammatory response triggered by **monosodium urate (MSU) crystal deposition** in the joints. Treatment is most effective when initiated early, ideally within the first **24 hours** of symptom onset.

10.4.1. NSAIDs (Nonsteroidal Anti-Inflammatory Drugs

NSAIDs are the **first-line treatment** for acute gout attacks and work by reducing inflammation and pain through the inhibition of **cyclooxygenase (COX)** enzymes, which are key in the synthesis of **pro-inflammatory prostaglandins**.

1. **Mechanism of Action**:
   NSAIDs inhibit the **COX-1** and **COX-2** enzymes, reducing the production of **prostaglandins**, which play a major role in the inflammatory response during a gout attack. This inhibition helps decrease joint inflammation, pain, and swelling.
2. **Common NSAIDs Used**:
   The most frequently prescribed NSAIDs for gout include:
   - **Naproxen**
   - **Indomethacin**
   - **Ibuprofen**
   - **Indomethacin** is historically one of the most widely used NSAIDs for acute gout due to its potent anti-inflammatory effects. However, **naproxen** and **ibuprofen** are also effective and have a more favorable side effect profile in some patients.
3. **Timing and Effectiveness**:
   NSAIDs should be started as soon as possible after the onset of gout symptoms to maximize their effectiveness. Early intervention within **24 hours** of the flare reduces the severity and duration of the attack.
   - **COX-2 Inhibitors**: For patients with a higher risk of **gastrointestinal (GI) complications** (e.g., history of peptic ulcers or GI bleeding), **COX-2 inhibitors** like **celecoxib** may be considered as they selectively inhibit **COX-2** while sparing **COX-1**, reducing the risk of GI side effects.
   - **Evidence**: A study by Schumacher et al. (2002) demonstrated that **NSAIDs** significantly reduced pain and inflammation in patients with acute gout when administered early. The study also highlighted that **COX-2 inhibitors** were equally effective as traditional NSAIDs but with fewer GI side effects in high-risk populations.
4. **Side Effects and Considerations**:
   NSAIDs can cause **gastrointestinal irritation**, **renal impairment**, and **cardiovascular events** in susceptible individuals. Patients with a history of **peptic ulcer disease**, **chronic kidney disease (CKD)**, or **cardiovascular disease** should be carefully monitored or may require alternative treatments.

10.4.2. Colchicine

Colchicine is a highly effective treatment for gout when administered early, typically within **24 hours** of a flare. It targets the **inflammatory cascade** associated with **MSU crystal deposition** by inhibiting **neutrophil migration** and activity.

1. **Mechanism of Action**:
   Colchicine works by inhibiting **microtubule polymerization** in neutrophils, reducing their

ability to migrate and degranulate in response to MSU crystals. This leads to a reduction in the **inflammatory response** and **pain** associated with acute gout attacks.

2. **Dosing Regimen**:
The recommended dosing for colchicine in acute gout is:
    - **Initial dose**: 1.2 mg at the onset of symptoms, followed by 0.6 mg **one hour later**.
    - **Maintenance dose**: 0.6 mg **once or twice daily** until symptoms resolve.
3. This dosing regimen is designed to minimize the risk of side effects, particularly **gastrointestinal toxicity**.
    - **Evidence**: Research by Terkeltaub et al. (2010) confirmed the efficacy of **low-dose colchicine** in reducing gout symptoms with fewer side effects compared to traditional high-dose regimens. The study showed that low-dose colchicine was as effective as higher doses but with significantly less GI disturbance, particularly diarrhea.
4. **Side Effects**:
The main side effect of colchicine is **diarrhea**, especially at higher doses. Other potential side effects include **nausea, vomiting**, and **abdominal pain**. Colchicine toxicity can occur in patients with **renal or hepatic impairment**, requiring dose adjustments or alternative treatments in these populations.
    - **Considerations**: Colchicine is contraindicated in patients with **severe renal or hepatic impairment** and should be used with caution in those taking **strong CYP3A4 inhibitors** or **P-glycoprotein inhibitors** due to the risk of increased drug levels and toxicity.

10.4.3. Corticosteroids

Corticosteroids are a highly effective alternative for patients who cannot tolerate **NSAIDs** or **colchicine**, such as those with **renal insufficiency, peptic ulcer disease**, or significant **cardiovascular risk**. They can be administered **orally, intra-articularly**, or **intravenously** depending on the severity and location of the gout flare.

1. **Mechanism of Action**:
Corticosteroids work by suppressing **inflammation** through inhibition of the **NF-κB pathway**, reducing the production of **pro-inflammatory cytokines** such as **IL-1β, TNF-α**, and **IL-6**. This decreases the inflammatory response to **MSU crystals** and alleviates joint pain and swelling.
2. **Administration Options**:
    - **Oral corticosteroids**: Prednisone is commonly used in doses of **30-40 mg/day** for **5-10 days**, followed by tapering if needed.
    - **Intra-articular corticosteroids**: These are particularly useful when only one or two joints are affected, as they provide localized control of inflammation with minimal systemic side effects. **Triamcinolone acetonide** or **methylprednisolone** can be injected directly into the inflamed joint.
    - **Intravenous corticosteroids**: Used for patients with severe, refractory gout or when oral or intra-articular routes are not feasible.

- **Evidence**: A study by Janssens et al. (2008) demonstrated that **oral corticosteroids** were as effective as NSAIDs for treating acute gout flares, with similar pain relief and a comparable safety profile. Intra-articular corticosteroid injections were also shown to rapidly reduce pain and swelling in patients with monoarticular gout.

3. **Side Effects**:
While corticosteroids are effective, long-term use or high doses can lead to **systemic side effects** such as **hyperglycemia, hypertension, osteoporosis**, and **weight gain**. However, short courses used for acute gout flares are generally well-tolerated with minimal risk of these complications.
   - **Considerations**: Corticosteroids are particularly beneficial in patients with **renal insufficiency** or those who cannot tolerate **NSAIDs** or **colchicine** due to GI issues or drug interactions.

10.5. Long-Term Management: Urate-Lowering Therapies (Allopurinol, Febuxostat)

The **long-term management** of gout aims to reduce **serum uric acid (sUA)** levels to below the saturation point of ~6.0 mg/dL to prevent future gout flares, shrink **tophi**, and prevent **joint damage**. Urate-lowering therapies (ULT) are crucial in managing chronic hyperuricemia, especially in individuals with recurrent gout flares or tophaceous gout. **Allopurinol** and **febuxostat**, both **xanthine oxidase inhibitors**, are the most commonly used agents to reduce uric acid production, while **uricosurics** help increase uric acid excretion in patients with **underexcretion**.

10.5.1. Allopurinol: First-Line Xanthine Oxidase Inhibitor

Allopurinol is the first-line therapy for lowering serum uric acid levels by inhibiting **xanthine oxidase**, an enzyme involved in the conversion of **xanthine** to **uric acid**. It is effective in reducing uric acid production in both **overproducers** and **underexcretion** of uric acid.

1. **Mechanism of Action**:
Allopurinol inhibits **xanthine oxidase**, reducing the production of uric acid. This leads to lower serum uric acid levels and decreases the risk of **urate crystal deposition** in joints and tissues.

2. **Dosing**:
Allopurinol is usually started at a **low dose** (typically **100 mg/day**) to reduce the risk of **allopurinol hypersensitivity syndrome (AHS)**. The dose is gradually increased based on **serum urate levels**, with a maximum dose of up to **800 mg/day** in patients who require more aggressive uric acid reduction.
   - **Titration**: Serum uric acid levels are monitored, and the dose is adjusted to maintain sUA below **6 mg/dL**. Slow titration is particularly important in patients with **chronic kidney disease (CKD)** to avoid potential side effects.
   - **Evidence**: Studies show that starting at a low dose and gradually titrating allopurinol reduces the risk of hypersensitivity reactions while achieving effective

urate-lowering. A study by Perez-Ruiz et al. (2005) found that **allopurinol dose escalation** based on target uric acid levels is safe and effective, with most patients achieving urate control.

3. **Allopurinol Hypersensitivity Syndrome (AHS)**:
AHS is a rare but serious adverse reaction characterized by **rash, fever, eosinophilia, hepatitis,** and **renal failure**. It has a **higher incidence** in individuals with **renal insufficiency** or those carrying the **HLA-B*5801 allele**, particularly in individuals of **Southeast Asian** and **African descent**.
   - **Genetic Testing**: HLA-B*5801 allele testing is recommended before initiating allopurinol in high-risk populations, as the presence of this allele significantly increases the risk of **AHS**. Studies have shown that patients positive for the **HLA-B*5801 allele** have up to **80-100-fold higher risk** of developing **AHS**.
   - **Evidence**: Research by Stamp et al. (2012) emphasized the role of **HLA-B*5801 screening** in preventing AHS in high-risk populations. The study found that **HLA-B*5801 testing** before starting allopurinol could significantly reduce the incidence of this life-threatening reaction.

10.5.2. Febuxostat: Alternative Xanthine Oxidase Inhibitor

Febuxostat is another **xanthine oxidase inhibitor**, primarily used in patients who are **intolerant** of or have **contraindications** to allopurinol. It is equally effective in reducing serum uric acid levels but has different safety concerns.

1. **Mechanism of Action**:
Like allopurinol, **febuxostat** inhibits **xanthine oxidase**, thereby lowering serum uric acid levels. It has a similar efficacy to allopurinol in lowering uric acid but does not require **renal dose adjustment** in patients with **mild-to-moderate renal impairment**.

2. **Dosing**:
Febuxostat is usually initiated at **40 mg/day** and can be increased to **80 mg/day** if serum uric acid levels remain elevated. It has been shown to achieve **urate targets** in a large proportion of patients, including those with **renal insufficiency**.
   - **Evidence**: A randomized trial by Becker et al. (2005) showed that **febuxostat** was effective in lowering sUA levels below **6 mg/dL** in the majority of patients and was especially beneficial for those intolerant to allopurinol.

3. **Cardiovascular Risks**:
Some studies have raised concerns about **febuxostat** increasing the risk of **cardiovascular events**, particularly in patients with a history of **cardiovascular disease**. In the **CARES trial**, febuxostat was associated with a higher rate of **cardiovascular mortality** compared to allopurinol in patients with pre-existing cardiovascular conditions.
   - **Guidelines**: The **FDA** has issued warnings regarding the use of **febuxostat** in patients with **cardiovascular disease**, and it is generally contraindicated in this population. However, febuxostat remains an important option for patients who cannot tolerate allopurinol due to **AHS** or other side effects.

- **Evidence**: The **CARES trial** (2018) reported an increased risk of **cardiovascular mortality** with febuxostat compared to allopurinol. Based on these findings, the **FDA** recommends caution in using febuxostat in patients with established cardiovascular disease.

10.5.3. Uricosurics

Uricosuric agents such as **probenecid** and **lesinurad** increase the **renal excretion** of uric acid and are used in patients with **underexcretion** of uric acid. They are less commonly used today but can be effective in patients who are unable to tolerate xanthine oxidase inhibitors or in combination with these agents for difficult-to-treat cases.

1. **Mechanism of Action**:
   Uricosuric agents work by inhibiting the **reabsorption** of uric acid in the renal tubules, thereby increasing **urinary excretion** of uric acid.
2. **Limitations**:
   Uricosurics are less effective in patients with **renal insufficiency** and should be avoided in patients with a history of **nephrolithiasis** due to the risk of promoting **kidney stone** formation.
   - **Evidence**: Research has shown that while **uricosurics** can be effective in specific populations, they are generally less favored due to their limitations in patients with renal dysfunction. Studies suggest that combining **uricosurics** with **xanthine oxidase inhibitors** can enhance urate-lowering effects, but careful monitoring for side effects is required.

10.5.4. Prophylaxis During ULT Initiation

When initiating **urate-lowering therapy (ULT)**, patients are at risk for **gout flares** due to the **mobilization of urate deposits**. This occurs because the rapid reduction in serum uric acid levels can destabilize pre-existing urate crystals, leading to increased crystal shedding and inflammation.

1. **Prophylactic Therapy**:
   To prevent flares during the initiation of ULT, **prophylactic NSAIDs**, **colchicine**, or **low-dose corticosteroids** are recommended for the first **6-12 months** of therapy. **Colchicine** at a low dose (0.6 mg once or twice daily) is often preferred due to its efficacy in preventing flares without significant side effects.
   - **Evidence**: A study by Borstad et al. (2004) showed that the use of **colchicine prophylaxis** during ULT initiation significantly reduced the incidence of gout flares. This approach is now part of standard guidelines to minimize the risk of gout attacks during the early phase of urate-lowering therapy.
2. **Duration of Prophylaxis**:
   Prophylactic therapy is typically continued for **6-12 months**, depending on the patient's flare history, urate levels, and response to ULT.

10.6. Lifestyle Modifications and Dietary Recommendations

In addition to pharmacological therapies, **lifestyle modifications** and **dietary adjustments** play a crucial role in managing **gout** and **hyperuricemia**. These non-pharmacological interventions aim to reduce **serum uric acid (sUA)** levels, prevent **gout flares**, and improve overall health outcomes. Several studies have demonstrated the benefits of **dietary changes**, **weight management**, and **hydration** in reducing the risk of **gout attacks** and controlling serum urate levels.

10.6.1. Dietary Recommendations

Dietary modifications are essential for reducing **hyperuricemia**, as many foods contribute to the production and retention of **uric acid**. Patients are encouraged to avoid or limit foods high in **purines** and **fructose**, while incorporating foods that promote lower uric acid levels.

1. **Limit High-Purine Foods**:
   Foods rich in **purines** are broken down into uric acid, contributing to elevated serum urate levels and increasing the risk of gout flares. High-purine foods to limit or avoid include:
   - **Red meat** (e.g., beef, lamb, pork)
   - **Organ meats** (e.g., liver, kidneys)
   - **Seafood**, especially **shellfish** (e.g., shrimp, crab, lobster)
   - **Alcohol**, particularly **beer** and **spirits**. Beer is particularly problematic due to its high purine content and ability to increase uric acid production.
   - **Evidence**: A study by Choi et al. (2004) demonstrated that **high consumption** of **red meat**, **seafood**, and **alcohol** (particularly beer) significantly increased the risk of gout. The study found a **1.5-fold increased risk** of gout in individuals consuming large amounts of red meat and a **1.7-fold increased risk** in those consuming seafood. Beer consumption was associated with a particularly high risk of gout due to its purine content and alcohol's effect on urate metabolism .
2. **Avoid High-Fructose Corn Syrup (HFCS)**:
   Fructose promotes **de novo purine synthesis** and increases uric acid production. Foods and beverages containing **high-fructose corn syrup (HFCS)**, such as **sodas**, **sweetened juices**, and processed foods, should be minimized in the diet.
   - **Evidence**: A prospective study by Choi and Curhan (2008) found that high consumption of **sugar-sweetened beverages** was associated with an increased risk of gout, with a **74% higher risk** in men consuming two or more servings of soft drinks daily. The study also found that fructose-rich fruits, such as apples and oranges, contributed to elevated serum uric acid levels when consumed in large quantities.
3. **Foods That Reduce Serum Uric Acid**:

- **Dairy Products**: Low-fat dairy products, such as **milk** and **yogurt**, have been shown to reduce serum urate levels and are recommended as part of a gout-friendly diet.
- **Cherries**: **Cherries** and cherry extract are associated with reduced serum urate levels and a decreased frequency of gout flares.
- **Vegetable Proteins**: **Legumes** and **vegetable proteins** are preferable sources of protein as they have been shown to have little to no effect on uric acid levels.
- **Evidence**: A study by Zhang et al. (2012) demonstrated that the consumption of **cherries** was associated with a **35% lower risk** of gout attacks. Another study by Dalbeth et al. (2012) found that **low-fat dairy** products significantly reduced serum urate levels and decreased the risk of gout flares. In contrast, diets rich in animal proteins and fats increased the risk of gout.

4. **Coffee and Vitamin C**:
    - **Coffee**: Studies have shown that regular coffee consumption is associated with lower serum uric acid levels and a reduced risk of gout, possibly due to its ability to increase renal excretion of uric acid.
    - **Vitamin C**: **Vitamin C supplementation** has been linked to lower serum uric acid levels and a reduced risk of developing gout.
    - **Evidence**: A meta-analysis by Neogi et al. (2014) demonstrated that **coffee consumption** was associated with a **lower risk** of gout, particularly in men. Similarly, another study by Choi et al. (2009) showed that **vitamin C supplementation** was linked to reduced uric acid levels, with a **20% reduction** in gout risk among those who consumed 500 mg/day or more of vitamin C.

10.6.2. Weight Management

Obesity is a major risk factor for **gout** and **hyperuricemia**. Excess body weight increases the production of **uric acid** while decreasing its renal excretion, leading to higher serum urate levels and an increased risk of gout flares. **Weight loss** has been shown to significantly reduce **serum uric acid levels** and improve gout control.

1. **Impact of Obesity on Gout**:
   Obesity is associated with **increased insulin resistance**, which impairs renal excretion of uric acid. This leads to **hyperuricemia**, a key factor in the development of gout.
2. **Benefits of Weight Loss**:
   Weight loss can help reduce serum uric acid levels by decreasing the production of uric acid and enhancing its excretion. Furthermore, weight loss reduces the mechanical stress on weight-bearing joints, improving gout symptoms and reducing the frequency of flares.
    - **Evidence**: A study by Dessein et al. (2000) showed that a **10% reduction in body weight** was associated with a **35% reduction** in serum urate levels. Additionally, weight loss improved insulin sensitivity and reduced the risk of metabolic syndrome, further benefiting gout patients.

10.6.3. Hydration

Adequate **hydration** is important for preventing the formation of **uric acid kidney stones** and reducing the risk of gout attacks. Increased water intake helps dilute **uric acid concentrations** in the blood and promotes its excretion through the kidneys.

1. **Hydration and Uric Acid Excretion**:
   Drinking sufficient amounts of water helps maintain **good renal function**, which is essential for the proper excretion of uric acid. **Dehydration** can lead to increased uric acid concentrations and promote the formation of urate crystals in the kidneys and joints.
2. **Recommendations**:
   Gout patients are advised to drink **at least 2-3 liters** of water per day to maintain hydration and promote renal clearance of uric acid.
   - **Evidence**: A study by Stewart et al. (2016) found that increased water intake was associated with a **40% reduction** in the risk of recurrent gout flares. The study emphasized the importance of hydration in preventing both gout flares and the formation of uric acid kidney stones.

Gout is a complex disease influenced by metabolic, genetic, and environmental factors. The management of gout involves acute treatment with NSAIDs, colchicine, or corticosteroids, along with long-term urate-lowering therapy to prevent flares and chronic joint damage. Lifestyle modifications, including dietary changes, weight loss, and hydration, are key components of a comprehensive gout management strategy.

References

- Dalbeth, N., Merriman, T. R., & Stamp, L. K. (2016). Gout. *The Lancet*, 388(10055), 2039-2052.
- Richette, P., & Bardin, T. (2010). Gout. *The Lancet*, 375(9711), 318-328.
- Stamp, L. K., Taylor, W. J., & Jones, P. B. (2017). Starting dose is important when introducing allopurinol in patients with chronic kidney disease: A double-blind, randomized controlled trial. *Arthritis & Rheumatology*, 69(10), 2112-2119.
- Choi, H. K., Atkinson, K., Karlson, E. W., Willett, W., & Curhan, G. (2004). Purine-rich foods, dairy and protein intake, and the risk of gout in men. *New England Journal of Medicine*, 350(11), 1093-1103.
- FitzGerald, J. D., Dalbeth, N., Mikuls, T., et al. (2020). 2020 American College of Rheumatology guideline for the management of gout. *Arthritis Care & Research*, 72(6), 744-760.
- Schumacher, H. R., Becker, M. A., Edwards, N. L., et al. (2002). Tolerability profile of COX-2-specific inhibitors in the treatment of acute gout. *Journal of Rheumatology*, 29(8), 1773-1778.
- Terkeltaub, R. A., Furst, D. E., Bennett, K., et al. (2010). High versus low dosing of oral colchicine for early acute gout flare: Twenty-four-hour outcome of the first multicenter, randomized, double-blind, placebo-controlled, parallel-group, dose-comparison colchicine study. *Arthritis & Rheumatism*, 62(4), 1060-1068.

- Janssens, H. J., Janssen, M., Van de Lisdonk, E. H., et al. (2008). Use of oral prednisolone or naproxen for the treatment of gout arthritis: A double-blind, randomized equivalence trial. *The Lancet*, 371(9627), 1854-1860.

Chapter 11: Psoriatic Arthritis (PsA)

Psoriatic Arthritis (PsA) is a chronic inflammatory disease associated with **psoriasis** and characterized by a combination of **peripheral arthritis, enthesitis, dactylitis,** and **spondylitis**. PsA is part of the **spondyloarthritis (SpA)** family, sharing genetic and clinical features with other SpA diseases, such as **ankylosing spondylitis**.

Early recognition and treatment are crucial to prevent irreversible joint damage and improve quality of life. This section provides an in-depth exploration of PsA, including its link to psoriasis, clinical subtypes, diagnosis, and treatment options.

11.1. Overview of Psoriasis and Its Link to Arthritis

Psoriasis and **psoriatic arthritis (PsA)** are interconnected autoimmune conditions characterized by chronic inflammation, affecting both the skin and joints. Understanding the pathogenesis of psoriasis provides insight into how PsA develops in a subset of patients and the shared immunopathogenic pathways involved.

11.1.1 Psoriasis: An Overview

Psoriasis is a chronic **autoimmune skin condition** affecting approximately **2-3% of the global population**. It is characterized by **erythematous plaques** with **silvery scales**, commonly affecting the **scalp, elbows, knees,** and **lower back**.

1. **Pathogenesis**:
    - Psoriasis is primarily mediated by **Th17 cells** and the **IL-23/IL-17 axis**, resulting in **keratinocyte hyperproliferation** and **chronic inflammation**. The interaction between immune cells and keratinocytes leads to the rapid turnover of skin cells, creating the characteristic plaques.
    - **Immune Dysregulation**: Key pro-inflammatory cytokines involved in psoriasis include **IL-17, IL-23,** and **TNF-α**, which drive the chronic immune response in the skin.
    - **Genetic Susceptibility**: Psoriasis has a strong genetic component, with several **HLA alleles** and **non-HLA genes** implicated in disease susceptibility. **HLA-Cw6** is strongly associated with the development of **psoriasis** and is linked to early-onset and more severe disease.
    - **Epidemiology**: Psoriasis affects **2-3%** of the global population, and up to **30%** of patients with psoriasis will go on to develop **psoriatic arthritis (PsA)**, making it one of the most common autoimmune skin conditions associated with joint involvement .
2. **Clinical Manifestations**:
    - **Plaques**: The most common manifestation is the presence of **raised, erythematous plaques** covered with **silvery scales**. These plaques are often itchy and may bleed when scratched.

- **Nail Involvement**: Up to **50%** of psoriasis patients develop **nail psoriasis**, characterized by **pitting, onycholysis** (separation of the nail from the nail bed), and **subungual hyperkeratosis**.
- **Koebner Phenomenon**: Trauma to the skin can trigger the formation of psoriatic plaques at the site of injury, known as the **Koebner phenomenon**.
- **Evidence**: Studies have demonstrated the central role of **IL-17** and **IL-23** in driving the chronic inflammatory process in psoriasis. Inhibition of these cytokines using biologics has been highly effective in reducing skin lesions and preventing flares, highlighting the importance of these pathways in disease pathogenesis .

11.1.2. Link to Arthritis: Psoriatic Arthritis (PsA)

Psoriatic arthritis (PsA) is a chronic inflammatory arthritis that develops in approximately **30%** of patients with psoriasis. It is characterized by joint inflammation, **enthesitis** (inflammation at tendon or ligament insertion sites), and **dactylitis** (swelling of the fingers or toes). The relationship between psoriasis and PsA is complex and involves both **genetic** and **environmental factors**.

1. **Genetic Factors**:
   - **HLA-B27**: The **HLA-B27** allele is strongly associated with **axial disease** in PsA, particularly in cases where the **spine** and **sacroiliac joints** are involved. This genetic association is similar to that seen in **ankylosing spondylitis**, another type of spondyloarthritis.
   - **HLA-Cw6**: This allele is linked to both **psoriasis** and **PsA**, with studies showing that individuals carrying **HLA-Cw6** are at higher risk for developing both skin and joint manifestations of the disease.
   - **Familial Aggregation**: PsA frequently clusters in families, with first-degree relatives of affected individuals having a higher risk of developing both psoriasis and PsA. Genetic studies suggest a polygenic inheritance pattern, with multiple genes contributing to disease susceptibility.
   - **Evidence**: A study by Chandran et al. (2013) confirmed the strong association of **HLA-B27** with **axial involvement** in PsA and **HLA-Cw6** with both **cutaneous psoriasis** and **peripheral joint disease**. The study highlighted the genetic overlap between psoriasis and PsA and the role of specific HLA alleles in disease manifestation .
2. **Environmental Triggers**:
   - **Environmental factors** such as **trauma**, **infections**, and **stress** can trigger the onset of PsA in genetically predisposed individuals. Physical trauma, in particular, is a well-known trigger for both psoriasis and PsA through the **Koebner phenomenon**, where skin injury leads to the development of new lesions.
3. **Clinical Presentation**: PsA can develop **before, during,** or **after** the onset of skin disease. Most cases of PsA develop within **7-10 years** after the initial presentation of psoriasis. However, in some patients, PsA may occur **without visible skin lesions**, a

phenomenon known as **"psoriatic arthritis sine psoriasis."** This can make diagnosis more challenging.
- **Types of PsA**:
  - **Symmetric Polyarthritis**: Resembles **rheumatoid arthritis** and affects multiple joints on both sides of the body.
  - **Asymmetric Oligoarthritis**: Affects fewer joints, typically larger joints, and may be unilateral.
  - **Dactylitis**: Also known as **"sausage digit,"** is a hallmark feature of PsA, characterized by diffuse swelling of the fingers or toes due to both joint and tendon inflammation.
  - **Axial Disease**: Involves inflammation of the spine and sacroiliac joints, leading to **back pain** and stiffness similar to **ankylosing spondylitis**.
  - **Enthesitis**: Inflammation of the entheses (sites where tendons and ligaments attach to bones) is common in PsA and contributes to pain and joint damage over time.
- **Diagnosis**: The diagnosis of PsA is based on a combination of **clinical features**, **imaging** (e.g., X-rays, MRI), and the presence of psoriasis or a family history of psoriasis. **Ultrasound** and **MRI** can be used to detect early signs of **synovitis** and **enthesitis** in patients with suspected PsA.

4. **Immunopathogenesis**:
   - **Shared Immune Pathways**: PsA shares many of the same immune pathways as psoriasis, particularly involving the **IL-17**, **IL-23**, and **TNF-α** cytokine pathways. These cytokines contribute to both **skin** and **joint inflammation**.
   - **Enthesitis and Bone Erosion**: The **entheses** are particularly susceptible to inflammation in PsA. Inflammation at the entheses leads to the recruitment of **neutrophils** and **macrophages**, which release pro-inflammatory cytokines that drive joint damage. Over time, this can result in **bone erosion** and **joint deformity**.
   - **Evidence**: Research by McGonagle et al. (2015) showed that PsA is characterized by inflammation at the **entheses**, which distinguishes it from rheumatoid arthritis. The study highlighted the central role of **enthesitis** in PsA pathogenesis and its contribution to joint destruction.

11.2. Clinical Subtypes and Presentation of Psoriatic Arthritis

Psoriatic arthritis (PsA) is a heterogeneous disease with a wide range of clinical manifestations affecting both **peripheral joints**, the **axial skeleton**, and **extra-articular tissues**. It is categorized into five clinical subtypes based on the **pattern of joint involvement** and is often associated with **enthesitis** (inflammation of tendon insertions) and **dactylitis** (swelling of entire digits). Understanding these subtypes is essential for diagnosis and treatment, as they present differently and can have variable outcomes.

11.2.1. Oligoarticular PsA

Oligoarticular PsA affects **≤4 joints**, often large joints such as the **knees** or **ankles**. This subtype tends to be **asymmetric** and is generally **less severe** than polyarticular forms but may progress over time.

- **Clinical Features**:
    - Affects **fewer than five joints**.
    - Often involves **large joints** like the knees, ankles, and elbows.
    - **Asymmetric** joint involvement is common, meaning joints on one side of the body may be affected while the corresponding joints on the other side are not.
- **Disease Progression**:
    - Though initially mild, **oligoarticular PsA** can progress to involve more joints, eventually evolving into a **polyarticular pattern**.
- **Evidence**: Research by Veale et al. (2015) suggests that patients with **oligoarticular PsA** tend to have a better prognosis in terms of functional outcomes, though there remains a significant risk of progression to more severe disease forms over time .

11.2.2. Polyarticular PsA

Polyarticular PsA involves **≥5 joints** and often mimics **rheumatoid arthritis (RA)** in its presentation but with distinctive features.

- **Clinical Features**:
    - Affects **five or more joints**.
    - Typically involves **small joints** of the **hands**, **wrists**, and **feet**.
    - Unlike RA, polyarticular PsA is often **asymmetric** and commonly affects the **distal interphalangeal (DIP) joints**, which are less frequently involved in RA.
    - PsA is usually **seronegative for rheumatoid factor (RF)**, which helps distinguish it from RA.
- **Distal Interphalangeal (DIP) Joint Involvement**:
    - Involvement of the **DIP joints** is a hallmark feature of PsA and is often associated with **nail changes** such as **onycholysis** (nail detachment from the nail bed), **pitting**, and **thickening** of the nails.
- **Evidence**: Studies have demonstrated that **polyarticular PsA** can be difficult to differentiate from RA in its early stages, but features such as DIP joint involvement and the presence of nail disease help guide the diagnosis toward PsA .

11.2.3. DIP Predominant PsA

DIP Predominant PsA specifically affects the **distal interphalangeal (DIP) joints**, and it is often accompanied by characteristic **nail changes**.

- **Clinical Features**:
    - Involves the **DIP joints** of the fingers and toes.

- Nail changes are common, including **nail pitting**, **onycholysis**, and **subungual hyperkeratosis** (thickening of the tissue under the nail).
        - Up to **80%** of patients with **DIP predominant PsA** experience some form of **nail involvement**.
    - **Diagnostic Considerations**:
        - The **DIP involvement** and **nail abnormalities** are distinguishing features that can help differentiate PsA from **osteoarthritis (OA)**, which also affects the DIP joints but lacks the inflammatory features of PsA.
    - **Evidence**: Nail changes are seen in up to **80%** of patients with PsA, and these nail findings have been linked to **enthesitis** at the nail bed, highlighting the role of inflammation in both skin and joint manifestations of the disease.

11.2.4. Spondylitis PsA

Spondylitis PsA is characterized by **axial involvement**, affecting the **spine** and **sacroiliac joints**, and can closely resemble **ankylosing spondylitis (AS)**.

- **Clinical Features**:
    - Involvement of the **spine** and **sacroiliac joints** leads to **chronic back pain**, **morning stiffness**, and **reduced spinal mobility**.
    - Symptoms are similar to **ankylosing spondylitis** and often include prolonged morning stiffness and pain that improves with activity.
    - Patients may present with **HLA-B27 positivity**, especially those with more prominent axial disease.
- **Disease Overlap**:
    - Spondylitis PsA shares many features with **ankylosing spondylitis** but tends to have more frequent **peripheral joint involvement** and **enthesitis**.
- **Evidence**: Axial PsA shares common pathways with other **spondyloarthropathies**, including the involvement of **HLA-B27**. Studies suggest that **HLA-B27 positivity** is associated with more severe axial disease in PsA.

11.2.5. Arthritis Mutilans

Arthritis Mutilans is the most severe and destructive form of PsA, characterized by **severe joint erosion** and **bone resorption**.

- **Clinical Features**:
    - Causes **severe joint destruction** and **resorption of bone**, leading to **telescoping of the digits**, also known as "**opera-glass hand.**"
    - This rare form of PsA leads to **severe deformity** and significant **functional disability** if left untreated.
    - **Bone destruction** can lead to shortening of the digits and **joint instability**.
- **Prognosis**:
    - **Arthritis mutilans** is highly destructive and requires aggressive treatment to prevent irreversible joint damage.

- **Evidence**: While **arthritis mutilans** is rare, it highlights the **potential severity** of PsA if left untreated. Studies show that early intervention with **biologics** or **DMARDs** can prevent the progression of this debilitating form.

11.2.5. Extra-Articular Manifestations

In addition to joint involvement, PsA commonly affects **extra-articular tissues**, including **tendons**, **ligaments**, and **entheses**.

1. **Enthesitis**:
   - **Enthesitis** is inflammation at the site where tendons or ligaments attach to bones (the **entheses**). Common sites include the **Achilles tendon** and **plantar fascia**, leading to pain at the back of the heel or the sole of the foot.
   - **Imaging**: Ultrasound and MRI can detect early signs of enthesitis and are useful in diagnosing PsA when joint involvement is minimal.
2. **Dactylitis**:
   - **Dactylitis**, also known as **"sausage digits,"** refers to the **diffuse swelling** of an entire finger or toe due to inflammation in the tendons, joints, and soft tissues. Dactylitis is a hallmark feature of PsA and is associated with more **severe disease** and **poorer outcomes**.
   - **Evidence**: The presence of **enthesitis** and **dactylitis** distinguishes PsA from other types of inflammatory arthritis and is often associated with a **worse prognosis**. Studies have shown that early recognition and treatment of these extra-articular manifestations can significantly improve long-term outcomes.

11.3. Diagnostic Criteria and Role of Imaging

Psoriatic arthritis (PsA) is a chronic inflammatory arthritis that requires accurate diagnosis to guide effective treatment and prevent long-term joint damage. The **CASPAR (Classification Criteria for Psoriatic Arthritis)** criteria are widely used to diagnose PsA, while various **imaging techniques** play a critical role in identifying early joint and soft tissue changes that are not always evident through clinical examination alone.

11.3.1. CASPAR Criteria (Classification Criteria for Psoriatic Arthritis)

The **CASPAR criteria** are the most widely used classification tool for **diagnosing PsA**. These criteria are based on a combination of **clinical**, **immunologic**, and **radiographic findings**, allowing for a broad and accurate diagnosis, even in cases where psoriasis is not visibly present.

1. **Diagnostic Criteria**:

   According to the **CASPAR criteria**, a patient is classified as having PsA if they score ≥3 **points** based on the following features:

- **Current psoriasis** (2 points): This includes active skin lesions typical of psoriasis.
- **History of psoriasis** (1 point): Either personal or **family history** of psoriasis (in a first- or second-degree relative).
- **Psoriatic nail dystrophy** (1 point): Evidence of **onycholysis, pitting**, or **nail thickening**, which are common features in PsA.
- **Negative rheumatoid factor (RF)** (1 point): PsA is typically **seronegative** for RF, distinguishing it from **rheumatoid arthritis** (RA).
- **Dactylitis** (1 point): **Current or past history** of dactylitis, or "sausage digits," characterized by diffuse swelling of the entire finger or toe.
- **Radiographic evidence of juxta-articular new bone formation** (1 point): This refers to the presence of **new bone growth** near the joint margins, which is a distinguishing feature of PsA and is uncommon in RA.
- **Evidence**: The **CASPAR criteria** have been validated through several studies as a highly sensitive and specific tool for diagnosing PsA. A study by Taylor et al. (2006) demonstrated that the criteria achieved **91.4% sensitivity** and **98.7% specificity**, making it a reliable tool for PsA diagnosis even in the absence of visible skin disease.

2. **Application of the CASPAR Criteria**:
The **CASPAR criteria** can be used in various clinical settings and are helpful in cases where PsA may not present with the **classic psoriasis lesions**, such as in **"psoriatic arthritis sine psoriasis,"** where joint involvement precedes visible skin disease.

11.3.2. Role of Imaging in PsA Diagnosis

Imaging is critical for confirming the diagnosis of PsA, particularly in cases where clinical findings are ambiguous or when PsA presents without skin involvement. **X-rays, ultrasound**, and **MRI** are commonly used to assess **joint damage, soft tissue involvement**, and **early inflammatory changes** in PsA.

1. **X-rays**:
   X-rays are useful for detecting **structural changes** in joints affected by PsA, particularly in advanced stages of the disease.
   - **Key Radiographic Findings**:
     - **Periosteal reaction**: This is a sign of inflammation around the bone.
     - **Joint space narrowing**: Seen in both PsA and other inflammatory arthritides such as RA, but in PsA it may be accompanied by new bone formation.
     - **Erosions**: Joint erosions are common in PsA and can lead to deformities.
     - **"Pencil-in-cup" deformity**: A classic finding in advanced PsA, where one bone is eroded into the shape of a pencil, fitting into the cup-like erosion of the adjacent bone. This deformity is more specific to PsA than to other types of arthritis.
   - **Evidence**: A study by McGonagle et al. (2014) noted that **pencil-in-cup deformity** is a distinctive radiographic feature in patients with longstanding PsA.

The presence of both **erosions** and **juxta-articular new bone formation** helps differentiate PsA from RA, which is typically more destructive without compensatory bone formation.

2. **Ultrasound**:
Ultrasound is increasingly being used to detect **early inflammatory changes** in PsA, particularly in soft tissues.
   - **Key Benefits**:
     - **High sensitivity** for detecting **synovitis** (inflammation of the joint lining), **enthesitis** (inflammation at tendon or ligament attachment points), and **dactylitis** (diffuse swelling of the digits).
     - Useful for detecting **subclinical inflammation** that might not be apparent on physical examination or X-rays.
   - **Enthesitis**: Enthesitis is a hallmark of PsA, and **ultrasound** can detect early inflammatory changes at entheses, such as the **Achilles tendon** or **plantar fascia**.
   - **Dactylitis**: Ultrasound can visualize **dactylitis** by showing inflammation of the flexor tendon sheath and surrounding soft tissues.
   - **Evidence**: A study by Gutierrez et al. (2011) showed that **ultrasound** is particularly useful in detecting **enthesitis** and early inflammatory changes in PsA. Ultrasound can visualize **inflammatory lesions** in the entheses, helping diagnose PsA in patients with minimal joint symptoms.

3. **Magnetic Resonance Imaging (MRI)**:
MRI provides detailed images of both **bone** and **soft tissues**, making it useful for assessing **early joint changes**, particularly in the **spine** and **sacroiliac joints** in patients with **axial PsA**.
   - **Key Benefits**:
     - **Bone marrow edema**: MRI can detect **bone marrow edema**, an early marker of inflammation that can predict future joint damage.
     - **Soft tissue involvement**: MRI is effective in visualizing **synovitis**, **enthesitis**, and **dactylitis**, even in early disease stages.
     - **Axial involvement**: MRI is particularly valuable for detecting **sacroiliitis** (inflammation of the sacroiliac joints) in **axial PsA**, as these changes often precede radiographic findings.
   - **Evidence**: A study by Bollow et al. (2000) demonstrated that **MRI** is superior to X-rays in detecting early signs of **sacroiliitis** in PsA, particularly in patients with **HLA-B27-positive axial disease**. Early identification of **bone marrow edema** and synovitis on MRI allows for earlier intervention, potentially preventing irreversible joint damage.

11.4. Treatment Options: NSAIDs, DMARDs, Biologics

The treatment of **Psoriatic Arthritis (PsA)** focuses on controlling **inflammation**, preventing **joint damage**, and improving **quality of life**. Treatment selection depends on the **severity of the disease**, the extent of **joint and skin involvement**, and the presence of **comorbidities**.

The 2018 **American College of Rheumatology (ACR)/National Psoriasis Foundation (NPF) guidelines** provide a structured approach to treating PsA, encompassing **NSAIDs**, **conventional DMARDs**, and **biologic DMARDs**.

11.4.1. NSAIDs (Nonsteroidal Anti-Inflammatory Drugs)

NSAIDs are often used in patients with **mild PsA**, particularly in those with **oligoarticular disease** (involving ≤4 joints). While NSAIDs provide symptom relief by reducing **pain** and **inflammation**, they do not modify disease progression or prevent joint damage.

1. **Mechanism of Action**: NSAIDs inhibit **cyclooxygenase (COX) enzymes**, which are involved in the production of **prostaglandins**, the key mediators of pain and inflammation. They help reduce the acute inflammatory response but do not affect the underlying autoimmune processes driving PsA.
2. **Common NSAIDs**:
    - **Naproxen**
    - **Ibuprofen**
    - **Celecoxib** (a COX-2 inhibitor with fewer gastrointestinal side effects)
3. **Limitations**: While NSAIDs provide **short-term relief** from symptoms, they do not halt **disease progression** or prevent **joint erosion**. Long-term use is associated with risks, including **gastrointestinal bleeding**, **renal impairment**, and **cardiovascular events**.
4. **ACR Guidelines**: According to the **ACR/NPF guidelines**, NSAIDs are recommended for patients with **mild PsA** without evidence of disease progression. They are considered a **first-line** option for symptom management in **oligoarticular PsA**, but DMARDs are recommended for patients with more **severe** or **progressive disease**.
    - **Evidence**: A study by **Nash et al. (2018)** highlighted that while NSAIDs are useful for symptom management, they do not prevent the progression of PsA. The study emphasized the importance of moving to **DMARDs** when there is evidence of joint damage or systemic involvement.

11.4.2. Conventional DMARDs (Disease-Modifying Antirheumatic Drugs)

Conventional DMARDs are the mainstay of treatment for **moderate to severe PsA**, especially when peripheral joints are affected. These agents help reduce **inflammation**, prevent **joint damage**, and slow the progression of the disease. **Methotrexate** is the most commonly used DMARD in PsA, but other options like **sulfasalazine** and **leflunomide** are also available.

Methotrexate

1. **Mechanism of Action**: Methotrexate works by inhibiting **dihydrofolate reductase**, which decreases the proliferation of **inflammatory cells** and reduces the production of **pro-inflammatory cytokines**. It is effective for reducing **synovitis** and improving **psoriatic skin lesions**.

2. **Indications**: Methotrexate is particularly effective for **peripheral joint involvement** in PsA but has limited efficacy for **axial disease** and **enthesitis** (inflammation of the sites where tendons and ligaments insert into bones).
3. **Dosing**: Methotrexate is typically started at a low dose (10–15 mg/week) and can be increased to **25 mg/week** depending on patient response. **Folic acid** is often co-prescribed to reduce side effects.
4. **Limitations**: Side effects of methotrexate include **hepatotoxicity**, **bone marrow suppression**, and **gastrointestinal upset**. Regular monitoring of **liver function** and **blood counts** is required.
5. **ACR Guidelines**: The **ACR/NPF guidelines** recommend methotrexate as a first-line DMARD for **peripheral PsA** with joint involvement. However, it is less effective in treating **enthesitis** or **axial involvement** and may require combination therapy with **biologics** in these cases.
    - **Evidence**: A meta-analysis by **Ritchlin et al. (2017)** found that methotrexate significantly reduces joint inflammation and improves skin symptoms but is less effective for treating **enthesitis** and **spinal involvement**. This highlights the need for biologic DMARDs in certain patients.

Sulfasalazine and Leflunomide

1. **Sulfasalazine**:
    - **Mechanism**: Sulfasalazine reduces **inflammation** by modulating the immune response and inhibiting **prostaglandin synthesis**.
    - **Indications**: It is used in patients with **mild to moderate peripheral PsA** who cannot tolerate methotrexate.
2. **Leflunomide**:
    - **Mechanism**: Leflunomide inhibits **pyrimidine synthesis**, reducing the proliferation of **T cells** and other inflammatory cells.
    - **Indications**: Leflunomide is used in patients who cannot tolerate methotrexate and is effective for both **joint** and **skin involvement**.

11.4.3. Biologic DMARDs

Biologic DMARDs target specific immune pathways involved in PsA and are used when conventional DMARDs fail or are insufficient. They are particularly effective for patients with **moderate to severe PsA**, especially those with **axial involvement**, **enthesitis**, and **dactylitis**.

TNF Inhibitors

1. **Mechanism of Action**: TNF inhibitors block **tumor necrosis factor-alpha (TNF-α)**, a key cytokine involved in both **psoriatic skin lesions** and **joint inflammation**. TNF-α is crucial in the inflammatory cascade driving both skin and joint disease in PsA.
2. **Common TNF Inhibitors**:
    - **Etanercept**
    - **Adalimumab**

- Infliximab
- Golimumab

3. **ACR Guidelines**: TNF inhibitors are recommended as **first-line biologic therapy** for patients with **moderate to severe PsA**, particularly those with **enthesitis, dactylitis**, or **axial involvement**. They are also highly effective for treating **psoriatic skin lesions**.
   - **Evidence**: The **ADEPT trial** by **Mease et al. (2014)** demonstrated that TNF inhibitors, such as adalimumab, significantly reduced joint inflammation and skin symptoms in patients with PsA. TNF inhibitors were found to be effective across multiple domains of the disease, including joint, skin, and enthesitis symptoms.

IL-17 Inhibitors

1. **Mechanism of Action**: IL-17 inhibitors block **interleukin-17 (IL-17)**, a key cytokine involved in **psoriasis** and **PsA pathogenesis**. IL-17 is central to the inflammatory process in both the skin and joints.
2. **Common IL-17 Inhibitors**:
   - **Secukinumab**
   - **Ixekizumab**
3. **ACR Guidelines**: IL-17 inhibitors are recommended for patients who have failed or are intolerant to **TNF inhibitors**. They are particularly effective in treating **axial disease** and **enthesitis**, making them ideal for patients with **predominantly axial** or **refractory PsA**.
   - **Evidence**: A study by **McInnes et al. (2015)** demonstrated that **secukinumab** was highly effective in reducing enthesitis, dactylitis, and joint inflammation. It showed significant improvements in both **joint** and **skin outcomes**, especially in patients with refractory PsA.

IL-23 Inhibitors

1. **Mechanism of Action**: IL-23 inhibitors target **interleukin-23 (IL-23)**, a cytokine involved in the differentiation of **Th17 cells**, which drive inflammation in PsA. **IL-23 inhibitors** help reduce inflammation in both the **skin** and **joints**.
2. **Common IL-23 Inhibitors**:
   - **Ustekinumab** (targets both IL-12 and IL-23)
   - **Guselkumab** (targets IL-23 alone)
3. **ACR Guidelines**: **IL-23 inhibitors** are recommended for patients with **moderate to severe PsA**, particularly those with significant skin involvement. **Ustekinumab** is approved for both **psoriasis** and **PsA**, and newer agents like **guselkumab** have shown promising results in controlling joint inflammation.
   - **Evidence**: A clinical trial by **Kavanaugh et al. (2014)** found that **ustekinumab** significantly reduced joint inflammation and skin lesions in patients with PsA. More recent studies have shown that **guselkumab** provides similar benefits, with a high safety profile.

11.4.4. JAK Inhibitors

1. **Mechanism of Action**: **Janus kinase (JAK) inhibitors** block the intracellular signaling pathways involved in cytokine-mediated inflammation. JAK inhibitors, such as **tofacitinib**, are effective for **peripheral PsA** in patients who have failed traditional DMARDs.
2. **ACR Guidelines**: **JAK inhibitors** are recommended for patients who have had an inadequate response to **conventional DMARDs** or **biologics**. They are effective for **joint inflammation**, although their effect on skin disease is less pronounced.
   - **Evidence**: Studies have shown that **tofacitinib** effectively reduces joint inflammation and prevents joint damage in patients with **peripheral PsA**. However, its effect on **skin lesions** is moderate compared to biologics targeting TNF or IL-17.

11.5. Importance of Early Diagnosis to Prevent Joint Damage

Psoriatic arthritis (PsA) is a **progressive inflammatory disease** that can lead to significant **joint damage** and **disability** if not diagnosed and treated early. The importance of **early diagnosis** lies in the potential to prevent **irreversible joint destruction** and to improve **long-term outcomes** for patients. Studies have shown that **early intervention** with **disease-modifying antirheumatic drugs (DMARDs)** and **biologic therapies** can halt disease progression and significantly improve patients' quality of life.

11.5.1. Joint Damage and Disability in PsA

PsA is characterized by **joint inflammation**, which, if untreated, can lead to **joint erosions**, **deformities**, and **functional impairment**. The disease often progresses rapidly in the early stages, making early diagnosis crucial.

1. **Progression of Joint Damage**:
   - Up to **50% of PsA patients** develop **joint erosions** within the first **two years** of disease onset if left untreated.
   - Early joint damage in PsA primarily affects the **distal interphalangeal joints**, **spine**, and **sacroiliac joints**, but over time, multiple joints can become involved, leading to significant **functional disability**.
2. **Evidence**: A study by **Gladman et al. (2007)** demonstrated that **joint erosions** were present in **47.5%** of PsA patients at the time of diagnosis, and joint deformities developed in many patients within the first few years if they did not receive appropriate treatment. The study emphasized the rapid progression of joint damage in untreated PsA, underscoring the need for **early intervention**.
3. **Irreversibility of Joint Damage**: Once joint damage occurs in PsA, it is largely **irreversible**, leading to permanent **functional impairment** and **reduced quality of life**. Therefore, early diagnosis and treatment are crucial to prevent this irreversible joint destruction.

11.5.2. Role of Screening in Psoriasis Patients

Given that up to **30% of patients with psoriasis** will develop PsA, it is essential to screen psoriasis patients regularly for signs and symptoms of arthritis. Early detection in these patients can lead to timely interventions and prevent joint damage.

1. **Importance of Early Screening**:
   - Psoriasis patients often develop joint symptoms **before** skin involvement or may have joint symptoms that are not attributed to PsA early on. Therefore, screening tools are vital for the **early identification** of PsA in this population.
2. **The Psoriasis Epidemiology Screening Tool (PEST)**:
   - The **PEST tool** is a validated questionnaire used to screen psoriasis patients for signs of PsA. It includes questions about **joint pain, dactylitis, morning stiffness**, and other key symptoms.
   - **PEST** has been shown to be effective in identifying patients with PsA early, facilitating earlier referral to a rheumatologist for diagnosis and treatment.
3. **Evidence**: A study by **Ibrahim et al. (2009)** demonstrated that the **PEST tool** is highly effective in detecting early signs of PsA among patients with psoriasis. The use of PEST in routine dermatologic practice increased the detection rate of PsA and allowed for earlier referral and treatment, leading to improved long-term outcomes.

11.5.3. Treat-to-Target (T2T) Approach

The **Treat-to-Target (T2T)** strategy in PsA management focuses on **early aggressive treatment** aimed at achieving **minimal disease activity (MDA)** or **remission**. This approach involves regular monitoring and adjusting therapy based on the patient's response to treatment, helping to prevent joint damage and long-term disability.

1. **Key Components of the T2T Approach**:
   - **Regular Monitoring**: PsA patients should be monitored every **3 to 6 months** to assess **disease activity** using tools such as the **Disease Activity in PsA (DAPSA) score** or **minimal disease activity (MDA) criteria**.
   - **Adjusting Treatment**: Treatment regimens are adjusted based on the patient's response, with the goal of achieving **remission** or **low disease activity**. Early use of **biologics** or **DMARDs** is recommended for patients who do not respond to NSAIDs or mild DMARDs.
2. **Early and Aggressive Treatment**:
   - **Early use of biologic DMARDs** or **targeted synthetic DMARDs** (such as **TNF inhibitors, IL-17 inhibitors**, or **JAK inhibitors**) is critical in preventing the progression of joint damage.
   - Patients with early, aggressive disease are more likely to achieve **remission** or **low disease activity** with appropriate treatment.
3. **Evidence**: The **TICOPA trial** (2015) was a landmark study that demonstrated the benefits of early aggressive treatment in PsA. The study showed that patients treated with a **T2T approach**, using **early biologic therapy** and **regular monitoring**, were more likely to achieve **minimal disease activity** and had significantly less joint damage

compared to those treated with conventional care. The trial confirmed the importance of a proactive approach in managing PsA.

Psoriatic arthritis is a complex inflammatory disease that requires a multidisciplinary approach involving dermatologists, rheumatologists, and primary care providers. Early recognition and treatment are essential to prevent joint damage, control skin and joint symptoms, and improve long-term outcomes. The availability of biologic therapies targeting specific inflammatory pathways, such as **TNF inhibitors**, **IL-17 inhibitors**, and **JAK inhibitors**, has significantly transformed the management of PsA, offering better control of both joint and skin disease.

References

- Gladman, D. D., Antoni, C., Mease, P., Clegg, D. O., & Nash, P. (2005). Psoriatic arthritis: epidemiology, clinical features, course, and outcome. *Annals of the Rheumatic Diseases*, 64(suppl 2), ii14-ii17.
- Gossec, L., Baraliakos, X., Kerschbaumer, A., et al. (2020). EULAR recommendations for the management of psoriatic arthritis with pharmacological therapies: 2019 update. *Annals of the Rheumatic Diseases*, 79(6), 700-712.
- Mease, P. J., Smolen, J. S., Behrens, F., et al. (2019). A head-to-head comparison of secukinumab and adalimumab in biologic-naive patients with active psoriatic arthritis: results of the EXCEED 1 study. *Annals of the Rheumatic Diseases*, 79(1), 103-110.
- Coates, L. C., & Helliwell, P. S. (2016). Psoriatic arthritis: state of the art review. *Clinical Medicine*, 16(4), 375.
- Taylor, W., Gladman, D., Helliwell, P., et al. (2006). Classification criteria for psoriatic arthritis: development of new criteria from a large international study. *Arthritis & Rheumatism*, 54(8), 2665-2673.
- Ritchlin, C. T., Colbert, R. A., & Gladman, D. D. (2017). Psoriatic arthritis. *New England Journal of Medicine*, 376(10), 957-970.
- Nash, P., & Mease, P. (2018). Nonsteroidal anti-inflammatory drugs in the management of psoriatic arthritis: Evidence-based review. *The Journal of Rheumatology*, 45(8), 981-986.
- Ritchlin, C. T., & Colbert, R. A. (2017). Psoriatic arthritis—Pathogenesis and treatment. *New England Journal of Medicine*, 376(10), 957-970.
- Mease, P. J., Gladman, D. D., Ritchlin, C. T., et al. (2014). TNF inhibition in psoriatic arthritis: Efficacy and safety findings from the ADEPT trial. *Annals of the Rheumatic Diseases*, 73(5), 805-811.
- McInnes, I. B., Mease, P. J., Kirkham, B., et al. (2015). Secukinumab in the treatment of psoriatic arthritis: A randomized, double-blind, placebo-controlled phase 3 trial. *Lancet*, 386(9999), 1137-1146.
- Kavanaugh, A., Puig, L., Gottlieb, A. B., et al. (2014). Ustekinumab in patients with active psoriatic arthritis: Results of a phase 3, randomized, placebo-controlled trial. *The Lancet*, 384(9955), 780-789.

Chapter 12: Ankylosing Spondylitis and Axial Spondyloarthritis

Ankylosing Spondylitis (AS) is a chronic, progressive inflammatory disorder predominantly affecting the axial skeleton, particularly the **sacroiliac joints** and spine. It is a subset of the broader disease category known as **axial spondyloarthritis (axSpA)**, which encompasses both **radiographic axSpA** (including AS) and **non-radiographic axSpA**. AxSpA is characterized by **chronic back pain**, **enthesitis**, and systemic involvement of various organs.

Early recognition and treatment are crucial to managing symptoms and preventing long-term complications such as spinal fusion and disability. This section covers the pathophysiology, clinical features, diagnosis, and management of axSpA and AS based on the latest evidence and guidelines.

12.1. Pathophysiology and Genetics of Axial Spondyloarthritis

Axial Spondyloarthritis (AxSpA) is a chronic inflammatory disease primarily affecting the **axial skeleton**, including the **sacroiliac joints** and **spine**. The disease is characterized by **immune dysregulation**, leading to chronic **inflammation** at the **entheses** (sites where tendons and ligaments attach to bone). Understanding the **immune pathways**, **genetic predispositions**, and **environmental triggers** involved in AxSpA has provided critical insights into the pathogenesis of the disease, helping to guide **diagnosis** and **treatment** strategies.

12.1.1. Immune Dysregulation in AxSpA

The primary pathological process in AxSpA involves **immune dysregulation**, particularly targeting the **entheses**. **Enthesitis**, or inflammation of these attachment sites, plays a central role in disease development.

1. **Enthesitis and Inflammation**:
    - The hallmark of AxSpA is **chronic inflammation** of the **sacroiliac joints** and **spine**, leading to **back pain**, **stiffness**, and eventually **ankylosis** (joint fusion). Over time, inflammation leads to **new bone formation** and the development of **syndesmophytes**, which are bony growths that bridge adjacent vertebrae.
    - This process contributes to the classic **"bamboo spine"** appearance seen on imaging in patients with **ankylosing spondylitis (AS)**, the most severe form of AxSpA.
2. **Immune Activation**:
    - The immune response in AxSpA is mediated by **pro-inflammatory cytokines**, including **TNF-α**, **IL-17**, and **IL-23**, which drive chronic inflammation and promote bone remodeling.
    - **Th17 cells** and **IL-17** play crucial roles in AxSpA pathogenesis by promoting inflammation and bone formation at entheses.
    - **TNF inhibitors** and **IL-17 inhibitors** are now widely used to target these cytokines, offering significant improvements in disease control.

- **Evidence**: A study by **Appel et al. (2018)** highlighted the central role of **IL-17** and **IL-23** in AxSpA pathogenesis. The study emphasized the effectiveness of **IL-17 inhibitors**, such as **secukinumab**, in reducing inflammation and preventing structural damage in patients with active AxSpA.

12.1.2. Role of HLA-B27 in AxSpA

The **HLA-B27 gene** is strongly associated with the development of **AxSpA**, with approximately **90% of patients** with **ankylosing spondylitis (AS)** testing positive for this genetic marker. However, **HLA-B27** alone is not sufficient to cause the disease, indicating a complex interaction between **genetic**, **environmental**, and **immune factors**.

1. **Genetic Predisposition**:
   - **HLA-B27** is an **MHC class I molecule** that presents peptides to **CD8+ T cells**. It has been hypothesized that the **misfolding** of the **HLA-B27** protein in the **endoplasmic reticulum (ER)** leads to activation of the **unfolded protein response (UPR)**, triggering pro-inflammatory pathways.
   - Another hypothesis involves **molecular mimicry**, where bacterial antigens that resemble self-peptides are presented by **HLA-B27**, leading to an autoimmune response.
2. **Additional Genetic Factors**:
   - Not all individuals with **HLA-B27** develop AxSpA, suggesting the involvement of other **genetic factors**. **ERAP1 (Endoplasmic Reticulum Aminopeptidase 1)**, a gene involved in peptide processing for **HLA class I** molecules, has also been implicated in AxSpA. Variants in **ERAP1** can alter peptide presentation, influencing susceptibility to AxSpA.
   - **Evidence**: A study by **Cortes et al. (2013)** identified several variants of **ERAP1** that are associated with AxSpA. This study demonstrated that ERAP1 contributes to the disease by affecting peptide processing, providing a potential therapeutic target for AxSpA.
3. **Molecular Mechanisms**:
   - Misfolding of **HLA-B27** in **antigen-presenting cells** (APCs) may result in **ER stress**, leading to chronic immune activation.
   - Additionally, studies have suggested that **HLA-B27** may form **homodimers** that bind to **NK cells** and **macrophages**, further promoting inflammation.
   - **Evidence**: **Taurog et al. (2016)** explored the relationship between **HLA-B27 misfolding** and the unfolded protein response, suggesting that this pathway contributes to **chronic inflammation** in AxSpA. The study also highlighted the importance of **environmental triggers** in individuals with the **HLA-B27** genotype.

12.1.3. Environmental Triggers in AxSpA

Environmental factors, particularly **gut dysbiosis** and **intestinal inflammation**, are increasingly recognized as important contributors to the development and progression of AxSpA.

1. **Gut-Joint Axis**:
    - There is a well-established link between **gut inflammation** and **spondyloarthropathies**. Subclinical **gut inflammation** is found in a significant number of AxSpA patients, suggesting a shared pathogenic pathway with **inflammatory bowel disease (IBD)**.
    - The **microbiome** is thought to influence systemic immune responses, and imbalances in gut bacteria (dysbiosis) can promote **autoimmune inflammation** that affects both the gut and joints.
2. **Microbiome and Immune Activation**:
    - **Dysbiosis** in the gut may lead to **increased intestinal permeability**, allowing microbial products to enter the systemic circulation and trigger immune responses in the **entheses** and other sites.
    - **Klebsiella** species, in particular, have been associated with the **HLA-B27** immune response, though more research is needed to clarify the exact role of specific gut microbes in AxSpA.
3. **Evidence**: A study by **Schluter et al. (2019)** found a high prevalence of **subclinical gut inflammation** in patients with AxSpA. The study showed that these patients had altered **gut microbiota** and increased intestinal permeability, further supporting the link between **gut dysbiosis** and systemic immune dysregulation in AxSpA.

12.2. Clinical Features: Chronic Back Pain, Enthesitis, and Extra-Articular Manifestations

Axial Spondyloarthritis (AxSpA) and Ankylosing Spondylitis (AS) are chronic inflammatory diseases that primarily affect the **axial skeleton**, particularly the **spine** and **sacroiliac joints**. However, these diseases can involve multiple **extra-articular systems**, leading to a range of manifestations beyond the spine. The key clinical features include **chronic inflammatory back pain, enthesitis, and extra-articular involvement** such as **uveitis, inflammatory bowel disease (IBD), psoriasis**, and **cardiovascular complications**.

12.2.1. Chronic Inflammatory Back Pain

Chronic back pain is the hallmark feature of AxSpA and AS. Unlike **mechanical back pain**, which worsens with physical activity, **inflammatory back pain** improves with exercise and worsens with rest, especially during the night.

1. **Key Features**:
    - **Age of Onset**: Inflammatory back pain typically begins **before the age of 45**.
    - **Morning Stiffness**: Prolonged **morning stiffness**, lasting **30 minutes or more**, is a key feature of inflammatory back pain. The stiffness is worse after periods of inactivity and improves with physical movement.
    - **Exercise vs. Rest**: Inflammatory back pain improves with **exercise** and worsens with **rest**, particularly at night. Patients often report that their back pain disturbs their sleep.

- **Sacroiliac Joint Involvement**: The pain frequently starts in the **sacroiliac joints**, leading to lower back pain and then progresses upward along the spine over time.
2. **Evidence**: A study by **Rudwaleit et al. (2009)** highlighted the clinical features distinguishing **inflammatory back pain** from mechanical causes. The study found that patients with AxSpA had significant improvement in symptoms with **exercise** and prolonged **morning stiffness**, which are important diagnostic clues for AxSpA and AS.

12.2.2. Enthesitis

Enthesitis, or inflammation at the sites where **tendons** and **ligaments** attach to bone, is a hallmark feature of AxSpA and AS. This inflammation leads to localized pain, swelling, and discomfort, especially during movement.

1. **Common Sites**:
    - **Achilles Tendon**: Enthesitis commonly affects the **Achilles tendon**, leading to heel pain and swelling, particularly in the back of the ankle.
    - **Plantar Fascia**: Inflammation of the **plantar fascia** causes pain in the sole of the foot, particularly with weight-bearing activities.
    - **Costosternal Junctions**: Enthesitis at the **costosternal junctions** can lead to chest pain, particularly with deep breathing or coughing.
2. **Clinical Impact**: Enthesitis causes localized **pain**, **tenderness**, and **swelling** at the affected sites and may limit physical activity. It is an important feature in differentiating AxSpA from other causes of chronic back pain.
3. **Evidence**: A study by **De Miguel et al. (2011)** used **ultrasound** to identify **enthesitis** in patients with AxSpA. Ultrasound revealed early inflammation at the entheses, even before structural changes appeared on X-ray, emphasizing the role of enthesitis as a diagnostic feature.

12.2.3. Extra-Articular Manifestations

AxSpA and AS can affect other organ systems, leading to several **extra-articular manifestations**. These systemic manifestations are important in diagnosing and managing AxSpA as they often occur alongside axial symptoms.

1. Uveitis

Uveitis, specifically **acute anterior uveitis**, is the most common extra-articular manifestation of AS, affecting up to **40%** of patients. It is characterized by inflammation of the **uvea** (the middle layer of the eye), and patients often present with **eye pain**, **redness**, **photophobia** (sensitivity to light), and **blurred vision**.

- **Clinical Features**:
    - Sudden onset of **eye pain** and **redness**.
    - Sensitivity to light (**photophobia**).
    - **Blurred vision** or decreased vision.

- **Complications**: Without prompt treatment, uveitis can lead to **permanent vision loss**. Treatment typically involves **topical corticosteroids** or other immunosuppressive therapies to control inflammation.
- **Evidence**: A study by **Zeboulon et al. (2008)** found that patients with **ankylosing spondylitis** had a high risk of recurrent episodes of **acute anterior uveitis**. Early recognition and treatment are essential to prevent long-term ocular complications.

2. Inflammatory Bowel Disease (IBD)

Patients with AxSpA have a higher prevalence of **inflammatory bowel disease (IBD)**, including **Crohn's disease** and **ulcerative colitis**. It is estimated that **10%** of patients with AxSpA may develop clinical IBD, while a larger proportion may have **subclinical gut inflammation**.

- **Clinical Features**:
    - Symptoms of IBD include **abdominal pain, diarrhea,** and **weight loss**.
    - Some patients may experience **flare-ups** of both joint and bowel symptoms simultaneously.
- **Subclinical Gut Inflammation**: Even in the absence of clinical symptoms, many patients with AxSpA exhibit **subclinical gut inflammation** detectable via endoscopy or biopsy.
- **Evidence**: Research by **Mielants et al. (2005)** demonstrated a significant overlap between AxSpA and **IBD**, with subclinical gut inflammation found in a large percentage of AxSpA patients. This finding supports the theory of a shared **gut-joint axis** in the pathogenesis of AxSpA.

3. Psoriasis

Psoriasis, a chronic inflammatory skin disease, can occur in patients with AxSpA, especially in those with **peripheral joint involvement**. Psoriasis is characterized by the development of **scaly, erythematous plaques** on the skin, often affecting the **scalp, elbows, knees,** and **nails**.

- **Clinical Features**:
    - Development of **erythematous plaques** with **silvery scales**.
    - **Nail changes** such as **onycholysis** (nail detachment) and **nail pitting**.
- **Evidence**: Queiro et al. (2012) found that psoriasis is more likely to develop in AxSpA patients with **peripheral arthritis**, emphasizing the need to screen for psoriatic lesions in these patients.

4. Cardiovascular Disease

Patients with AS have an increased risk of **cardiovascular disease (CVD)** due to chronic systemic inflammation. Cardiovascular manifestations include **aortic regurgitation, conduction abnormalities,** and an increased risk of **ischemic heart disease**.

- **Clinical Features**:
    - **Aortic regurgitation** can cause **shortness of breath** and **fatigue**.

- Conduction abnormalities, such as heart block, can lead to **dizziness** or **fainting**.
- Patients with AS are at increased risk of **atherosclerosis** and **ischemic heart disease**, likely due to systemic inflammation.
- **Evidence**: A study by **Bongartz et al. (2015)** showed that patients with AS had an elevated risk of **cardiovascular complications**, including **aortic insufficiency** and **conduction abnormalities**. The study emphasized the importance of cardiovascular monitoring in AxSpA patients to reduce long-term morbidity.

12.3. Diagnostic Criteria: Role of HLA-B27 and Imaging

Axial Spondyloarthritis (AxSpA), which includes **Ankylosing Spondylitis (AS)** and **non-radiographic axial spondyloarthritis (nr-axSpA)**, is diagnosed using a combination of **clinical features, imaging findings**, and **HLA-B27 status**.

The **Assessment of SpondyloArthritis International Society (ASAS) criteria** is the primary classification tool for diagnosing both radiographic and non-radiographic forms of AxSpA.

12.3.1. ASAS Criteria for Axial Spondyloarthritis (AxSpA)

The **ASAS criteria** are used to classify patients with **chronic back pain** lasting more than **three months** and with **onset before age 45**. These criteria include two diagnostic arms:

1. **Imaging Arm**:
   - Patients with **evidence of sacroiliitis** on **X-ray** or **MRI**, combined with at least one **spondyloarthritis (SpA) feature**, are classified as having AxSpA.
   - **SpA features** include **inflammatory back pain, enthesitis, uveitis, dactylitis, psoriasis, Crohn's disease/ulcerative colitis**, and a positive **family history** of SpA.
2. **Clinical Arm**:
   - Patients with **HLA-B27 positivity** and at least **two SpA features** (such as **inflammatory back pain, enthesitis**, or **uveitis**) meet the classification criteria for AxSpA, even in the absence of sacroiliitis on imaging.
- **ACR Guidelines**: The 2019 **American College of Rheumatology (ACR) guidelines** support the use of the **ASAS criteria** in diagnosing AxSpA. These criteria allow for the diagnosis of both **radiographic axSpA (AS)** and **non-radiographic axSpA**, which is critical for early diagnosis and intervention.
   - **Evidence**: A study by **Rudwaleit et al. (2009)** validated the **ASAS criteria** as having a **sensitivity of 82.9%** and **specificity of 84.4%** in diagnosing axial spondyloarthritis, highlighting its utility in both clinical and research settings.

12.3.2. Role of Imaging in AxSpA Diagnosis

Imaging plays a pivotal role in diagnosing **axSpA**, particularly in distinguishing between **radiographic axSpA (AS)** and **non-radiographic axSpA**. The two primary imaging modalities are **X-rays** and **MRI**.

X-rays (Radiographic AxSpA)

X-rays are the primary imaging modality for diagnosing **radiographic axSpA**, also known as **Ankylosing Spondylitis (AS)**. X-rays are essential for detecting structural damage in the **sacroiliac joints** and **spine**.

1. **Key Findings on X-ray**:
   - **Bilateral Sacroiliitis**: The hallmark finding in **radiographic axSpA** is **bilateral sacroiliitis**, characterized by **sclerosis**, **erosions**, and **joint space narrowing** in the **sacroiliac joints**.
   - **Syndesmophytes**: In advanced AS, **syndesmophytes** (bony outgrowths) form between vertebrae, eventually leading to the characteristic **"bamboo spine"** appearance.
   - **Joint Fusion**: Over time, chronic inflammation can lead to **ankylosis** (fusion) of the **sacroiliac joints** and the spine.
2. **ACR Guidelines**: The **2019 ACR/Spondylitis Association of America/Spondyloarthritis Research and Treatment Network (SPARTAN)** guidelines recommend the use of **X-rays** as the first imaging modality for diagnosing **radiographic axSpA (AS)** in patients with **chronic back pain** and suspected spondyloarthritis.
   - **Evidence**: A study by **Braun et al. (2002)** demonstrated that X-rays are the gold standard for detecting **sacroiliitis** and are critical for diagnosing **AS**, especially in the later stages of the disease when structural changes are more apparent.

MRI (Non-Radiographic AxSpA)

Magnetic Resonance Imaging (MRI) is more sensitive than X-rays for detecting **early inflammatory changes** in patients with **non-radiographic axSpA**. MRI can visualize inflammation before structural damage is evident on X-rays, making it crucial for early diagnosis, particularly in younger patients.

1. **Key Findings on MRI**:
   - **Bone Marrow Edema (BME)**: **Bone marrow edema** at the **sacroiliac joints** is a hallmark of early **axSpA** and is often present in patients with **non-radiographic axSpA**. BME reflects active inflammation and is detectable on **STIR (short tau inversion recovery)** or **T2-weighted** MRI sequences.
   - **Subchondral Inflammation**: MRI can also detect **subchondral inflammation** and early **erosions** in the sacroiliac joints before these changes become visible on X-rays.
2. **ACR Guidelines**: According to the 2019 **ACR/SPARTAN guidelines**, **MRI** should be used in patients with **chronic back pain** and suspected axSpA, especially in those with

normal X-rays but clinical features suggestive of the disease. MRI is particularly valuable in diagnosing **non-radiographic axSpA**.

- **Evidence**: A study by **Weber et al. (2010)** showed that MRI detected **sacroiliac joint inflammation** in 88% of patients with early axSpA, compared to only 43% detected by X-ray. This finding underscores the sensitivity of MRI in diagnosing **non-radiographic axSpA** and supports its use in early disease detection.

12.3.3. HLA-B27 in AxSpA Diagnosis

HLA-B27 is a genetic marker that plays a critical role in the diagnosis of AxSpA. Although **HLA-B27 positivity** is strongly associated with **Ankylosing Spondylitis (AS)**, it is not exclusive to the disease. The presence of HLA-B27, combined with clinical features and imaging, significantly increases the likelihood of a diagnosis of AxSpA.

1. **Prevalence of HLA-B27**:
   - **HLA-B27** is present in up to **90%** of patients with **AS** and around **50-70%** of patients with **non-radiographic axSpA**.
   - Not all individuals with **HLA-B27** develop AxSpA, suggesting that **other genetic and environmental factors** contribute to disease pathogenesis.
2. **Diagnostic Role**:
   - In the **clinical arm** of the **ASAS criteria**, **HLA-B27 positivity** combined with **two or more SpA features** (e.g., **inflammatory back pain**, **uveitis**, or **enthesitis**) is sufficient for classifying AxSpA, even in the absence of imaging evidence of sacroiliitis.
   - The absence of **HLA-B27** does not exclude AxSpA, but its presence increases the diagnostic certainty, especially in patients with unclear clinical presentations.
3. **ACR Guidelines**: The **2019 ACR/SPARTAN guidelines** recommend **HLA-B27 testing** in patients with suspected AxSpA, particularly in those with **chronic back pain** and other SpA features. The presence of HLA-B27 can help guide diagnostic and treatment decisions, especially in cases where imaging findings are inconclusive.
   - **Evidence**: A study by **Khan et al. (2017)** confirmed the strong association between **HLA-B27** and AxSpA, with the gene present in **85-90%** of patients with AS. The study highlighted that **HLA-B27 positivity** should prompt further investigation, particularly in patients with early or mild symptoms.

12.4. Evidence-Based Pharmacologic Treatments: NSAIDs, TNF Inhibitors, IL-17 Inhibitors

The treatment of **Axial Spondyloarthritis (AxSpA)**, including **Ankylosing Spondylitis (AS)**, focuses on controlling **inflammation**, **alleviating symptoms**, and **preventing disease progression**. Pharmacologic treatment options include **NSAIDs, TNF inhibitors**, and **IL-17 inhibitors**, with selection based on disease severity, response to initial treatments, and the presence of extra-articular manifestations. Below is an overview of the evidence supporting these therapies.

12.4.1. NSAIDs (Nonsteroidal Anti-Inflammatory Drugs)

NSAIDs are considered the **first-line treatment** for both acute and chronic management of **AxSpA**. These drugs are effective in reducing **pain**, **stiffness**, and **inflammation**, and improving **quality of life** in patients with AxSpA. Continuous NSAID therapy may also have a **disease-modifying effect** by slowing **radiographic progression** in Ankylosing Spondylitis (AS).

1. **Mechanism of Action**:
   - NSAIDs inhibit **cyclooxygenase (COX) enzymes**, thereby reducing the production of **prostaglandins**, which are mediators of pain and inflammation.
2. **Effectiveness**:
   - **Symptom Relief**: NSAIDs have been shown to reduce **back pain** and **morning stiffness** in AxSpA patients. Regular NSAID use improves **mobility** and **physical function**.
   - **Radiographic Progression**: Some studies suggest that long-term use of NSAIDs may reduce **radiographic progression** of spinal damage in AS by inhibiting the inflammatory process involved in **syndesmophyte** formation.
3. **Common NSAIDs**:
   - **Naproxen**
   - **Diclofenac**
   - **Indomethacin**
4. **Safety and Monitoring**:
   - Long-term use of NSAIDs requires careful monitoring for potential **gastrointestinal (GI)** side effects, including **GI bleeding**, and **renal impairment**, particularly in older adults.
   - **Evidence**: A study by **Wanders et al. (2005)** found that continuous NSAID use significantly reduced radiographic progression in patients with **AS** compared to on-demand use. However, the risk of long-term NSAID-related side effects necessitates careful patient selection and monitoring.

TNF Inhibitors

When NSAIDs fail to control disease symptoms or when patients experience significant disease progression, **TNF inhibitors** are the next line of treatment. **TNF inhibitors** target **tumor necrosis factor (TNF)-α**, a central cytokine in the inflammatory process of **AxSpA**. These drugs are highly effective in reducing **disease activity**, improving **physical function**, and preventing **spinal fusion** in **AS**.

1. **Mechanism of Action**:
   - TNF inhibitors block **TNF-α**, a key pro-inflammatory cytokine involved in the immune response that drives **joint inflammation, syndesmophyte formation**, and **spinal fusion** in AxSpA.
2. **Effectiveness**:

- **Symptom Control**: TNF inhibitors significantly reduce **back pain**, **morning stiffness**, and improve **spinal mobility**.
- **Prevention of Joint Damage**: Studies have shown that TNF inhibitors can **slow disease progression** and reduce the risk of **spinal fusion** in AS, which is associated with long-term disability.
- **Extra-Articular Manifestations**: TNF inhibitors are also effective in treating extra-articular manifestations such as **uveitis**, **psoriasis**, and **inflammatory bowel disease (IBD)**, which commonly occur in AxSpA patients.

3. **Common TNF Inhibitors**:
   - **Etanercept**
   - **Adalimumab**
   - **Infliximab**
   - **Golimumab**
4. **Safety and Monitoring**:
   - While TNF inhibitors are generally well-tolerated, they can increase the risk of **infections** (especially **latent tuberculosis**) and **malignancies**. Regular monitoring is recommended for all patients receiving TNF inhibitors.
   - **Evidence**: The **ASSERT trial** (2005) demonstrated that **infliximab** significantly improved **spinal mobility** and reduced **inflammation** on MRI in patients with AS. Additionally, a meta-analysis by **Sieper et al. (2013)** confirmed the long-term efficacy and safety of **adalimumab, etanercept**, and **infliximab** in reducing both radiographic and clinical progression of AS.

IL-17 Inhibitors

IL-17 inhibitors represent a newer class of biologic therapies for **AxSpA**, specifically targeting **interleukin-17 (IL-17)**, a pro-inflammatory cytokine that plays a crucial role in both **AS** and **psoriasis**. These drugs are particularly beneficial for patients who have an inadequate response to **TNF inhibitors** or those with coexisting **psoriasis**.

1. **Mechanism of Action**:
   - **IL-17 inhibitors** block **IL-17**, a cytokine produced by **Th17 cells**, which is involved in the pathogenesis of AxSpA by promoting **inflammation** and **bone destruction**.
2. **Effectiveness**:
   - **Reduction in Joint Inflammation**: **IL-17 inhibitors** reduce **inflammation** at the **sacroiliac joints** and **spine**, improving **pain**, **stiffness**, and **mobility**.
   - **Coexisting Psoriasis**: Patients with both **AxSpA** and **psoriasis** benefit significantly from **IL-17 inhibitors** as these drugs are effective for both **joint** and **skin** inflammation.
   - **Efficacy after TNF Failure**: IL-17 inhibitors are an important option for patients who have **failed TNF inhibitors** or have experienced **adverse effects** from TNF inhibitors.
3. **Common IL-17 Inhibitors**:
   - **Secukinumab** (approved for AS and psoriasis)

- **Ixekizumab** (approved for AS and psoriasis)
4. **Safety and Monitoring**:
    - IL-17 inhibitors have a good safety profile, though they may increase the risk of **infections** such as **upper respiratory tract infections. Monitoring for infections** and **autoimmune diseases** is recommended during therapy.
    - **Evidence**: The **MEASURE trials** (2015) demonstrated that **secukinumab** significantly reduced **spinal inflammation** and improved **physical function** in patients with **active AS**. **Secukinumab** has also shown efficacy in patients with **psoriasis** and **AxSpA**, providing a dual benefit for patients with both conditions. **Ixekizumab** has shown similar efficacy in reducing **axial inflammation** and improving quality of life in patients with AS.

12.5. Non-Pharmacological Management: Physical Therapy, Exercise

Non-pharmacological interventions, particularly **physical therapy (PT)** and **exercise**, are essential components of managing **Axial Spondyloarthritis (AxSpA)**. These interventions help maintain **joint mobility**, reduce **pain**, and prevent **deformity**, such as **kyphosis** (spinal curvature). Regular physical activity, along with **patient education** and **lifestyle modifications**, has been shown to significantly improve **long-term outcomes** for patients with AxSpA.

12.5.1. Physical Therapy (PT) in AxSpA Management

Physical therapy is considered a **cornerstone** of AxSpA management. The primary goals of PT are to maintain **spinal mobility**, improve **posture**, and enhance **physical function**.

1. **Key Components of Physical Therapy**:
    - **Spinal Mobility Exercises**: Exercises that promote **flexibility** and **mobility** of the spine are critical to prevent the development of **kyphosis** and **joint stiffness**.
    - **Posture Correction**: Correcting and maintaining **upright posture** helps prevent spinal deformities that can develop over time, particularly **kyphosis**. Therapists work with patients to maintain proper **postural alignment** through targeted exercises.
    - **Stretching**: Stretching exercises are used to maintain the flexibility of the spine and surrounding joints, preventing contractures and promoting full range of motion.
2. **Benefits of Physical Therapy**:
    - **Preventing Spinal Deformity**: Early and regular PT can prevent or delay the progression of **kyphosis** and **spinal fusion** in patients with advanced disease.
    - **Improving Quality of Life**: By enhancing **flexibility**, **strength**, and **posture**, PT helps reduce **pain** and improve **physical function**, allowing patients to maintain an active lifestyle.
3. **Evidence**: A study by **Zochling et al. (2006)** demonstrated that structured **physical therapy** improved **spinal mobility** and **posture** in patients with **ankylosing spondylitis**. Patients who participated in supervised PT programs had better outcomes

in terms of **spinal mobility** and **quality of life** compared to those who relied solely on pharmacological treatment.
4. **ACR Guidelines**: The **American College of Rheumatology (ACR) guidelines** emphasize the importance of **physical therapy** in the comprehensive management of AxSpA. The guidelines recommend **regular PT** to help maintain spinal flexibility and prevent disability.

12.5.2. Exercise in AxSpA

Regular exercise is one of the most important non-pharmacological strategies for managing AxSpA. **Low-impact exercises**, such as **swimming**, **cycling**, and **walking**, help to improve **joint function**, reduce **stiffness**, and enhance **overall physical fitness**.

1. **Types of Exercise**:
   - **Swimming**: Swimming is particularly beneficial because it is a **low-impact** activity that engages multiple muscle groups while minimizing stress on the joints.
   - **Cycling**: Cycling helps maintain **hip** and **spinal mobility** while improving cardiovascular fitness.
   - **Walking**: Regular walking helps improve **flexibility** and reduce **joint stiffness**, especially in the spine and hips.
2. **Core Strengthening**: Strengthening the **core muscles** (abdominal and back muscles) helps support the spine and maintain **postural stability**. Exercises like **planks**, **bridges**, and **pelvic tilts** are commonly recommended to improve **core strength** in AxSpA patients.
3. **Impact on Disease Activity**:
   - **Exercise Reduces Disease Activity**: Studies have shown that consistent exercise reduces **disease activity** and improves **physical function** in patients with AxSpA. Exercise helps reduce **inflammation**, increase **flexibility**, and improve **cardiovascular health**.
   - **Prevention of Spinal Fusion**: Regular exercise can prevent or delay the progression of **spinal fusion** by maintaining **joint mobility** and reducing the risk of deformity.
4. **Evidence**: A study by **Fernández-de-Las-Peñas et al. (2016)** found that patients with **ankylosing spondylitis** who engaged in regular exercise experienced significant improvements in **pain**, **stiffness**, and **overall physical function**. The study also demonstrated that exercise helped reduce **fatigue** and improved **mental well-being** in AxSpA patients.
5. **ACR Guidelines**: The **ACR guidelines** recommend **regular, low-impact physical activity** as part of a comprehensive treatment plan for AxSpA. **Exercise programs** should be individualized based on the patient's disease severity and physical capabilities, but regular activity is encouraged to maintain **spinal mobility** and **prevent disability**.

12.5.3. Patient Education and Lifestyle Modifications

In addition to PT and exercise, **patient education** and **lifestyle modifications** play a crucial role in AxSpA management.

1. **Educating Patients**:
   - Patients should be educated about the importance of maintaining **physical activity** and **good posture** to prevent long-term complications.
   - **Posture maintenance** exercises are important for preventing **spinal deformities** like **kyphosis**, which can develop in advanced disease stages.
2. **Smoking Cessation**:
   - **Smoking** is a known risk factor for **increased disease activity** and **faster progression** in AxSpA. Smoking contributes to chronic inflammation and has been linked to **worse outcomes** in patients with **ankylosing spondylitis**.
   - **Evidence**: A study by **Poddubnyy et al. (2012)** found that smoking is associated with **higher disease activity**, more severe **radiographic progression**, and **reduced response** to biologic therapy in patients with AS. Smoking cessation is a critical lifestyle modification for improving outcomes in AxSpA.
3. **Encouraging Core Strengthening**:
   - **Core strengthening exercises** are recommended to improve **spinal support** and **stability**, reducing the risk of spinal deformities and improving overall mobility.

Ankylosing Spondylitis and Axial Spondyloarthritis are chronic, progressive diseases that primarily affect the axial skeleton but can involve multiple organ systems. Early diagnosis, aided by HLA-B27 testing and imaging modalities such as MRI, is crucial to prevent irreversible spinal damage and disability. Evidence-based treatments, including NSAIDs, TNF inhibitors, and IL-17 inhibitors, are effective in controlling inflammation and preserving joint function. Non-pharmacological management, particularly physical therapy and regular exercise, is equally important in maintaining mobility and improving quality of life.

References

- Sieper, J., Poddubnyy, D., & Braun, J. (2017). Axial spondyloarthritis. *The Lancet*, 390(10089), 73-84.
- Van der Heijde, D., Ramiro, S., Landewe, R., et al. (2017). 2016 update of the ASAS-EULAR management recommendations for axial spondyloarthritis. *Annals of the Rheumatic Diseases*, 76(6), 978-991.
- Braun, J., & Sieper, J. (2007). Ankylosing spondylitis. *The Lancet*, 369(9570), 1379-1390.
- Baraliakos, X., Haibel, H., Listing, J., et al. (2014). Continuous treatment with infliximab leads to inhibition of radiographic progression in patients with ankylosing spondylitis. *Annals of the Rheumatic Diseases*, 73(1), 117-123.
- van der Heijde, D., Cheng-Chung Wei, J., Dougados, M., et al. (2019). Ixekizumab, an interleukin-17A inhibitor, in patients with ankylosing spondylitis (COAST-V): a

randomised, double-blind, active-controlled phase 3 trial. *The Lancet*, 394(10214), 37-47.
- Wanders, A., Heijde, D. V. D., Landewé, R., et al. (2005). Nonsteroidal anti-inflammatory drugs reduce radiographic progression in patients with ankylosing spondylitis: A randomized clinical trial. *Arthritis & Rheumatism*, 52(6), 1756-1765.
- Braun, J., Brandt, J., Listing, J., et al. (2005). Treatment of active ankylosing spondylitis with infliximab: A randomised controlled multicentre trial. *Lancet*, 359(9313), 1187-1193.
- Sieper, J., Poddubnyy, D., & Miossec, P. (2013). The IL-23–IL-17 pathway as a therapeutic target in axial spondyloarthritis. *Nature Reviews Rheumatology*, 9(8), 485-493.
- Baeten, D., Sieper, J., Braun, J., et al. (2015). Secukinumab, an interleukin-17A inhibitor, in ankylosing spondylitis. *New England Journal of Medicine*, 373(26), 2534-2548.

Chapter 13: Fibromyalgia

Fibromyalgia (FM) is a chronic disorder characterized by **widespread musculoskeletal pain**, **fatigue**, **sleep disturbances**, and **cognitive dysfunction**. The condition is believed to result from **central sensitization**, where the central nervous system amplifies pain signals. Fibromyalgia is not a disease of the joints or muscles themselves but rather a dysfunction in how the brain processes pain. The complexity of its symptoms and overlap with other conditions make diagnosis and management challenging. This section provides a detailed overview of fibromyalgia's pathogenesis, risk factors, diagnosis, and evidence-based treatments.

13.1. Pathogenesis and Risk Factors for Fibromyalgia

Fibromyalgia (FM) is a chronic pain disorder characterized by widespread musculoskeletal pain, fatigue, and cognitive disturbances. The pathogenesis is complex and involves both **central nervous system (CNS) dysfunction** and **genetic and environmental factors**. Understanding the mechanisms and risk factors that contribute to the development of fibromyalgia is essential for developing effective treatment strategies.

13.1.1. Central Sensitization in Fibromyalgia

The **primary mechanism** underlying **fibromyalgia** is **central sensitization**, where the CNS becomes hypersensitive to pain signals, leading to an exaggerated response to both painful and non-painful stimuli.

1. **Central Sensitization**:
    - **Central sensitization** refers to a heightened sensitivity to sensory stimuli, particularly pain, due to abnormal processing within the CNS. This results in two hallmark symptoms in FM:
        - **Allodynia**: Pain resulting from stimuli that are not normally painful (e.g., light touch).
        - **Hyperalgesia**: Exaggerated pain response to typically painful stimuli.
2. **Abnormal Neurotransmitter Levels**:
    - Studies suggest that patients with fibromyalgia have altered levels of key **neurotransmitters** involved in pain modulation, including:
        - **Serotonin** and **norepinephrine**, which are involved in descending pain inhibition.
        - **Glutamate**, which plays a role in pain transmission and can lead to neuronal excitability.
        - **Substance P**, a neuropeptide that enhances pain perception and is elevated in the cerebrospinal fluid of fibromyalgia patients.
3. **Brain Imaging Findings**:
    - **Functional imaging studies** using **functional MRI (fMRI)** and **positron emission tomography (PET)** have shown increased activity in pain-processing regions of the brain, such as the **insula, anterior cingulate cortex, thalamus**,

and **brainstem** in fibromyalgia patients. This suggests that fibromyalgia involves dysfunctional pain processing at multiple levels of the CNS.
- **Evidence**: A study by **Gracely et al. (2002)** used fMRI to demonstrate increased neural activity in the **pain-processing regions** of fibromyalgia patients in response to both painful and non-painful stimuli, supporting the concept of **central sensitization** as a key mechanism in fibromyalgia.

13.1.2. Genetic and Environmental Factors

Both **genetic predisposition** and **environmental triggers** contribute to the development of fibromyalgia.

1. **Genetic Predisposition**:
    - Fibromyalgia has a **heritable component**, with first-degree relatives of fibromyalgia patients having a higher risk of developing the condition.
    - Genetic studies have identified several genes that may increase susceptibility to fibromyalgia and chronic pain, including:
        - **5-HTTLPR**: A polymorphism in the **serotonin transporter gene** that affects serotonin reuptake and is associated with altered pain perception.
        - **COMT (catechol-O-methyltransferase)**: Variants of this gene, which affect **catecholamine metabolism**, have been implicated in pain sensitivity and stress response.
2. **Environmental Triggers**:
    - Genetics alone do not fully account for the development of fibromyalgia. Environmental factors often play a **triggering role** in the onset of symptoms. Common **precipitating events** include:
        - **Physical trauma**: Injury or physical stress can precipitate fibromyalgia in genetically susceptible individuals.
        - **Infections**: Certain viral infections, such as **Epstein-Barr virus (EBV)** or **hepatitis C**, have been associated with the onset of fibromyalgia.
        - **Emotional stress**: Significant emotional or psychological stress, such as the loss of a loved one or experiencing trauma, can trigger the onset of fibromyalgia.
    - **Evidence**: A study by **Kato et al. (2006)** found that specific variants of the **COMT gene** were associated with increased pain sensitivity in fibromyalgia patients, providing further evidence for a genetic basis in fibromyalgia. Environmental triggers, such as **stressful life events**, were found to interact with these genetic factors to exacerbate pain symptoms.

13.1.3. Risk Factors for Fibromyalgia

Several factors increase the risk of developing fibromyalgia:

1. **Sex**:

- **Women** are significantly more likely to develop fibromyalgia than men, with a **female-to-male ratio** of approximately **9:1**.
- **Hormonal differences**, particularly related to **estrogen**, are thought to contribute to this gender disparity, although the exact mechanism is not fully understood.

2. **Sleep Disturbances**:
   - Non-restorative sleep is a **common feature** of fibromyalgia, and disrupted sleep has been shown to contribute to **central sensitization** and **pain amplification**.
   - **Evidence**: Research by **Moldofsky et al. (1993)** found that **sleep deprivation** led to increased pain sensitivity in healthy individuals, mimicking the symptoms of fibromyalgia, indicating that sleep disturbances play a role in **pain modulation** in fibromyalgia patients.

3. **Mood Disorders**:
   - There is a strong association between fibromyalgia and **mood disorders** such as **depression, anxiety**, and **post-traumatic stress disorder (PTSD)**.
   - These **comorbidities** can exacerbate pain perception and interfere with the body's **coping mechanisms**, leading to a **vicious cycle** of worsening pain and mood dysfunction.
   - **Evidence**: A meta-analysis by **Løge-Hansen et al. (2012)** highlighted the strong association between **depression** and **fibromyalgia**, suggesting that mood disorders not only increase the risk of developing fibromyalgia but also contribute to worsening symptoms and reduced quality of life.

13.2. Diagnosis: Differentiating Fibromyalgia from Inflammatory Diseases

Fibromyalgia (FM) presents a diagnostic challenge due to its overlap with symptoms of other **inflammatory diseases**, such as **rheumatoid arthritis (RA)** and **systemic lupus erythematosus (SLE)**. Both fibromyalgia and inflammatory diseases share common features like **widespread pain, fatigue**, and **stiffness**, which can complicate the clinical picture. However, fibromyalgia is distinct in that it is a **non-inflammatory** disorder and lacks the objective inflammatory findings typically seen in diseases like RA or SLE. Differentiating fibromyalgia from these conditions requires a careful clinical evaluation based on symptom patterns, physical examination, and laboratory results.

13.2.1. Diagnostic Criteria for Fibromyalgia (2016 ACR Criteria)

The **American College of Rheumatology (ACR)** updated its diagnostic criteria for **fibromyalgia** in 2016. These criteria focus on **symptom severity** and the **distribution of pain**, moving away from the previous emphasis on tender points. The criteria aim to capture the **chronic, diffuse pain** and associated symptoms that characterize fibromyalgia.

1. **Widespread Pain Index (WPI)**:
   - The **WPI** is a score based on the number of body areas where the patient has experienced pain over the past week. It assesses **19 specific body regions**, with scores ranging from **0 to 19**, depending on how many areas are affected.

2. **Symptom Severity Scale (SSS)**:
   - The **SSS** assesses the severity of the patient's **fatigue, unrefreshing sleep, cognitive symptoms**, and **other somatic symptoms** (e.g., headaches, gastrointestinal issues). The score ranges from **0 to 12**, with higher scores indicating more severe symptoms.
3. **Chronicity of Symptoms**:
   - For a diagnosis of fibromyalgia, the symptoms must have been present at a similar level for at least **three months**.
4. **Absence of Other Explanations**:
   - The diagnosis of fibromyalgia is confirmed when **no other disorder** can explain the pain and symptoms.
5. **Key Difference from Previous Criteria**:
   - Unlike the earlier **ACR 1990 criteria**, which required the presence of **tender points** (pain in 11 of 18 specific points on the body), the **2016 criteria** focus more on the **patient's subjective experience** of pain and symptom severity.
   - **Evidence**: A study by **Wolfe et al. (2016)** evaluated the **2016 ACR criteria** and found them to be more **sensitive** and **specific** in identifying fibromyalgia compared to the older tender-point-based criteria. The study also emphasized that the newer criteria better reflect the **multisystemic nature** of fibromyalgia, incorporating cognitive and somatic symptoms.

13.2.2. Differentiating Fibromyalgia from Inflammatory Diseases

Fibromyalgia can mimic **inflammatory diseases**, but there are several important distinctions that help differentiate it from conditions like **rheumatoid arthritis (RA)** and **systemic lupus erythematosus (SLE)**:

1. **Absence of Inflammatory Findings**:
   - **Fibromyalgia** does not cause **objective signs of inflammation**, such as **joint swelling, redness**, or **synovitis**. In contrast, **RA** and **SLE** often present with **synovial inflammation** (visible as swelling or warmth of the joints) and other inflammatory markers.
   - **Physical Exam**: In fibromyalgia, **physical examination** is typically unremarkable except for **diffuse tenderness**. There is **no joint swelling** or **deformity**, while in RA or SLE, examination often reveals **swollen joints** and possibly **joint deformities** in advanced cases.
2. **Laboratory Tests**:
   - In **fibromyalgia**, laboratory tests such as **erythrocyte sedimentation rate (ESR), C-reactive protein (CRP)**, and **autoantibodies** (e.g., **antinuclear antibodies (ANA)** or **rheumatoid factor (RF)**) are typically **normal**.
   - RA and SLE are associated with abnormal laboratory findings, such as:
     - **Elevated ESR or CRP** in cases of inflammation.
     - **Positive rheumatoid factor (RF)** or **anti-cyclic citrullinated peptide (anti-CCP)** in RA.
     - **Positive ANA** or **anti-dsDNA antibodies** in SLE.

- **Evidence**: A study by **Garrity et al. (2017)** emphasized the importance of distinguishing fibromyalgia from inflammatory diseases by relying on **normal inflammatory markers** and the **lack of synovitis** on physical examination, underscoring that fibromyalgia is a non-inflammatory disorder.

3. **Pain Distribution**:
    - **Fibromyalgia** typically presents with **diffuse pain** affecting multiple areas of the body, often involving both the **upper** and **lower extremities** on both sides. The pain is described as widespread and does not correspond to specific joints.
    - **RA** usually affects **specific joints**, especially the **small joints** of the hands, wrists, and feet, with a **symmetrical pattern** of involvement. **Morning stiffness** lasting more than an hour, which improves with activity, is a hallmark of inflammatory arthritis.
    - **SLE** may involve **migratory joint pain** that affects multiple joints but is usually **episodic** and associated with other systemic symptoms like **rash**, **photosensitivity**, and **renal involvement**.

4. **Fatigue and Systemic Symptoms**:
    - While both **fibromyalgia** and **inflammatory diseases** like SLE can present with **fatigue**, the nature of the fatigue differs. In fibromyalgia, fatigue is often linked to **non-restorative sleep** and is persistent.
    - In contrast, fatigue in inflammatory diseases like **RA** and **SLE** is often associated with **active systemic inflammation** and may fluctuate depending on disease activity.

5. **Morning Stiffness**:
    - In **fibromyalgia**, **morning stiffness** is common but tends to resolve **more quickly** and is not as prolonged as in inflammatory diseases. In RA, morning stiffness lasting **more than one hour** is a common diagnostic clue.
    - **Evidence**: A study by **Wolfe et al. (2009)** compared patients with **fibromyalgia** and **RA**, finding that **morning stiffness** in fibromyalgia patients was less severe and resolved more quickly compared to those with RA, where the stiffness typically persisted for longer periods.

13.3. Evidence-Based Treatment: Pharmacologic (Antidepressants, Anticonvulsants) and Nonpharmacologic (Cognitive Behavioral Therapy, Exercise)

The treatment of **fibromyalgia** requires a **multimodal approach** that targets both **central pain processing** abnormalities and the **physical and psychological** components of the disorder. **Pharmacologic treatments** aim to modulate neurotransmitters involved in **pain regulation**, while **non-pharmacologic strategies** focus on improving **coping mechanisms**, **physical function**, and **mental health**. Studies support the combined use of these approaches to achieve optimal symptom relief and improved quality of life in fibromyalgia patients.

13.3.1. Pharmacologic Treatment

The primary goal of pharmacologic therapy is to address the **central sensitization** that underlies fibromyalgia, particularly by targeting neurotransmitters like **serotonin**, **norepinephrine**, and **glutamate**.

1. Antidepressants

Antidepressants are widely used in fibromyalgia management due to their ability to modulate **serotonin** and **norepinephrine**, which are key neurotransmitters in the **descending inhibitory pain pathways**. These drugs not only alleviate pain but also improve associated symptoms such as **fatigue** and **sleep disturbances**.

Serotonin-Norepinephrine Reuptake Inhibitors (SNRIs)

1. **Duloxetine** and **milnacipran** are **FDA-approved** for the treatment of fibromyalgia.
   - **Duloxetine**: This SNRI has been shown to significantly reduce **pain** and **fatigue** in fibromyalgia patients while also improving **sleep** and **overall quality of life**. It is particularly effective in individuals with coexisting **depression** or **anxiety**.
     - **Study Evidence**: A study by **Arnold et al. (2012)** demonstrated that **duloxetine** significantly reduced pain and improved mood in fibromyalgia patients, with a sustained effect over 12 weeks.
   - **Milnacipran**: Another SNRI approved for fibromyalgia, milnacipran, has shown efficacy in reducing **pain** and improving **physical function**.
     - **Study Evidence**: In a randomized controlled trial by **Clauw et al. (2008)**, **milnacipran** was associated with significant improvements in **pain** and **global patient impression** scores, particularly in patients with moderate-to-severe fibromyalgia.

Tricyclic Antidepressants (TCAs)

2. **Amitriptyline**: Although not FDA-approved for fibromyalgia, low doses of **amitriptyline** have been used off-label to reduce **pain**, **improve sleep**, and alleviate **fatigue**. However, **side effects** such as **dry mouth**, **drowsiness**, and **weight gain** can limit its long-term use.
   - **Study Evidence**: A review by **Moore et al. (2015)** found that **amitriptyline** provided pain relief in approximately 30% of fibromyalgia patients. However, dropout rates due to side effects were significant, highlighting the need for careful patient selection.

2. Anticonvulsants

Anticonvulsants are effective in fibromyalgia treatment due to their ability to inhibit **calcium channels** in the central nervous system, which reduces **neurotransmitter release** involved in pain signaling.

1. **Pregabalin** and **gabapentin** are **gabapentinoids** that have shown efficacy in reducing **widespread pain**, improving **sleep**, and reducing **anxiety** symptoms in fibromyalgia patients.
    - **Pregabalin**: **FDA-approved** for fibromyalgia, pregabalin works by binding to **alpha-2-delta subunits** of voltage-gated calcium channels, inhibiting the release of excitatory neurotransmitters.
        - **Study Evidence**: In a pivotal trial by **Crofford et al. (2005)**, **pregabalin** significantly reduced pain and improved **sleep quality** in fibromyalgia patients over a 12-week period. Side effects included **dizziness, somnolence**, and **peripheral edema**.
    - **Gabapentin**: Similar to pregabalin, gabapentin has shown benefits in reducing pain and improving sleep. It is often used off-label for fibromyalgia.
        - **Study Evidence**: A study by **Arnold et al. (2007)** found that **gabapentin** improved pain and sleep disturbances in fibromyalgia patients, though side effects such as **dizziness** and **fatigue** were common.

3. Other Pharmacologic Treatments

1. **Cyclobenzaprine**: A **muscle relaxant** with central effects, **cyclobenzaprine** is structurally similar to **TCAs** and has been used for short-term relief of fibromyalgia symptoms, particularly improving **sleep** and reducing **pain**.
    - **Study Evidence**: A study by **Tofferi et al. (2004)** found that **cyclobenzaprine** improved **sleep quality** and reduced pain in fibromyalgia patients, with fewer side effects than amitriptyline.
2. **Acetaminophen and NSAIDs**: These medications are not generally effective in fibromyalgia because they target **peripheral pain mechanisms**, whereas fibromyalgia is primarily a **central pain disorder**. However, they may provide **symptomatic relief** in patients with **concurrent conditions** like **osteoarthritis** or **other musculoskeletal pain**.

13.3.2. Non-Pharmacologic Treatment

Non-pharmacologic interventions are critical in fibromyalgia management. They focus on improving **physical function, mental health**, and overall **coping mechanisms**.

1. Cognitive Behavioral Therapy (CBT)

Cognitive Behavioral Therapy (CBT) is a well-established psychological intervention for fibromyalgia that aims to change **negative thought patterns** and improve **coping strategies**.

1. **Benefits of CBT**:
    - CBT helps patients understand the connection between **thoughts, emotions**, and **pain perception**, allowing them to develop healthier **coping mechanisms**.
    - It has been shown to reduce **pain intensity, improve mood**, and increase **physical activity**.

2. **Study Evidence**:
    - A meta-analysis by **Bernardy et al. (2010)** found that **CBT** provided significant improvements in **pain**, **sleep**, and **quality of life** in fibromyalgia patients. The study highlighted that the benefits of CBT were often sustained long after therapy completion.

2. Exercise

Regular **exercise** is a cornerstone of non-pharmacologic fibromyalgia treatment. Exercise improves **physical function**, reduces **pain**, and combats **fatigue**.

1. **Types of Exercise**:
    - **Low-impact aerobic exercises**, such as **walking**, **swimming**, and **cycling**, are effective in reducing **pain** and improving **overall function**.
    - **Strength training** and **flexibility exercises** also help reduce **stiffness** and increase **muscle strength**.
2. **Impact on Disease Activity**:
    - **Exercise** has been shown to reduce **pain** and **fatigue**, as well as improve **sleep** quality and **mood**. Regular physical activity also addresses the **deconditioning** that can occur in fibromyalgia patients due to reduced mobility.
3. **Study Evidence**:
    - A systematic review by **Busch et al. (2011)** concluded that **aerobic exercise** consistently led to reductions in pain and improved **physical function** in patients with fibromyalgia. The review emphasized the importance of **individualized exercise programs** to optimize results.
    - Another study by **McLoughlin et al. (2011)** found that **strength training** improved **muscle strength** and **endurance**, leading to a decrease in **pain** and **fatigue**..

13.5. Managing Chronic Pain and Mental Health

Managing **fibromyalgia** is complex due to its multisystemic nature, which includes both **chronic pain** and significant **mental health comorbidities** like **depression** and **anxiety**. Effective management involves a **multidisciplinary approach** that combines **physical therapy**, **psychological support**, **patient education**, and **lifestyle modifications**.

This integrative approach addresses both the physical and mental aspects of the condition, helping patients improve **quality of life** and better manage their symptoms.

13.5.1. Multidisciplinary Approach

A **multidisciplinary approach** to managing fibromyalgia is key, involving collaboration between various healthcare providers:

- **Rheumatologists** often oversee the treatment of fibromyalgia, particularly when co-occurring with other rheumatic diseases.

- **Primary care physicians** coordinate overall patient care, including medication management and addressing comorbidities such as **diabetes** or **cardiovascular disease**.
- **Physical therapists** guide exercise programs to improve **mobility** and reduce **pain**.
- **Psychologists** or **mental health professionals** provide therapy, such as **cognitive behavioral therapy (CBT)**, to address **depression**, **anxiety**, and **pain-related catastrophizing**.

This comprehensive approach allows for the treatment of **physical symptoms** (pain, stiffness, fatigue) as well as **mental health concerns** (depression, anxiety), which frequently coexist in fibromyalgia patients.

- **Evidence**: A review by **Bernardy et al. (2013)** demonstrated that multidisciplinary care, including physical therapy, psychological support, and patient education, significantly improved **pain** and **quality of life** in fibromyalgia patients compared to pharmacologic interventions alone.

13.5. 2. Sleep Hygiene

Nonrestorative sleep is a hallmark of fibromyalgia, and poor sleep exacerbates pain and fatigue. Thus, addressing **sleep disturbances** is critical for effective symptom management.

1. **Sleep Hygiene Education**:
   - **Maintaining a regular sleep schedule**: Patients are encouraged to go to bed and wake up at the same time every day to regulate their sleep-wake cycle.
   - **Avoiding stimulants**: Caffeine, nicotine, and other stimulants should be avoided in the evening as they can interfere with sleep quality.
   - **Creating a comfortable sleep environment**: Patients should ensure their sleep environment is **cool**, **dark**, and **quiet**, and avoid electronic devices before bed.
2. **Impact on Pain**:
   - Improving sleep quality directly impacts **pain perception**, as poor sleep is linked to increased **pain sensitivity** and **fatigue**.
3. **Evidence**: A study by **Moldofsky et al. (2011)** highlighted that improving sleep quality in fibromyalgia patients reduced **pain intensity** and improved **cognitive function**, emphasizing the importance of sleep management in reducing the overall symptom burden of the disease.

13.5.3. Mindfulness and Relaxation Techniques

Mindfulness-based stress reduction (MBSR) and other **relaxation techniques** are increasingly used in fibromyalgia management to reduce stress and improve well-being.

1. **Techniques**:
   - **Deep breathing exercises**: Focusing on slow, controlled breathing to calm the nervous system.

- **Guided imagery**: Visualization techniques that help shift focus away from pain and stress.
- **Progressive muscle relaxation**: Tensing and relaxing muscles systematically to reduce physical tension and promote relaxation.
2. **Impact of Stress on Pain**:
    - Stress exacerbates **pain** and other symptoms of fibromyalgia, such as **fatigue** and **cognitive dysfunction**. Teaching patients how to manage stress through **mindfulness** and **relaxation** techniques can reduce symptom severity.
3. **Evidence**: A systematic review by **Cash et al. (2015)** found that **mindfulness-based interventions**, including **MBSR**, led to significant reductions in **pain**, **depression**, and **anxiety** in fibromyalgia patients, with improvements sustained over several months.

13.5.4. Support Groups and Patient Education

Patient education and **peer support** play essential roles in the long-term management of fibromyalgia.

1. **Support Groups**:
    - Participating in **support groups** allows fibromyalgia patients to share their experiences and strategies for managing chronic pain. It also reduces the sense of **isolation** often felt by those living with chronic illness.
    - Peer support can lead to **improved coping strategies** and greater adherence to treatment regimens.
2. **Patient Education**:
    - Educating patients about the nature of **fibromyalgia** helps empower them to manage their symptoms more effectively. Understanding the chronic nature of the condition and the importance of **self-management** can improve adherence to both **pharmacologic** and **non-pharmacologic** therapies.
    - Patients should be informed about the **biopsychosocial model** of fibromyalgia, which explains that pain is influenced by biological, psychological, and social factors, all of which need to be addressed.
3. **Evidence**: A study by **Schaefer et al. (2015)** demonstrated that participation in **fibromyalgia support groups** improved **self-efficacy** and **quality of life**. In addition, **patient education programs** increased **treatment adherence** and reduced **feelings of helplessness** related to chronic pain.

Fibromyalgia is a complex disorder of chronic pain amplification with a wide range of symptoms that significantly affect quality of life. The pathogenesis involves central sensitization, and a combination of genetic, environmental, and psychological factors contribute to its onset. Diagnosis requires careful differentiation from inflammatory diseases, as fibromyalgia lacks the objective signs of inflammation seen in conditions like RA or SLE.

A multimodal treatment approach, including pharmacologic therapies such as antidepressants and anticonvulsants, alongside non-pharmacologic interventions like cognitive behavioral therapy and exercise, is essential for effective symptom management. Addressing both chronic pain and mental health is key to improving outcomes in patients with fibromyalgia.

References

- Clauw, D. J. (2014). Fibromyalgia: A clinical review. *JAMA*, 311(15), 1547-1555.
- Häuser, W., Sarzi-Puttini, P., & Fitzcharles, M. A. (2019). Fibromyalgia syndrome: Under-, over- and misdiagnosis. *Clinical and Experimental Rheumatology*, 37(Suppl 116), 90-97.
- Arnold, L. M., Choy, E., Clauw, D. J., et al. (2012). Fibromyalgia and chronic pain syndromes: A white paper detailing current challenges in the field. *The Journal of Pain*, 13(2), 111-120.
- Wolfe, F., Clauw, D. J., Fitzcharles, M. A., et al. (2010). The American College of Rheumatology preliminary diagnostic criteria for fibromyalgia and measurement of symptom severity. *Arthritis Care & Research*, 62(5), 600-610.
- Goldenberg, D. L., Clauw, D. J., & Palmer, R. E. (2020). Improving the recognition and diagnosis of fibromyalgia. *Mayo Clinic Proceedings*, 95(7), 1348-1361.
- Häuser, W., Bernardy, K., Arnold, B., Offenbächer, M., & Schiltenwolf, M. (2009). Efficacy of multicomponent treatment in fibromyalgia syndrome: A meta-analysis of randomized controlled clinical trials. *Arthritis Care & Research*, 61(2), 216-224.

Chapter 14: Vasculitis Syndromes

Vasculitis refers to a group of disorders characterized by **inflammation of blood vessels**, leading to vessel wall damage, ischemia, and tissue injury. Vasculitis can affect vessels of different sizes, ranging from small capillaries to large arteries. It is classified based on the size of the affected vessels into **small-vessel**, **medium-vessel**, and **large-vessel vasculitis**. Early diagnosis and treatment are critical in preventing irreversible organ damage and improving patient outcomes. This section provides an overview of vasculitis, diagnostic approaches, treatment strategies, and long-term management.

14.1. Overview of Vasculitis: Small, Medium, and Large Vessel Types

Vasculitis refers to inflammation of the blood vessels, and it can affect vessels of various sizes, leading to organ damage due to compromised blood flow. Vasculitis is broadly classified into **small-vessel**, **medium-vessel**, and **large-vessel** vasculitis based on the size of the affected vessels. Each type of vasculitis has distinct clinical features, pathophysiology, and treatment considerations. Below is an overview of each type of vasculitis, highlighting common syndromes within each category.

14.1.1. Small-Vessel Vasculitis

Small-vessel vasculitis primarily affects **capillaries**, **venules**, and **small arterioles**. This form of vasculitis involves inflammation and immune complex deposition in the walls of small vessels, leading to tissue damage and organ involvement.

1. **ANCA-Associated Vasculitis (AAV)**:
   - **ANCA-associated vasculitis (AAV)** is a group of disorders involving **anti-neutrophil cytoplasmic antibodies (ANCA)**, which target proteins like **proteinase 3 (PR3)** or **myeloperoxidase (MPO)** on neutrophils, leading to vascular inflammation. Common syndromes include **granulomatosis with polyangiitis (GPA)** and **microscopic polyangiitis (MPA)**.
   - **Granulomatosis with Polyangiitis (GPA)**:
     - GPA is characterized by **granulomatous inflammation** affecting the **respiratory tract** and **kidneys**. Patients may present with **sinusitis, pulmonary hemorrhage**, and **glomerulonephritis**. The presence of **PR3-ANCA** is often diagnostic.
     - **Study Evidence**: A study by **Luqmani et al. (2011)** showed that **PR3-ANCA** positivity is associated with more severe disease and increased likelihood of pulmonary involvement in GPA.
   - **Microscopic Polyangiitis (MPA)**:
     - MPA is similar to GPA but lacks granulomatous inflammation. It primarily affects the **kidneys**, leading to **rapidly progressive glomerulonephritis**. **MPO-ANCA** is typically present in MPA.
2. **IgA Vasculitis (Henoch-Schönlein Purpura)**:

- This form of vasculitis is more common in children and involves **IgA-containing immune complexes** depositing in vessel walls. It typically presents with **cutaneous purpura**, **arthritis**, **abdominal pain**, and **glomerulonephritis**.
- **Study Evidence**: Research by **Pillebout et al. (2016)** found that children with IgA vasculitis often have self-limited disease, while adults are more likely to develop renal involvement, requiring long-term monitoring.
3. **Cryoglobulinemic Vasculitis**:
   - This form of vasculitis is associated with **cryoglobulins**, proteins that precipitate at cold temperatures. It can occur in patients with **hepatitis C** or autoimmune disorders, leading to **skin lesions**, **renal disease**, and **neuropathy**.

14.1.2. Medium-Vessel Vasculitis

Medium-vessel vasculitis affects **muscular arteries**, including the **renal** and **mesenteric arteries**, resulting in **organ ischemia**. The most common forms include **polyarteritis nodosa (PAN)** and **Kawasaki disease**.

1. **Polyarteritis Nodosa (PAN)**:
   - **PAN** is characterized by **necrotizing inflammation** of medium-sized arteries without **glomerulonephritis** or ANCA involvement. It presents with **systemic symptoms** such as **fever**, **weight loss**, **myalgia**, and signs of **organ ischemia**, including **hypertension**, **abdominal pain**, and **neuropathy**.
   - **Clinical Features**:
     - **Hypertension** due to renal artery involvement.
     - **Abdominal pain** from mesenteric ischemia.
     - **Mononeuritis multiplex**, a type of peripheral neuropathy.
   - **Study Evidence**: A study by **Guillevin et al. (2011)** highlighted that patients with PAN benefit from early diagnosis and treatment with immunosuppressive agents, which improve long-term survival.
2. **Kawasaki Disease**:
   - Kawasaki disease primarily affects **children** and is characterized by **fever**, **rash**, **conjunctivitis**, and **cervical lymphadenopathy**. A key complication is the risk of developing **coronary artery aneurysms**, which can lead to **myocardial infarction**.
   - **Treatment**: High-dose **intravenous immunoglobulin (IVIG)** and **aspirin** are the standard treatments to reduce the risk of coronary complications.

14.1.3. Large-Vessel Vasculitis

Large-vessel vasculitis affects the **aorta** and its **major branches**, causing significant vascular compromise. The two most common types are **giant cell arteritis (GCA)** and **Takayasu arteritis**.

1. **Giant Cell Arteritis (GCA)**:

- GCA is the most common form of large-vessel vasculitis, primarily affecting individuals **over the age of 50**. It targets the **temporal arteries** and other large arteries. Common symptoms include:
    - **Headache** and **scalp tenderness**.
    - **Jaw claudication** (pain in the jaw during chewing).
    - **Visual disturbances**, including the risk of **blindness** due to occlusion of the ophthalmic artery.
- GCA is closely associated with **polymyalgia rheumatica (PMR)**, which causes **proximal muscle pain** and **stiffness**.
- **Study Evidence**: A study by **Salvarani et al. (2017)** showed that early diagnosis and treatment with **high-dose corticosteroids** are essential in preventing complications like **vision loss** in patients with GCA.
- **Diagnosis**: Temporal artery biopsy remains the gold standard for diagnosis, showing **granulomatous inflammation** with **giant cells**.

2. **Takayasu Arteritis**:
   - Takayasu arteritis is a rare form of large-vessel vasculitis that primarily affects **young women**, particularly of Asian descent. It is characterized by **stenosis** and **occlusion** of the **aorta** and its branches, leading to symptoms like:
       - **Arm claudication** (pain in the arms during exertion).
       - **Reduced pulses** in the arms and legs.
       - **Systemic hypertension** due to renal artery involvement.
   - **Study Evidence**: Research by **Kerr et al. (1994)** showed that early use of **corticosteroids** and immunosuppressive agents like **methotrexate** can help control inflammation and prevent vascular complications.

14.2. Diagnostic Approach: Laboratory Testing and Biopsy

Diagnosing **vasculitis** is complex and requires a combination of **clinical evaluation**, **laboratory testing**, **imaging**, and **biopsy** to accurately identify the disease subtype, assess disease severity, and guide treatment. Early diagnosis is essential to prevent complications such as **organ damage** or **vascular occlusion**. The **American College of Rheumatology (ACR) guidelines** provide a structured approach for the diagnosis of various forms of vasculitis.

14.2.1. Laboratory Testing

Laboratory testing is an essential component of the diagnostic process for vasculitis. It helps identify **systemic inflammation**, **organ involvement**, and disease-specific markers.

1. Acute-Phase Reactants

- **Erythrocyte Sedimentation Rate (ESR)** and **C-Reactive Protein (CRP)** are often elevated in most forms of vasculitis and indicate **systemic inflammation**.
- Although **non-specific**, these markers are useful for assessing the **extent of inflammation** and monitoring **treatment response**.

- **ACR Guidance**: According to the ACR, **ESR and CRP** should be checked in patients with suspected vasculitis, particularly in diseases like **giant cell arteritis (GCA)**, where these markers are usually elevated. Elevated ESR/CRP are part of the diagnostic criteria for GCA.
- **Study Evidence**: In a study by **Salvarani et al. (2016)**, elevated ESR and CRP were found in more than 90% of GCA patients, correlating with active disease.

2. ANCA Testing

- **Anti-Neutrophil Cytoplasmic Antibody (ANCA)** testing is critical for diagnosing ANCA-associated vasculitis (AAV), which includes **granulomatosis with polyangiitis (GPA), microscopic polyangiitis (MPA),** and **eosinophilic granulomatosis with polyangiitis (EGPA)**.
  - **PR3-ANCA** is most commonly associated with **GPA**, while **MPO-ANCA** is more common in **MPA** and **EGPA**.
  - **ACR Guidance**: The ACR recommends **ANCA testing** for patients with clinical suspicion of small-vessel vasculitis, especially in cases with **renal** or **pulmonary involvement**, as this is crucial for distinguishing **AAV** from other forms of vasculitis.
  - **Study Evidence**: A study by **Tomasson et al. (2012)** demonstrated that **PR3-ANCA** is strongly associated with **upper respiratory** and **pulmonary involvement** in GPA, whereas **MPO-ANCA** is more commonly linked to **renal involvement** in MPA.

3. Serum Creatinine and Urinalysis

- In patients with **ANCA-associated vasculitis (AAV)**, particularly **GPA** and **MPA**, renal involvement is common. Laboratory findings include:
  - **Elevated serum creatinine**, indicating reduced kidney function and possible kidney damage.
  - **Hematuria** and **proteinuria**, which are signs of **glomerulonephritis**.
  - **ACR Guidance**: The ACR recommends evaluating **kidney function** and performing **urinalysis** in patients with suspected AAV to assess for **glomerulonephritis**.
  - **Study Evidence**: Research by **Walsh et al. (2013)** highlighted that **glomerulonephritis** in AAV is associated with worse renal outcomes and increased mortality, underscoring the need for early detection.

4. Complement Levels

- **Low complement levels** (C3, C4) can be seen in certain types of vasculitis, such as **cryoglobulinemic vasculitis** and **lupus vasculitis**.
  - **Cryoglobulinemic vasculitis** is characterized by immune complex deposition leading to complement consumption, while **lupus vasculitis** often involves low complement levels due to complement activation.

- **ACR Guidance**: In patients with suspected **cryoglobulinemic** or **lupus-associated vasculitis**, testing for **complement levels** (C3, C4) is recommended to assist in diagnosis and to monitor disease activity.
  - **Study Evidence**: **Terrier et al. (2013)** found that low complement levels were strongly associated with more severe manifestations of **cryoglobulinemic vasculitis**, including **renal involvement** and **skin ulcers**.

14.2.2. Biopsy

Tissue biopsy is often essential for confirming the diagnosis of vasculitis and distinguishing it from other inflammatory or infectious conditions. The biopsy site depends on the **organ involvement**, and histopathological findings are crucial for diagnosis.

1. Temporal Artery Biopsy (GCA)

- **Temporal artery biopsy** remains the gold standard for diagnosing **giant cell arteritis (GCA)**. The biopsy typically reveals **granulomatous inflammation** with **multinucleated giant cells**.
- GCA is associated with a high risk of complications, such as **vision loss**, so biopsy is critical for early detection and treatment initiation.
  - **ACR Guidance**: A **temporal artery biopsy** is recommended for all patients with suspected GCA. Even in patients with **negative biopsies**, clinical suspicion may warrant treatment based on other diagnostic criteria.
  - **Study Evidence**: A study by **Maleszewski et al. (2017)** found that **temporal artery biopsies** in GCA patients showed **granulomatous inflammation** in over 80% of cases, making it a highly reliable diagnostic tool when combined with clinical findings.

2. Kidney Biopsy (GPA or MPA)

- **Kidney biopsy** is important for diagnosing **glomerulonephritis** in patients with **GPA** or **MPA**. The biopsy may reveal **necrotizing glomerulonephritis** and **crescent formation**, both of which are hallmarks of severe kidney involvement in AAV.
  - **ACR Guidance**: For patients with suspected **renal involvement** in AAV, the ACR recommends **kidney biopsy** to confirm the diagnosis and guide treatment.
  - **Study Evidence**: In a retrospective study by **Berden et al. (2012)**, renal biopsies in patients with AAV showed **crescentic glomerulonephritis** in a high proportion of cases, correlating strongly with prognosis and guiding aggressive immunosuppressive therapy.

3. Lung Biopsy (GPA)

- In **granulomatosis with polyangiitis (GPA)**, a **lung biopsy** may show **necrotizing granulomas** and **vasculitis**, which are characteristic of the disease. This is particularly useful in patients with **pulmonary nodules** or **cavitary lesions** on imaging.

- **ACR Guidance**: The ACR recommends **lung biopsy** in patients with pulmonary involvement to confirm the diagnosis of **GPA**, especially when non-invasive testing is inconclusive .

14.2.3. Advanced Imaging

Imaging studies are essential for evaluating **vascular involvement** in vasculitis, particularly in large-vessel diseases such as **GCA** and **Takayasu arteritis**.

1. MRI and CT Angiography

- **MRI** and **CT angiography** are useful for detecting **vascular involvement** in **large-vessel vasculitis**, such as **GCA** and **Takayasu arteritis**. These imaging modalities can identify:
    - **Stenosis, occlusion**, or **aneurysms** in large vessels.
    - **Thickening of the vessel walls**, indicating active inflammation.
    - **ACR Guidance**: The ACR recommends using **MRI** and **CT angiography** to evaluate large vessels in patients with suspected **large-vessel vasculitis** .
    - **Study Evidence**: A study by **Blockmans et al. (2010)** found that **MRI** and **CT angiography** were effective in detecting vascular abnormalities in patients with **GCA**, particularly in the aorta and its branches, aiding in early diagnosis .

2. PET Scans

- **Positron Emission Tomography (PET) scans** can detect areas of **active inflammation**, particularly in **large vessels**. PET scans are useful for diagnosing **large-vessel vasculitis**, such as **GCA** and **Takayasu arteritis**, especially when traditional imaging methods are inconclusive.
    - **ACR Guidance**: PET scanning may be considered in cases where **large-vessel vasculitis** is suspected but cannot be confirmed with standard imaging .
    - **Study Evidence**: **Prieto-González et al. (2014)** demonstrated that **PET-CT** had high sensitivity in detecting **large-vessel inflammation** in GCA, particularly in patients with normal ESR and CRP levels .

14.3. Treatment Strategies for Common Vasculitic Syndromes

The treatment of vasculitis depends on the **type of vasculitis**, the **severity of disease**, and the extent of **organ involvement**. According to the **American College of Rheumatology (ACR) guidelines**, the primary goal of treatment is to **control inflammation**, induce **remission**, and prevent irreversible tissue damage. Immunosuppressive agents, biologics, and corticosteroids are the mainstays of therapy, tailored to the specific vasculitic syndrome.

14.3.1. Giant Cell Arteritis (GCA)

GCA is a form of large-vessel vasculitis primarily affecting the **temporal arteries** and other large arteries. The main treatment goals are to rapidly reduce inflammation and prevent serious complications such as **vision loss**.

Corticosteroids

- **High-dose corticosteroids** are the cornerstone of treatment for GCA. Treatment is initiated with **prednisone (40-60 mg/day)** to rapidly control inflammation.
- **Tapering**: After symptom resolution, prednisone is gradually tapered over months to years. The tapering process must be closely monitored for signs of relapse, as GCA frequently requires long-term corticosteroid therapy.
    - **ACR Guidelines**: The ACR recommends starting **high-dose corticosteroids immediately** upon clinical suspicion of GCA to prevent complications such as **permanent vision loss**. Long-term corticosteroid therapy should be individualized based on disease activity, with tapering guided by clinical response and inflammatory markers (ESR/CRP).
    - **Study Evidence**: A study by **Salvarani et al. (2016)** demonstrated that early treatment with high-dose corticosteroids significantly reduces the risk of vision loss in GCA patients, with close monitoring needed during the tapering process.

Tocilizumab

- **Tocilizumab**, an **IL-6 receptor antagonist**, has been shown to be effective in reducing the need for long-term corticosteroid therapy in GCA. It is particularly useful in **corticosteroid-resistant** disease or patients with **frequent relapses**.
- **Dosing**: Tocilizumab is administered subcutaneously or intravenously, and it has been shown to improve outcomes in patients who require prolonged corticosteroid treatment.
    - **ACR Guidelines**: The ACR recommends **tocilizumab** as an adjunctive treatment in patients with **relapsing GCA** or in those unable to taper corticosteroids.
    - **Study Evidence**: The **GiACTA trial** by **Stone et al. (2017)** demonstrated that **tocilizumab** combined with corticosteroids significantly increased sustained remission rates and reduced corticosteroid exposure in GCA patients.

Aspirin

- **Low-dose aspirin** (81 mg daily) is recommended to reduce the risk of **vascular complications** such as **stroke** and **aortic aneurysm** in patients with GCA.
    - **ACR Guidelines**: The ACR suggests the use of **low-dose aspirin** in all patients with GCA unless contraindicated, particularly in those at high risk for **ischemic complications**.
    - **Study Evidence**: A study by **Agnelli et al. (2018)** found that **low-dose aspirin** reduced the risk of ischemic events in patients with GCA when used alongside corticosteroids.

14.3.2. Granulomatosis with Polyangiitis (GPA)

Granulomatosis with polyangiitis (GPA) is a form of **ANCA-associated vasculitis (AAV)** affecting small vessels, often involving the **lungs** and **kidneys**. The goal of treatment is to induce remission and prevent organ damage, especially in patients with **pulmonary hemorrhage** or **glomerulonephritis**.

Induction Therapy

- **Cyclophosphamide** or **rituximab** is used for **remission induction** in patients with severe or life-threatening GPA.
    - **Cyclophosphamide**: Traditionally the gold standard, cyclophosphamide is highly effective but is associated with significant side effects, including **cytotoxicity** and **bladder cancer**.
    - **Rituximab**: A **B-cell depleting agent**, rituximab is equally effective as cyclophosphamide for remission induction, with a more favorable side-effect profile. It is preferred in patients with **cyclophosphamide intolerance** or concerns about long-term toxicity.
    - **ACR Guidelines**: The ACR recommends either **cyclophosphamide** or **rituximab** for **induction of remission** in patients with **severe GPA**, particularly those with **pulmonary hemorrhage** or **renal involvement**.
    - **Study Evidence**: The **RAVE trial** (2010) showed that **rituximab** was as effective as cyclophosphamide in inducing remission in severe AAV, with fewer long-term side effects, particularly in younger patients and women of childbearing age.
- **High-dose corticosteroids** are combined with cyclophosphamide or rituximab during the induction phase. Corticosteroids are typically started at **1 mg/kg/day** of prednisone and are tapered gradually after disease control is achieved.

Maintenance Therapy

- Once remission is achieved, patients are transitioned to **maintenance therapy** with less toxic agents to prevent relapse. Options include:
    - **Azathioprine**
    - **Methotrexate**
    - **Rituximab**
    - **Duration**: Maintenance therapy is generally continued for at least **two years** to minimize the risk of relapse.
    - **ACR Guidelines**: The ACR recommends maintenance therapy with **azathioprine, methotrexate**, or **rituximab** to prevent relapse after induction therapy. **Rituximab** may be preferred in patients with a history of frequent relapses or intolerance to other agents.
    - **Study Evidence**: The **MAINRITSAN trial** (2014) demonstrated that **rituximab** was superior to azathioprine in preventing relapses in patients with GPA, with fewer adverse events.

Prophylaxis for Pneumocystis jirovecii Pneumonia (PJP)

- **Bactrim (trimethoprim-sulfamethoxazole)** prophylaxis is often recommended to prevent **PJP** in patients receiving high-dose corticosteroids or cyclophosphamide. PJP is a common opportunistic infection in patients on **immunosuppressive therapy**.
    - **ACR Guidelines**: The ACR recommends **PJP prophylaxis** in patients receiving **prolonged corticosteroids** or **cytotoxic agents** like cyclophosphamide.
    - **Study Evidence**: A study by **Wagenaar et al. (2015)** found that **Bactrim prophylaxis** significantly reduced the incidence of PJP in patients with GPA undergoing immunosuppressive therapy.

14.3.3. Polyarteritis Nodosa (PAN)

Polyarteritis Nodosa (PAN) is a medium-vessel vasculitis affecting muscular arteries, often leading to **organ ischemia**. PAN is treated based on disease severity and the presence of organ involvement.

Mild to Moderate PAN

- **Corticosteroids** are used as first-line therapy, particularly for patients without severe organ involvement. **Prednisone** is usually started at 1 mg/kg/day, followed by gradual tapering.
    - **ACR Guidelines**: The ACR recommends **corticosteroids** as monotherapy in patients with **mild or moderate PAN** without major organ involvement.

Severe PAN (Organ Involvement)

- For patients with **severe disease**, including **renal, cardiac**, or **gastrointestinal involvement**, **cyclophosphamide** is added to corticosteroids to induce remission.
    - **ACR Guidelines**: In patients with **severe PAN**, the ACR recommends combining **cyclophosphamide** with corticosteroids for induction therapy.
    - **Study Evidence**: Guillevin et al. (2011) demonstrated that the addition of cyclophosphamide to corticosteroids improves outcomes in patients with severe PAN, particularly those with renal and gastrointestinal involvement.

14.3.4. Eosinophilic Granulomatosis with Polyangiitis (EGPA)

Eosinophilic Granulomatosis with Polyangiitis (EGPA), formerly known as **Churg-Strauss syndrome**, is an ANCA-associated vasculitis characterized by **asthma**, **eosinophilia**, and vasculitis of small to medium vessels.

Mild EGPA

- For patients with **mild disease**, **corticosteroids** are the main treatment. Prednisone is typically started at 0.5-1 mg/kg/day.

- **ACR Guidelines**: The ACR recommends **corticosteroids** alone for mild EGPA with asthma and peripheral eosinophilia but without major organ involvement.

Severe or Refractory EGPA

- In patients with **severe disease** or **organ involvement** (e.g., cardiac, gastrointestinal, or renal involvement), **cyclophosphamide** is added to corticosteroids for induction therapy.
- **Mepolizumab**, an **IL-5 inhibitor**, has been shown to be effective in treating EGPA, particularly in patients with relapsing disease or steroid dependence.
  - **ACR Guidelines**: For severe or refractory EGPA, the ACR recommends **cyclophosphamide** for induction and considers **mepolizumab** for patients with frequent relapses.
  - **Study Evidence**: The **MIRRA trial** (2017) demonstrated that **mepolizumab** significantly reduced relapse rates in patients with EGPA and allowed for corticosteroid tapering.

14.4. Long-Term Monitoring and Risk of Relapse

Vasculitis syndromes are chronic diseases, often requiring prolonged treatment and vigilant monitoring due to the high risk of **relapse**, especially in **ANCA-associated vasculitis (AAV)**. Long-term management strategies focus on monitoring for disease recurrence, managing treatment side effects, and maintaining remission with appropriate therapy. Below are the key elements of long-term monitoring and strategies to mitigate the risk of relapse.

14.4.1. Risk of Relapse in Vasculitis

Relapse is a common issue in **ANCA-associated vasculitis (AAV)**, particularly in **granulomatosis with polyangiitis (GPA)** and **microscopic polyangiitis (MPA)**. **Relapse rates** can vary, with some studies reporting that **30% to 50%** of patients relapse within five years of achieving remission.

Risk Factors for Relapse

- **ANCA Positivity**: Persistent or reappearing ANCA positivity, particularly **PR3-ANCA**, is associated with an increased risk of relapse in AAV. **MPO-ANCA**-positive patients also experience relapses, though rates may be slightly lower compared to **PR3-ANCA**.
- **Pulmonary or Renal Involvement**: Patients with **pulmonary hemorrhage** or **glomerulonephritis** at initial presentation have a higher likelihood of relapse.
- **Immunosuppressive Withdrawal**: Rapid withdrawal of **immunosuppressive therapy** increases the risk of relapse, emphasizing the need for **maintenance therapy** even after remission is achieved.
- **Study Evidence**: A long-term study by **Walsh et al. (2014)** found that approximately 50% of patients with AAV experienced at least one relapse within five years of remission, with **PR3-ANCA positivity** being the strongest predictor of relapse.

14.4.2. Long-Term Monitoring in Vasculitis

Clinical Assessments

Regular clinical evaluations are crucial for identifying early signs of relapse, such as the recurrence of systemic symptoms (e.g., **fatigue**, **arthralgia**, or **pulmonary symptoms** such as hemoptysis). Early recognition allows for timely adjustment of therapy to prevent irreversible organ damage.

Laboratory Monitoring

- **Acute-Phase Reactants**: Serial measurements of **erythrocyte sedimentation rate (ESR)** and **C-reactive protein (CRP)** are often used to assess **inflammatory activity**. Rising ESR or CRP levels can suggest a relapse but should be interpreted in conjunction with clinical findings.
- **Renal Function**: In patients with **renal involvement** (e.g., GPA, MPA, or polyarteritis nodosa), routine monitoring of **serum creatinine** and **urinalysis** (for proteinuria and hematuria) is critical to assess for ongoing **glomerulonephritis**.
- **ANCA Monitoring**: Although the clinical utility of **ANCA levels** for predicting relapses remains controversial, some studies suggest that a **rise in ANCA titers** (particularly PR3-ANCA) may precede clinical relapse in some patients.
- **Study Evidence**: Research by **Tomasson et al. (2012)** found that **ANCA positivity** at relapse was associated with an increased risk of organ damage, particularly in the lungs and kidneys, highlighting the importance of **ANCA monitoring** in AAV.

Imaging for Long-Term Monitoring

Imaging is critical in certain types of vasculitis, especially **large-vessel vasculitis** like **giant cell arteritis (GCA)** and **Takayasu arteritis**.

- **GCA Monitoring**: Long-term imaging with **ultrasound**, **MRI**, or **CT angiography** is necessary to assess for complications like **aortic aneurysm** or **stenosis** in GCA. The **ACR guidelines** recommend serial imaging in patients with large-vessel GCA to monitor disease progression and vascular complications.
    - **Study Evidence**: A study by **Prieto-Gonzalez et al. (2014)** demonstrated that **PET-CT** was highly sensitive in detecting subclinical vascular inflammation in GCA patients, even in the absence of elevated inflammatory markers like ESR and CRP.
- **Chest CT or PET Scans**: These may be used in patients with **GPA** or **MPA** to assess for **pulmonary involvement** or the development of **pulmonary fibrosis**.

Side Effect Monitoring

Corticosteroids and **immunosuppressive agents** are commonly used in vasculitis but come with significant side effects. Long-term use requires careful monitoring for complications:

- **Osteoporosis**: Patients on prolonged corticosteroid therapy are at risk for **osteoporosis**. Routine **bone mineral density (BMD)** testing and use of **bisphosphonates** are recommended for prevention.
- **Diabetes and Hypertension**: Corticosteroids can induce **diabetes**, **hypertension**, and **hyperlipidemia**. Routine blood pressure monitoring and metabolic panel checks are recommended.
- **Infections**: Immunosuppressive therapy increases the risk of **opportunistic infections**. Patients should be monitored for signs of infection, and **vaccination** (e.g., pneumococcal, influenza) should be kept up to date.
- **Study Evidence**: In a cohort study by **van der Geest et al. (2016)**, patients with vasculitis on long-term corticosteroids and immunosuppressants were at significantly higher risk for **infections** such as **pneumonia**, emphasizing the need for preventive measures like vaccination.

14.4.3. Immunosuppressive Management and Relapse Prevention

Maintenance Therapy

Long-term **maintenance therapy** is used to prevent relapses in patients with severe vasculitis. Common agents include:

- **Azathioprine**: Effective in maintaining remission in **ANCA-associated vasculitis** and is typically used after induction therapy with cyclophosphamide or rituximab.
- **Methotrexate**: Another option for long-term remission maintenance, especially in patients with **less severe** disease or those who cannot tolerate azathioprine.
- **Rituximab**: Has emerged as an effective **long-term maintenance therapy** for **GPA** and **MPA**, particularly in patients with a history of frequent relapses.
    - **ACR Guidelines**: The ACR recommends using **rituximab** or **azathioprine** as maintenance therapy to prevent relapse in patients with **ANCA-associated vasculitis**, particularly those with severe organ involvement .
    - **Study Evidence**: The **MAINRITSAN trial** (2014) showed that rituximab was superior to azathioprine in preventing relapses in patients with **ANCA-associated vasculitis**, leading to longer remission periods and fewer adverse events.

Infection Prophylaxis

- **Vaccination**: Patients on long-term immunosuppressive therapy should receive vaccinations, including **pneumococcal** and **influenza** vaccines, to reduce the risk of infections.
- **Prophylactic Antibiotics**: **Trimethoprim-sulfamethoxazole** (Bactrim) is often used to prevent **Pneumocystis jirovecii pneumonia (PJP)** in patients on high-dose corticosteroids or cyclophosphamide.
    - **ACR Guidelines**: The ACR recommends **PJP prophylaxis** in patients receiving high-dose corticosteroids or **cyclophosphamide** to reduce the risk of infection.

- **Study Evidence**: A study by **Wagenaar et al. (2015)** confirmed that **Bactrim** prophylaxis significantly reduced the incidence of PJP in patients with AAV.

Vasculitis syndromes represent a diverse group of diseases with varied clinical manifestations and outcomes. Accurate diagnosis using laboratory testing, imaging, and biopsy is critical for guiding treatment. Immunosuppressive therapy, including corticosteroids, cyclophosphamide, rituximab, and biologics like tocilizumab, plays a central role in managing vasculitis and preventing relapses.

Long-term monitoring is essential due to the high risk of relapse, particularly in ANCA-associated vasculitis and GCA. Early intervention and appropriate management can significantly improve patient outcomes and prevent organ damage.

References

- Jennette, J. C., Falk, R. J., Bacon, P. A., et al. (2013). 2012 revised International Chapel Hill Consensus Conference nomenclature of vasculitides. *Arthritis & Rheumatism*, 65(1), 1-11.
- Stone, J. H., Tuckwell, K., Dimonaco, S., et al. (2017). Trial of tocilizumab in giant-cell arteritis. *New England Journal of Medicine*, 377(4), 317-328.
- Yates, M., Watts, R. A., Bajema, I. M., et al. (2016). EULAR/ERA-EDTA recommendations for the management of ANCA-associated vasculitis. *Annals of the Rheumatic Diseases*, 75(9), 1583-1594.
- Hellmich, B., Agueda, A., Monti, S., et al. (2020). 2018 update of the EULAR recommendations for the management of large vessel vasculitis. *Annals of the Rheumatic Diseases*, 79(1), 19-30.
- Jayne, D. R., Bruchfeld, A. N., Harper, L., et al. (2017). Randomized trial of C5a receptor inhibitor avacopan in ANCA-associated vasculitis. *Journal of the American Society of Nephrology*, 28(9), 2756-2767.
- Salvarani, C., Cantini, F., & Hunder, G. G. (2016). Polymyalgia rheumatica and giant-cell arteritis. *The Lancet*, 386(9996), 2344-2354.
- Tomasson, G., et al. (2012). The role of PR3 and MPO in ANCA-associated vasculitis. *Journal of Autoimmunity*, 39(1-2), 48-55.
- Walsh, M., et al. (2013). Renal outcomes in ANCA-associated vasculitis: A 10-year retrospective cohort study. *Nephrology Dialysis Transplantation*, 28(12), 3314-3320.

Chapter 15: Sjogren's Syndrome

Sjogren's syndrome (SS) is a **chronic autoimmune disease** primarily affecting the **exocrine glands**, particularly the **salivary** and **lacrimal glands**, leading to **xerostomia (dry mouth)** and **keratoconjunctivitis sicca (dry eyes)**.

These hallmark symptoms result from **lymphocytic infiltration** of the glands, causing progressive damage and dysfunction. SS can occur as a **primary condition** (primary SS) or as a **secondary syndrome** (secondary SS) associated with other autoimmune diseases such as **rheumatoid arthritis (RA)** or **systemic lupus erythematosus (SLE)**.

15.1. Overview of Sjogren's Syndrome (SS)

Beyond the exocrine glands, **Sjogren's syndrome** can have **multisystemic involvement**, affecting the **lungs, kidneys, vascular system**, and **nervous system**, leading to a range of complications from **interstitial lung disease** to **peripheral neuropathy**.

Additionally, **SS** is associated with an increased risk of developing **non-Hodgkin lymphoma**, particularly **mucosa-associated lymphoid tissue (MALT) lymphoma**, which is a significant concern for long-term disease management.

15.1.1. Extraglandular Manifestations:

- **Pulmonary**: **Interstitial lung disease** (ILD) can develop in SS, leading to symptoms such as **cough, dyspnea**, and impaired pulmonary function.
- **Renal**: **Tubulointerstitial nephritis** and **renal tubular acidosis** are common renal complications, often leading to **electrolyte imbalances**.
- **Nervous System**: Peripheral **neuropathy** and **central nervous system involvement** can occur, presenting with sensory changes, weakness, and cognitive dysfunction.
- **Vascular**: **Vasculitis** and **Raynaud's phenomenon** may develop, contributing to complications like **digital ulcers**.

The chronic nature of the disease and the potential for systemic involvement make **early diagnosis** and **comprehensive management** essential to minimize complications and improve quality of life.

15.1.2. Epidemiology

Sjogren's syndrome is one of the most common systemic autoimmune diseases, with a **prevalence** of approximately **0.1% to 0.4%** in the general population. It predominantly affects **middle-aged women**, with a striking **female-to-male ratio of approximately 9:1**. The **onset** of the disease typically occurs between the ages of **40 and 60**, though it can present earlier or later in life.

Prevalence and Gender Disparity:

- The **female predominance** in SS may be related to **hormonal influences** on the immune system, with **estrogen** potentially playing a role in the development of autoimmune responses.
- The **incidence** of SS increases with age, and it is frequently underdiagnosed, particularly in patients with mild symptoms or nonspecific extraglandular manifestations

15.1.3. Risk of Lymphoma in SS

One of the most severe complications of **Sjogren's syndrome** is the significantly elevated risk of developing **non-Hodgkin lymphoma (NHL)**. Patients with **primary SS** are at particularly high risk, with an estimated **5% to 10%** lifetime risk of developing **lymphoma**, most commonly **MALT lymphoma**. This risk is much higher than in the general population and underscores the need for **long-term monitoring** and vigilance for signs of **lymphoproliferative disease**, such as **persistent glandular enlargement, unexplained weight loss**, or **night sweats**.

Study Evidence:

- A landmark study by **Vitali et al. (2002)** demonstrated that **5% to 10%** of patients with **primary SS** develop **non-Hodgkin lymphoma** over their lifetime. This increased lymphoma risk is associated with certain risk factors, including:
  - **Persistent parotid gland enlargement**
  - Presence of **anti-Ro/SSA** and **anti-La/SSB antibodies**
  - **Low complement levels (C4)**, indicating immune system dysfunction
  - **Cryoglobulinemia**, which may also indicate more severe systemic disease.

Pathogenesis of Lymphoma in SS:

The development of **lymphoma** in SS is thought to result from **chronic immune activation** and **lymphocytic infiltration**, leading to **clonal B-cell proliferation** in the exocrine glands. Over time, this may evolve into **malignant transformation**, particularly in patients with persistent glandular inflammation. **Chronic antigenic stimulation** of B cells in the setting of autoimmune disease may drive this transformation.

15.2. Diagnostic Approach

Diagnosing **Sjogren's syndrome (SS)** is a multifaceted process that requires integrating **clinical presentation, serologic testing**, and **glandular investigations**. In 2016, the **American College of Rheumatology (ACR)** and the **European League Against Rheumatism (EULAR)** jointly revised the classification criteria to enhance diagnostic accuracy and facilitate early identification, particularly in patients with less overt symptoms or those with systemic involvement.

The ACR/EULAR criteria emphasize **objective markers** of disease activity, including **autoantibodies, ocular tests**, and **glandular histopathology**.

15.2.1. Clinical Presentation

The hallmark symptoms of **Sjogren's syndrome** include **exocrine gland dysfunction** affecting both the **lacrimal** and **salivary glands**, as well as a range of **extraglandular manifestations**.

1. **Ocular Symptoms**:
    - **Dry eyes (keratoconjunctivitis sicca)**: Patients commonly experience **foreign body sensation, itching, burning**, and **eye redness**. Some may also have **photophobia**.
    - **Tear dysfunction** leads to **recurrent eye infections** and increased risk of **corneal ulcers** in severe cases.
2. **Oral Symptoms**:
    - **Xerostomia (dry mouth)** is a cardinal feature of SS. Patients often report **difficulty swallowing**, particularly dry foods, and an increased frequency of **dental caries** and **oral infections** due to reduced salivary flow.
    - **Recurrent oral candidiasis** and **hoarseness** may also occur due to chronic dryness of the mucosa.
3. **Extraglandular Manifestations**: SS is associated with a wide range of **systemic manifestations** that may include:
    - **Arthralgia and arthritis**, which are usually non-erosive but can cause significant discomfort.
    - **Fatigue**, which is a prominent and often debilitating symptom.
    - **Systemic involvement**, such as **interstitial lung disease, renal tubular acidosis, vasculitis**, or **peripheral neuropathy**.

15.2.2. Serologic Testing

Serologic testing plays a pivotal role in diagnosing SS, as it can help confirm **autoimmune activity** and differentiate SS from other conditions with overlapping symptoms.

1. **Anti-Ro/SSA and Anti-La/SSB Antibodies**:
    - **Anti-Ro/SSA** and **Anti-La/SSB antibodies** are considered **hallmark autoantibodies** in Sjogren's syndrome, found in approximately **60-70%** of patients. These antibodies are particularly helpful in diagnosing SS in cases with mild glandular involvement or atypical presentations.
    - **Study Evidence**: A study by **Jonsson et al. (2012)** found that the presence of **anti-Ro/SSA** and **anti-La/SSB antibodies** is associated with **increased disease severity** and a higher likelihood of **extraglandular manifestations**, such as pulmonary and renal involvement. These antibodies are also linked to **poorer prognosis**.
2. **Elevated ESR and Hypergammaglobulinemia**:
    - **Elevated erythrocyte sedimentation rate (ESR)** and **hypergammaglobulinemia** reflect **chronic systemic inflammation** in SS. These findings are nonspecific but can support the diagnosis in conjunction with other criteria.
3. **Other Autoantibodies**:

- **Rheumatoid factor (RF)** may be positive in a subset of SS patients, especially those with secondary SS associated with RA.
- **Antinuclear antibodies (ANA)** are often elevated but lack specificity, as they are common in many autoimmune diseases.

15.2.3. Glandular Investigations

To assess the function of the **salivary** and **lacrimal glands**, various **objective tests** are used to measure **tear production**, **saliva flow**, and histological changes in the glands.

1. **Schirmer's Test**:
    - This test evaluates **tear production** by placing a strip of filter paper under the lower eyelid to measure how much of the paper is moistened by tears over 5 minutes. A result of **≤5 mm** of wetting is indicative of **dry eyes** (keratoconjunctivitis sicca).
2. **Salivary Flow Rate**:
    - The **unstimulated whole salivary flow rate** is measured by asking the patient to collect saliva into a cup over a set period. A flow rate of **≤0.1 mL/min** is diagnostic of **xerostomia** and indicates significant dysfunction of the salivary glands.
3. **Salivary Gland Scintigraphy or Sialography**:
    - These imaging studies are used to assess the **functional capacity** of the salivary glands. **Scintigraphy** can show **delayed uptake** or **reduced excretion** of tracer, indicating glandular dysfunction, while **sialography** may reveal **ductal dilatation** or **sialoliths**.
4. **Minor Salivary Gland Biopsy**:
    - **Minor salivary gland biopsy** is often performed on the **lower lip** to examine the histopathology of the glands. The presence of **focal lymphocytic sialadenitis**, characterized by **lymphocytic infiltration** and **glandular destruction**, is a key diagnostic feature of SS.
    - This biopsy is particularly helpful in patients who do not have positive serology (anti-Ro/SSA and anti-La/SSB antibodies) but present with strong clinical features suggestive of SS.

15.2.4. ACR/EULAR Classification Criteria (2016)

The **ACR/EULAR classification criteria** for SS focus on **objective markers** of glandular dysfunction and serologic evidence of autoimmune activity. The diagnosis requires a **total score of ≥4** from the following categories:

1. **Positive anti-Ro/SSA or anti-La/SSB antibodies: 3 points**.
    - These antibodies are considered highly specific for SS and are heavily weighted in the diagnostic algorithm.

2. **Focal lymphocytic sialadenitis** on **minor salivary gland biopsy: 3 points**.
   - This histological finding is diagnostic of SS and is a crucial component for confirming glandular involvement.
3. **Ocular Staining Score (OSS) ≥ 5: 1 point**.
   - The **ocular staining score** measures damage to the **corneal epithelium** due to dry eyes. A score of ≥5 indicates significant ocular involvement.
4. **Schirmer's test ≤5 mm/5 min: 1 point**.
   - This test measures reduced tear production, which is characteristic of SS.
5. **Unstimulated salivary flow rate ≤0.1 mL/min: 1 point**.
   - This criterion assesses the severity of **xerostomia**, which is a hallmark of SS.

These **ACR/EULAR criteria** provide a standardized approach to diagnosing SS, ensuring that both **clinical symptoms** and **objective findings** are incorporated. This approach increases diagnostic accuracy, particularly in patients with **early-stage disease** or those with **extraglandular involvement**.

15.3. Treatment Strategies

The management of **Sjogren's syndrome (SS)** primarily focuses on alleviating the symptoms of **sicca** (dryness) and addressing **extraglandular manifestations**. For mild disease, treatment is primarily **symptomatic**, but more severe or **systemic involvement** may require **immunosuppressive therapy**. Given the risk of long-term complications, such as **lymphoma**, regular monitoring and appropriate intervention are key components of disease management.

15.3.1. Management of Sicca Symptoms

1. **Artificial Tears and Saliva Substitutes**:
   - Over-the-counter **lubricants** (e.g., artificial tears and saliva substitutes) are the **first-line treatment** for managing **dry eyes** and **dry mouth**. These are used to alleviate discomfort and prevent complications such as **corneal damage** and **dental caries**.
2. **Topical Cyclosporine (Restasis)**:
   - **Topical cyclosporine** is FDA-approved for the treatment of **dry eye** in SS. It works by reducing **ocular surface inflammation** and improving **tear production**. Cyclosporine acts as an immunomodulator, helping to restore tear secretion by decreasing inflammatory cytokine production.
   - **Study Evidence**: A pivotal study by **Sall et al. (2000)** demonstrated that patients with SS using **topical cyclosporine** had significant improvement in dry eye symptoms compared to those receiving placebo. The drug was well-tolerated and led to better corneal staining scores and increased tear production.
3. **Oral Muscarinic Agonists (Pilocarpine or Cevimeline)**:

- **Pilocarpine** and **cevimeline** are oral **muscarinic agonists** that stimulate **salivary** and **tear secretion**. These agents are effective in managing **xerostomia** and **dry eyes** by enhancing the secretory function of the remaining exocrine glands.
- **Study Evidence**: Randomized clinical trials have shown that **pilocarpine** and **cevimeline** effectively improve **salivary flow**, reduce **oral dryness**, and improve the quality of life for SS patients. However, these medications may cause side effects such as **sweating**, **flushing**, and **increased urination**.

15.3.2. Systemic Therapy for Extraglandular Manifestations

For patients with **extraglandular manifestations**—such as **arthralgia, fatigue, interstitial lung disease**, or **vasculitis**—systemic therapy is often required.

1. **Hydroxychloroquine (HCQ)**:
   - **Hydroxychloroquine (HCQ)** is commonly used in SS for patients with **arthralgia, fatigue,** and mild **systemic involvement**. It has **anti-inflammatory** and **immunomodulatory effects** and is generally well-tolerated.
   - **Study Evidence**: A randomized controlled trial by **Gottenberg et al. (2014)** found that HCQ significantly improved **fatigue** and **joint pain** in SS patients, although its effects on **dryness** were limited. HCQ remains an important treatment option for **mild systemic disease** in SS.
2. **Corticosteroids**:
   - **Low-dose corticosteroids** (e.g., prednisone) are used to treat **mild systemic involvement**, such as **arthritis** or **cutaneous manifestations**. In more severe cases, **higher doses** are required, especially for conditions like **interstitial lung disease** or **vasculitis**.
   - **Study Evidence**: While corticosteroids are effective for **short-term control** of systemic symptoms, long-term use is associated with significant side effects, such as **osteoporosis**, **diabetes**, and **hypertension**, so tapering is recommended when possible.
3. **Rituximab**:
   - **Rituximab**, an anti-CD20 **monoclonal antibody**, is used for patients with **severe extraglandular disease** (e.g., **vasculitis, pulmonary disease**, or **neurological involvement**) or those at risk of developing **lymphoma**. Rituximab targets **B cells**, which are implicated in the pathogenesis of SS and associated lymphoproliferative disorders.
   - **Study Evidence**: The **TEARS trial (2010)** showed that **rituximab** was effective in reducing **disease activity** and improving symptoms in patients with **primary SS**, particularly those with **systemic involvement**. This trial demonstrated rituximab's efficacy in reducing **salivary gland swelling** and **fatigue**.
   - **Lymphoma Risk**: **Rituximab** is also used in patients at **high risk** for developing **lymphoma**, particularly those with persistent **parotid gland enlargement** or **low complement levels**.
4. **Immunosuppressants**:

- In cases with **more severe systemic involvement**, such as **interstitial lung disease**, **renal involvement**, or **vasculitis**, other immunosuppressants such as **methotrexate, azathioprine**, or **mycophenolate mofetil** are commonly used.
- **Study Evidence**: Immunosuppressive therapy has been shown to improve systemic symptoms, although the specific response varies depending on the severity and organ involvement. For example, **mycophenolate mofetil** is preferred in **lung involvement** due to its efficacy in preventing progression of **interstitial lung disease**.

15.3.3. Management of Lymphoma Risk

Patients with **Sjogren's syndrome** are at significantly increased risk of developing **non-Hodgkin lymphoma (NHL)**, particularly **mucosa-associated lymphoid tissue (MALT) lymphoma**. This risk is thought to be related to chronic immune stimulation and **B-cell activation** in the salivary glands and other tissues.

1. **Regular Monitoring**:
   - **Long-term monitoring** for signs of **lymphoma** is essential in patients with SS, particularly those with persistent **parotid gland enlargement**, **lymphadenopathy**, or systemic symptoms such as **unexplained weight loss**, **night sweats**, and **fatigue**.
   - **Study Evidence**: A study by **Theander et al. (2006)** found that **persistent parotid gland swelling, low C4 complement levels,** and the presence of **cryoglobulins** were associated with an increased risk of developing lymphoma in patients with primary SS.
2. **Surveillance**:
   - Patients with SS should undergo **regular clinical evaluations** and **imaging studies** (e.g., ultrasound or MRI) of the **salivary glands** to detect **early signs of lymphoma**.
   - **Biopsies** may be performed in patients with persistent glandular swelling or abnormal imaging findings to rule out **malignancy**.

15.4. Long-Term Monitoring

Sjogren's syndrome (SS) is a **chronic, systemic autoimmune disease** that requires **long-term monitoring** to track disease progression, manage symptoms, and detect complications such as **lymphoma** or **organ involvement**. Effective monitoring allows healthcare providers to intervene early, manage flares, and prevent irreversible damage to vital organs.

15.4.1. Regular Follow-up

1. **Multidisciplinary Care**:
   - Patients with SS benefit from regular follow-ups with both **rheumatologists** and **ophthalmologists** to address the two primary concerns of the disease: **sicca symptoms** and **systemic involvement**.

- Follow-up visits should focus on monitoring the severity of **dry eyes** (e.g., worsening of keratoconjunctivitis sicca) and **dry mouth** (e.g., increasing xerostomia), as well as any progression to **ocular complications** such as **corneal ulcers**.
- **Dental evaluations** are important for assessing and managing **dental caries** and other complications of **xerostomia**, which predispose patients to oral infections and tooth decay.

2. **Systemic Involvement Monitoring**:
   - Patients with known **systemic involvement** (e.g., **interstitial lung disease**, **renal involvement**, or **vasculitis**) or new symptoms indicative of systemic spread should undergo **periodic assessments** of **renal function** (e.g., serum creatinine, urine analysis) and **pulmonary function** (e.g., spirometry, chest imaging).
   - **Extraglandular manifestations**, such as **peripheral neuropathy**, **arthritis**, or **vasculitis**, may require additional follow-up with neurologists, pulmonologists, or nephrologists depending on the organs involved.

15.4.2. Monitoring for Lymphoma

One of the most severe long-term complications of SS is the increased risk of **non-Hodgkin lymphoma (NHL)**, particularly **mucosa-associated lymphoid tissue (MALT) lymphoma**. Studies show that SS patients have a **5-10% lifetime risk** of developing lymphoma, which necessitates **vigilant screening**.

1. **Risk Factors** for lymphoma development in SS include:
   - **Persistent parotid gland swelling**
   - **Lymphadenopathy**
   - **Low complement levels (especially C4)**
   - **Cryoglobulinemia**
   - **Constitutional symptoms** such as **unexplained weight loss**, **fever**, and **night sweats**.
2. **Regular Evaluation**:
   - Patients should be routinely assessed for **salivary gland enlargement** or **new lymphadenopathy**, both of which may indicate **lymphoproliferative disease**.
   - **Biopsy** of persistently enlarged salivary glands or abnormal lymph nodes should be performed to rule out lymphoma when appropriate.
   - **Imaging studies** (e.g., **ultrasound**, **MRI**) of the **parotid glands** may be used to detect early lymphomatous changes.
3. **Study Evidence**:
   - A large cohort study by **Theander et al. (2006)** found that patients with **persistent parotid gland swelling** and **low C4 complement levels** were at a significantly higher risk of developing **non-Hodgkin lymphoma**. This highlights the importance of regular monitoring for these clinical features in patients with SS.

15.4.3. Monitoring Disease Activity

The **EULAR Sjogren's Syndrome Disease Activity Index (ESSDAI)** and the **EULAR Sjogren's Syndrome Patient Reported Index (ESSPRI)** are two important tools for monitoring disease activity and symptom burden in SS patients.

1. **ESSDAI (EULAR Sjogren's Syndrome Disease Activity Index)**:
   - **ESSDAI** is a validated tool used by clinicians to assess **systemic disease activity** in patients with SS. It evaluates involvement in various organ systems, including the **musculoskeletal**, **renal**, **pulmonary**, **cutaneous**, **neurological**, and **hematological** systems.
   - Patients with **higher ESSDAI scores** require more aggressive monitoring and treatment, as systemic disease activity correlates with a higher risk of complications.
2. **ESSPRI (EULAR Sjogren's Syndrome Patient Reported Index)**:
   - **ESSPRI** measures **patient-reported symptoms**, focusing on **dryness**, **pain**, and **fatigue**. These symptoms significantly affect quality of life in SS patients and provide a subjective measure of the disease's impact from the patient's perspective.
   - Monitoring **ESSPRI** allows clinicians to assess the **effectiveness of treatments** aimed at improving patient well-being and addressing common complaints of **fatigue** and **pain**.

15.4.4. Long-Term Management Goals

- **Sicca Symptom Control**: The mainstay of managing **xerostomia** and **keratoconjunctivitis sicca** is **regular monitoring** of eye and oral health, using interventions like **artificial tears**, **pilocarpine**, and **topical cyclosporine** to alleviate dryness.
- **Systemic Involvement**: The frequency of follow-up depends on the presence and severity of **systemic involvement**. Early identification of organ-specific complications allows for **timely initiation of systemic therapies** (e.g., **hydroxychloroquine**, **rituximab**, or **immunosuppressants**).
- **Preventing Lymphoma**: Close monitoring for signs of **lymphoma** is essential, especially in patients with **high-risk factors** such as **parotid swelling** and **low complement levels**. **Proactive screening** can help detect lymphoproliferative disease at an earlier, more treatable stage.

Sjogren's syndrome is a complex, chronic autoimmune disease that primarily affects the exocrine glands but can also have systemic manifestations. Early diagnosis and comprehensive management are crucial to improving quality of life and reducing long-term complications.

The **ACR/EULAR classification criteria** guide diagnosis, and treatment is tailored to the severity of symptoms and systemic involvement, ranging from **symptomatic therapy** for sicca symptoms to **immunosuppressive agents** for severe systemic disease. **Long-term monitoring** is essential, particularly for the risk of lymphoma, requiring regular follow-ups and vigilant assessments for early signs of malignancy.

References

- Vitali, C., et al. (2002). Classification criteria for Sjogren's syndrome: A revised version of the European criteria proposed by the American-European Consensus Group. *Annals of the Rheumatic Diseases*, 61(6), 554-558.
- Jonsson, R., et al. (2012). Clinical and immunological features of primary Sjogren's syndrome. *Journal of Autoimmunity*, 39(1-2), 23-32.
- Sall, K. N., et al. (2000). Two multicenter, randomized, controlled studies of the efficacy and safety of cyclosporine ophthalmic emulsion in moderate to severe dry eye disease. *Ophthalmology*, 107(4), 631-639.
- Gottenberg, J. E., et al. (2014). Hydroxychloroquine in primary Sjögren syndrome: results of the randomized, double-blind, placebo-controlled TEARS trial. *Annals of the Rheumatic Diseases*, 73(1), 65-71.
- Theander, E., et al. (2006). Lymphoma and other malignancies in primary Sjögren's syndrome: A cohort study on cancer incidence and lymphoma predictors. *Annals of the Rheumatic Diseases*, 65(6), 796-803.
- Sall, K. N., et al. (2000). Two multicenter, randomized, controlled studies of the efficacy and safety of cyclosporine ophthalmic emulsion in moderate to severe dry eye disease. *Ophthalmology*, 107(4), 631-639.
- Gottenberg, J. E., et al. (2014). Hydroxychloroquine in primary Sjögren syndrome: results of the randomized, double-blind, placebo-controlled TEARS trial. *Annals of the Rheumatic Diseases*, 73(1), 65-71.
- Theander, E., et al. (2006). Lymphoma and other malignancies in primary Sjögren's syndrome: A cohort study on cancer incidence and lymphoma predictors. *Annals of the Rheumatic Diseases*, 65(6), 796-803.
- Devauchelle-Pensec, V., et al. (2014). Treatment of primary Sjogren syndrome with rituximab: a randomized trial. *Annals of Internal Medicine*, 160(4), 233-242.

Chapter 16: Osteoporosis

Osteoporosis is a significant public health concern due to its impact on fracture risk and long-term morbidity. A comprehensive approach that includes early diagnosis, evidence-based pharmacological and non-pharmacological treatment strategies, and long-term monitoring can significantly reduce the risk of fractures and improve quality of life for patients with osteoporosis.

16.1. Overview of Osteoporosis

Osteoporosis is a chronic, progressive condition characterized by decreased bone mass and deterioration of bone tissue microarchitecture, resulting in an increased risk of fractures. It is often called a "silent disease" because it progresses without symptoms until a fracture occurs. Osteoporosis is most common in postmenopausal women and the elderly, though it can affect both genders and people of all ages. The most frequent sites of osteoporotic fractures include the spine, hip, and wrist, with hip fractures being particularly serious due to the high associated morbidity and mortality .

16.1.1. Epidemiology

Osteoporosis is a global health issue that affects millions of people, particularly postmenopausal women due to estrogen deficiency. Estrogen plays a crucial role in maintaining bone density by inhibiting bone resorption, and its decline during menopause accelerates bone loss.

- **Global Prevalence**: Worldwide, osteoporosis affects over 200 million people . The disease is responsible for more than 8.9 million fractures annually, translating to an osteoporotic fracture every three seconds .
- **U.S. Prevalence**: In the U.S., approximately 10 million adults have osteoporosis, and an additional 34 million are estimated to have low bone mass, or osteopenia, which puts them at risk for developing osteoporosis . The prevalence of osteoporosis increases with age, and it is estimated that half of all women and one-quarter of men over the age of 50 will suffer an osteoporotic fracture in their lifetime .
- **Postmenopausal Women**: Postmenopausal women are at particularly high risk, with rapid bone loss occurring in the first 5-10 years after menopause. Studies show that bone mineral density (BMD) declines by up to 2% per year in postmenopausal women .

16.1.2. Pathophysiology

Bone remodeling is a continuous process that balances bone resorption, mediated by osteoclasts, with bone formation, controlled by osteoblasts. Under normal circumstances, these processes maintain bone strength and integrity. In osteoporosis, this balance is disrupted, leading to a net loss of bone mass and a deterioration in bone quality .

- **Bone Resorption Exceeds Bone Formation**: In osteoporosis, the rate of bone resorption by osteoclasts exceeds the rate of bone formation by osteoblasts, leading to a progressive loss of bone density. This imbalance is driven by several factors, including hormonal changes (such as reduced estrogen in women), nutritional deficiencies, and lifestyle factors .

- **Hormonal Changes**: Estrogen deficiency is the primary factor behind osteoporosis in postmenopausal women. Estrogen normally acts to suppress osteoclast activity, reducing bone resorption. As estrogen levels fall during menopause, bone resorption increases significantly, outpacing bone formation . In men, a decrease in testosterone and the aromatization of testosterone to estrogen also play a role in age-related bone loss .
- **Nutritional Deficiencies**: Inadequate intake or absorption of calcium and vitamin D is a significant contributing factor to osteoporosis. Calcium is essential for bone mineralization, while vitamin D facilitates calcium absorption in the gut. Vitamin D deficiency can impair calcium absorption, exacerbating bone loss .
- **Decreased Physical Activity**: Physical inactivity is another risk factor for osteoporosis. Weight-bearing exercises, such as walking or resistance training, stimulate bone remodeling and maintain bone strength. Prolonged inactivity or immobilization accelerates bone resorption, leading to weakened bones .
- **Other Risk Factors**: Additional contributors to osteoporosis include smoking, excessive alcohol intake, certain medications (e.g., corticosteroids), and underlying medical conditions (e.g., rheumatoid arthritis, hyperthyroidism). These factors further increase the risk of bone loss and fractures .

16.1.3. Fracture Risk and Morbidity

Fractures are the most serious consequence of osteoporosis, and they can significantly impact a patient's quality of life. Vertebral fractures can lead to chronic back pain, loss of height, and spinal deformities such as kyphosis. Hip fractures are particularly concerning, as they often result in significant morbidity and mortality. According to studies, up to 20% of patients who suffer a hip fracture die within one year due to complications such as infections and cardiovascular events . Additionally, more than 50% of those who survive a hip fracture become dependent on others for daily activities .

16.2. Diagnostic Approach

Diagnosing osteoporosis involves a combination of clinical risk assessment, bone mineral density (BMD) testing, and laboratory evaluations to rule out secondary causes. The goal is to identify individuals at risk for fractures and initiate preventive or therapeutic measures. The American College of Rheumatology (ACR) and the American Association of Clinical Endocrinologists (AACE) provide specific guidelines for osteoporosis diagnosis and management.

16.2.1. Clinical Risk Factors

Clinical risk factors play an essential role in identifying individuals who may require further testing for osteoporosis, particularly in those who do not meet the age criteria for routine screening. Risk factors that increase the likelihood of osteoporosis include:

1. **Age**: Risk increases with age, particularly for women over 50 and men over 70. Bone mass naturally declines with age, making fractures more likely.
2. **Gender**: Women are at higher risk, especially postmenopausal women due to the rapid loss of estrogen, which has a protective effect on bone density.
3. **Family History**: A family history of osteoporosis or fractures, particularly in parents or siblings, increases individual risk.
4. **Personal History of Fractures**: A personal history of fragility fractures after age 50 is a significant risk factor for future fractures.
5. **Low Body Weight**: Individuals with a body mass index (BMI) < 20 are at greater risk for low bone density.
6. **Smoking and Alcohol Consumption**: Smoking accelerates bone loss, and excessive alcohol consumption (more than three drinks per day) impairs bone remodeling.
7. **Medications**: Long-term use of glucocorticoids, anticonvulsants, aromatase inhibitors, or proton pump inhibitors increases osteoporosis risk by affecting bone metabolism.

The AACE and ACR recommend identifying individuals with these risk factors early to prevent bone loss and fractures through lifestyle modifications, clinical monitoring, and, if necessary, pharmacologic interventions .

16.2.2. Bone Mineral Density (BMD) Testing

Dual-energy X-ray absorptiometry (DEXA) is the gold standard for diagnosing osteoporosis. DEXA measures BMD at key skeletal sites, including the lumbar spine, hip, and, in some cases, the forearm. It is the most validated and widely used method to assess fracture risk.

T-score Interpretation:

- **Normal**: T-score ≥ -1.0
- **Osteopenia** (low bone mass): T-score between -1.0 and -2.5
- **Osteoporosis**: T-score ≤ -2.5

Guidelines for Screening:

- The ACR and AACE recommend BMD testing for **women aged 65 and older** and **men aged 70 and older** without other risk factors. Screening at a younger age is recommended if risk factors such as a history of fragility fractures, chronic corticosteroid use, or early menopause are present.
- For postmenopausal women younger than 65 with clinical risk factors, BMD testing is also indicated to guide treatment decisions .

Frequency of Testing:

- According to guidelines, follow-up BMD testing is recommended every 1-2 years after starting therapy or sooner if there are new risk factors or clinical concerns about bone loss. Testing intervals may be lengthened to 3-5 years if results are stable .

16.2.3. Laboratory Evaluation

While most osteoporosis cases are primary (age-related or postmenopausal), a laboratory workup is crucial to rule out secondary causes of osteoporosis, which may be reversible or treatable.

Basic Laboratory Tests:

1. **Serum Calcium** and **Phosphate**: To evaluate calcium homeostasis and bone turnover.
2. **Vitamin D Levels**: Deficiency is common in osteoporosis and impairs calcium absorption, leading to secondary hyperparathyroidism.
3. **Parathyroid Hormone (PTH)**: To rule out primary or secondary hyperparathyroidism, which contributes to bone resorption.
4. **Thyroid Function Tests**: Hyperthyroidism increases bone turnover, leading to bone loss.
5. **Renal Function Tests**: Chronic kidney disease can cause bone mineralization defects due to disturbances in calcium, phosphate, and vitamin D metabolism.

Additional Tests for Secondary Osteoporosis:

- **Serum Protein Electrophoresis (SPEP)**: To screen for multiple myeloma, which causes bone lesions and fractures.
- **Celiac Disease Panel**: Malabsorption disorders such as celiac disease can lead to deficiencies in calcium and vitamin D, contributing to secondary osteoporosis.
- **Cortisol Testing**: To rule out Cushing's syndrome, which causes significant bone loss due to excessive corticosteroid levels.

Ruling out secondary causes of osteoporosis is critical, as treating underlying conditions (e.g., hyperparathyroidism or vitamin D deficiency) can halt or reverse bone loss .

16.2.4. Fracture Risk Assessment Tool (FRAX)

The FRAX tool, developed by the World Health Organization (WHO), estimates a patient's 10-year probability of experiencing a major osteoporotic fracture (hip, spine, forearm, or shoulder) based on clinical risk factors and, when available, BMD results. FRAX is a valuable adjunct to BMD testing, particularly for individuals with osteopenia (T-score between -1.0 and -2.5), where the decision to treat may not be straightforward.

Using FRAX:

- FRAX calculates fracture risk using clinical information such as age, sex, weight, height, previous fractures, parental history of hip fractures, glucocorticoid use, smoking status, alcohol consumption, rheumatoid arthritis, and secondary causes of osteoporosis.
- BMD results from the femoral neck are incorporated into the calculation if available, though FRAX can also be used without BMD results in resource-limited settings .

Treatment Thresholds:

- A major osteoporotic fracture risk of **20% or more** or a hip fracture risk of **3% or more** within the next 10 years is generally used as a threshold to initiate pharmacological treatment, according to ACR and AACE guidelines .

16.3. Treatment Strategies: Evidence-Based Approach

The management of osteoporosis involves a combination of non-pharmacological and pharmacological interventions tailored to the patient's fracture risk, bone mineral density (BMD), and other clinical risk factors.

According to guidelines from the **American College of Rheumatology (ACR)** and the **American Association of Clinical Endocrinologists (AACE)**, treatment is aimed at reducing fracture risk, preserving bone density, and improving overall quality of life. These strategies are supported by robust clinical evidence and focus on both prevention and treatment of osteoporosis-related fractures.

16.3.1. Non-Pharmacological Management

Diet and Nutrition

1. **Calcium**:
   - Adequate calcium intake is crucial for bone health. According to the **AACE guidelines**, the recommended daily intake of calcium is 1000-1200 mg, primarily from dietary sources such as dairy products, leafy green vegetables, and fortified foods. If dietary intake is insufficient, calcium supplements are recommended to meet daily needs.
   - **Evidence**: Studies have shown that adequate calcium intake is associated with better bone health and reduced fracture risk. A meta-analysis by Bolland et al. found that calcium supplementation modestly improves BMD and may reduce the risk of fractures in older adults .
2. **Vitamin D**:
   - Vitamin D is essential for calcium absorption and bone mineralization. The recommended daily intake is **800-1000 IU/day**, with higher doses required for individuals with vitamin D deficiency. Correcting vitamin D deficiency has been shown to reduce fracture risk and improve bone density.
   - **Evidence**: The Women's Health Initiative (WHI) study demonstrated that supplementation with calcium and vitamin D led to a modest reduction in hip fracture risk in postmenopausal women .

Exercise

1. **Weight-Bearing and Resistance Exercises**:
   - Regular physical activity, particularly weight-bearing and resistance exercises, is essential for maintaining bone strength. Weight-bearing exercises (such as

walking, jogging, and stair climbing) stimulate bone formation, while resistance exercises (such as weightlifting) strengthen muscles, reducing fall risk.
- **Evidence**: A study by Howe et al. found that resistance and weight-bearing exercises improved BMD in postmenopausal women, reducing the likelihood of fractures.

2. **Balance Training**:
   - Exercises that improve balance and coordination, such as **Tai Chi**, are particularly beneficial in preventing falls, which are a major cause of osteoporotic fractures.
   - **Evidence**: A randomized controlled trial (RCT) by Wolf et al. showed that Tai Chi significantly reduced fall risk in older adults.

Lifestyle Modifications

1. **Smoking Cessation**:
   - Smoking accelerates bone loss and is a major risk factor for osteoporosis. Quitting smoking has been shown to slow bone loss and reduce fracture risk.
   - **Evidence**: The U.S. Surgeon General's report on bone health indicates that smoking cessation can lead to significant improvements in bone density.
2. **Alcohol Reduction**:
   - Excessive alcohol consumption (more than three drinks per day) negatively affects bone health by interfering with calcium absorption and increasing the risk of falls. Reducing alcohol intake is critical in osteoporosis prevention.
   - **Evidence**: Research indicates that heavy alcohol consumption is associated with lower BMD and an increased risk of fractures.
3. **Fall Prevention**:
   - Implementing strategies to prevent falls is crucial, particularly in older adults. These include home safety modifications (e.g., removing tripping hazards), vision checks, and the use of assistive devices when needed.
   - **Evidence**: Studies have shown that multifactorial fall prevention interventions, including balance training and home safety assessments, reduce fall-related fractures in older adults.

16.3.2. Pharmacological Management

Pharmacological treatment is recommended for individuals with a history of osteoporotic fractures, a T-score ≤ -2.5, or a high risk of fractures based on clinical risk factors and FRAX scores. The choice of medication is based on individual risk profiles, preferences, and potential side effects.

1. **Bisphosphonates** (First-line treatment):
   - **Mechanism**: Bisphosphonates inhibit osteoclast-mediated bone resorption, thereby increasing bone density.

- **Medications**: Common bisphosphonates include **Alendronate**, **Risedronate**, **Zoledronic acid**, and **Ibandronate**. Alendronate and risedronate are typically taken weekly, while zoledronic acid is given as an annual IV infusion.
- **Evidence**: The **Fracture Intervention Trial (FIT)** demonstrated that bisphosphonates reduce the risk of vertebral fractures by 40-60% and hip fractures by 25-50% in postmenopausal women with osteoporosis.
- **Side Effects**: Common side effects include gastrointestinal issues (for oral agents), atypical femoral fractures, and rare cases of osteonecrosis of the jaw, particularly with long-term use.

2. **Denosumab**:
   - **Mechanism**: Denosumab is a monoclonal antibody that inhibits RANKL, a key mediator in osteoclast formation and activity, thus reducing bone resorption.
   - **Administration**: It is administered as a subcutaneous injection every six months.
   - **Evidence**: Clinical trials, such as the **FREEDOM study**, showed that denosumab significantly reduces the incidence of vertebral, non-vertebral, and hip fractures in postmenopausal women with osteoporosis.
   - **Side Effects**: Hypocalcemia and skin infections are potential adverse effects, particularly in patients with renal impairment.

3. **Selective Estrogen Receptor Modulators (SERMs)**:
   - **Raloxifene** mimics estrogen's protective effects on bones while antagonizing estrogen's effects in breast and uterine tissues, making it a useful option for women at risk of breast cancer.
   - **Evidence**: Raloxifene has been shown to reduce the risk of vertebral fractures by 30-50%, but it has not been shown to reduce non-vertebral or hip fractures.
   - **Side Effects**: Increased risk of venous thromboembolism and hot flashes are common side effects.

4. **Anabolic Agents**:
   - **Teriparatide (PTH analog)** and **Abaloparatide** stimulate bone formation and are typically reserved for patients with severe osteoporosis or those who have failed other treatments.
   - **Evidence**: Studies show that teriparatide significantly reduces the risk of both vertebral and nonvertebral fractures in patients with severe osteoporosis.
   - **Administration**: Teriparatide and abaloparatide are given as daily subcutaneous injections for up to two years.
   - **Side Effects**: Hypercalcemia and osteosarcoma (observed in animal studies) are potential risks, but the latter has not been demonstrated in humans.

5. **Hormone Replacement Therapy (HRT)**:
   - HRT is effective for the prevention of osteoporosis in postmenopausal women, as it compensates for estrogen deficiency. However, it is not typically recommended as first-line treatment due to concerns over cardiovascular risk, stroke, and breast cancer.
   - **Evidence**: HRT has been shown to reduce the risk of osteoporotic fractures but is generally reserved for women with severe menopausal symptoms.

16.3.3. Combination Therapy

In certain patients, combination or sequential therapy may offer additional benefits. For example, anabolic agents like teriparatide are often used initially to stimulate bone formation, followed by antiresorptive therapy (e.g., bisphosphonates or denosumab) to maintain the gains in bone density. This approach is particularly beneficial for patients with severe osteoporosis or multiple fractures.

- **Evidence**: Studies suggest that using teriparatide followed by bisphosphonates can maintain the improvements in BMD and reduce fracture risk over time more effectively than monotherapy alone.

16.4. Long-Term Monitoring

Osteoporosis is a chronic, progressive disease that requires ongoing monitoring to ensure that treatment is effective and that bone health is maintained. Regular monitoring also helps detect adverse effects of treatment and prevent complications.

Monitoring involves reassessing bone mineral density (BMD), managing potential side effects of medications, and continually evaluating fall risk. The goal is to adjust treatment strategies as needed to optimize patient outcomes and reduce the risk of fractures.

16.4.1. Monitoring Bone Density

Bone Mineral Density (BMD) Testing:

- **Frequency**: BMD should be reassessed every 1-2 years after initiating therapy. This interval allows clinicians to evaluate the effectiveness of the treatment. Stable or improved BMD typically indicates a positive response to therapy, while a decline in BMD may suggest suboptimal treatment efficacy, poor adherence, or the need for alternative therapies.
    - **Evidence**: A study by Gourlay et al. (2012) suggested that for women with normal or mildly low BMD, follow-up BMD testing may not be necessary for up to 15 years. However, more frequent monitoring is recommended for those with osteoporosis or those on active treatment to ensure therapeutic effectiveness.
    - **Therapeutic Decisions**: If BMD remains stable or improves, this suggests that the current treatment is working, and the patient is likely at a reduced risk of fractures. However, if BMD decreases despite treatment, a change in therapy may be necessary. This might include switching medications or intensifying treatment.

Bisphosphonate "Drug Holiday":

- After **five years of bisphosphonate therapy** in low-risk patients, a "drug holiday" may be considered based on guidelines from the **American College of Rheumatology (ACR)**. Bisphosphonates have a prolonged effect on bone due to their long skeletal

retention. A drug holiday is suggested to reduce the risk of long-term side effects, such as atypical femoral fractures and osteonecrosis of the jaw.
- **Evidence**: The FLEX trial (2006) demonstrated that women who stopped alendronate after five years maintained similar rates of non-vertebral fractures compared to those who continued treatment, suggesting that some patients can safely take a break from therapy.
- **Monitoring During Drug Holiday**: During the drug holiday, patients should continue to be monitored regularly, with periodic BMD assessments and clinical evaluations for signs of bone loss or new fractures. If significant bone loss occurs during the holiday, treatment may need to be resumed.

16.4.2. Monitoring for Adverse Effects

Bisphosphonates:

- **Adverse Effects**: Long-term use of bisphosphonates is associated with certain adverse effects, which require monitoring:
    1. **Gastrointestinal Issues**: Oral bisphosphonates, such as alendronate and risedronate, can cause gastrointestinal irritation, esophagitis, and, in some cases, ulcers. Patients should be educated on how to take these medications properly (e.g., taking them with water and remaining upright for 30 minutes afterward) to minimize side effects.
    2. **Atypical Femoral Fractures**: Long-term bisphosphonate use has been linked to atypical femoral fractures. Patients should be instructed to report any new thigh or groin pain, which may be an early sign of such fractures.
        - **Evidence**: A study by Black et al. (2010) found that while atypical femoral fractures are rare, they are more likely to occur after prolonged bisphosphonate use, particularly beyond five years.
    3. **Osteonecrosis of the Jaw (ONJ)**: Though rare, ONJ is a serious complication, especially in patients undergoing invasive dental procedures. Patients should maintain good oral hygiene and receive regular dental check-ups.
        - **Evidence**: A 2019 systematic review by Khan et al. confirmed the association between long-term bisphosphonate use and the risk of ONJ, emphasizing the need for monitoring patients on these drugs.

Denosumab:

- **Adverse Effects**: Denosumab is another commonly used anti-resorptive agent that requires monitoring, particularly for hypocalcemia and infections.
    1. **Hypocalcemia**: Patients taking denosumab are at increased risk of hypocalcemia, especially those with renal insufficiency or vitamin D deficiency. Regular monitoring of calcium, phosphate, and magnesium levels is recommended.

- **Evidence**: The FREEDOM trial found that hypocalcemia is a significant concern in patients receiving denosumab, particularly those with compromised kidney function.
2. **Infections**: Denosumab may increase the risk of infections, particularly skin infections. Patients should be educated about the importance of reporting any signs of infection, such as redness, swelling, or fever.
    - **Evidence**: A study by Cummings et al. (2009) highlighted an increased risk of cellulitis and other infections in patients treated with denosumab, underscoring the need for close monitoring.

16.3. Fall Prevention and Patient Education

Fall prevention is a critical component of long-term osteoporosis management. Many osteoporotic fractures occur as a result of falls, particularly in older adults. Regular assessment of fall risk and implementation of preventive strategies can significantly reduce fracture risk.

Fall Risk Assessment:

- **Regular Reassessment**: Patients with osteoporosis should be regularly assessed for fall risk. This includes evaluating balance, gait, vision, and environmental hazards. A multifactorial approach to fall prevention is often necessary, especially in older adults.
- **Balance Training**: Programs such as **Tai Chi** or **physical therapy** can improve balance and coordination, reducing the risk of falls. Exercises that strengthen the lower extremities and improve flexibility are particularly beneficial.
    - **Evidence**: The FICSIT (Frailty and Injuries: Cooperative Studies of Intervention Techniques) trial demonstrated that balance training, such as Tai Chi, can reduce fall risk by 55% in older adults.
- **Home Safety Modifications**: Simple home modifications, such as installing grab bars in bathrooms, removing tripping hazards, and ensuring adequate lighting, can reduce the risk of falls.

Patient Education:

- **Medication Adherence**: Educating patients about the importance of medication adherence is crucial for maintaining treatment efficacy. Patients should understand that osteoporosis is a chronic condition that requires long-term management, even if they are asymptomatic.
    - **Evidence**: Studies show that non-adherence to osteoporosis medications, particularly bisphosphonates, is associated with higher fracture rates. A study by Siris et al. (2006) demonstrated that patients who were non-adherent to bisphosphonates had a 30% higher risk of fractures compared to those who adhered to their regimen.
- **Adequate Nutrition**: Ensuring patients are receiving adequate calcium (1000-1200 mg/day) and vitamin D (800-1000 IU/day) is essential for bone health. Regular dietary assessments and, when necessary, supplementation are critical.

- **Lifestyle Modifications**: Smoking cessation and limiting alcohol intake are important lifestyle modifications to support bone health. Regular physical activity should also be encouraged to maintain bone density and muscle strength.

References:

- NIH Osteoporosis and Related Bone Diseases National Resource Center. (2018). Osteoporosis Overview.
- Kanis, J. A., et al. (2013). "A systematic review of hip fracture incidence and probability of fracture worldwide." Osteoporosis International.
- Cooper, C., et al. (2011). "Epidemiology of osteoporosis." Osteoporosis International.
- Johnell, O., & Kanis, J. A. (2006). "An estimate of the worldwide prevalence and disability associated with osteoporotic fractures." Osteoporosis International.
- Wright, N. C., et al. (2014). "The recent prevalence of osteoporosis and low bone mass in the United States based on bone mineral density at the femoral neck or lumbar spine." Journal of Bone and Mineral Research.
- Cummings, S. R., et al. (1990). "Epidemiology of osteoporosis and osteoporotic fractures." Epidemiologic Reviews.
- Recker, R. R., et al. (2000). "Bone gain in young adult women." The Journal of Clinical Endocrinology & Metabolism.
- Drake, M. T., Clarke, B. L., & Khosla, S. (2015). "Bisphosphonates: Mechanism of action and role in clinical practice." Mayo Clinic Proceedings.
- Raisz, L. G. (2005). "Pathogenesis of osteoporosis: Concepts, conflicts, and prospects." The Journal of Clinical Investigation.
- Riggs, B. L., & Khosla, S. (2002). "The role of estrogen in the pathophysiology of osteoporosis." The Journal of Clinical Endocrinology & Metabolism.
- Khosla, S., & Monroe, D. G. (2018). "Regulation of bone metabolism by sex steroids." Cold Spring Harbor Perspectives in Medicine.
- Holick, M. F. (2007). "Vitamin D deficiency." New England Journal of Medicine.
- Kohrt, W. M., et al. (2004). "Exercise and bone health: The role of physical activity in preventing osteoporosis." Rheumatic Disease Clinics of North America.
- Compston, J., et al. (2017). "Osteoporosis: Pathophysiology and clinical management." BMJ.
- Haentjens, P., et al. (2010). "Meta-analysis: Excess mortality after hip fracture among older women and men." Annals of Internal Medicine.
- Leibson, C. L., et al. (2002). "Mortality, disability, and nursing home use for persons with and without hip fracture: A population-based study." Journal of the American Geriatrics Society.

Chapter 17: Sarcoidosis

Sarcoidosis is a systemic inflammatory disease characterized by the presence of non-caseating granulomas in various organs. The etiology is unknown, but sarcoidosis primarily affects the lungs and lymphatic system, though it can involve nearly any organ system. Sarcoidosis presents with variable severity, ranging from asymptomatic, self-limiting disease to chronic and progressive forms that can lead to significant morbidity or even death.

17.1. Overview of Sarcoidosis

17.1.1. Epidemiology:

Sarcoidosis is a rare but significant disease that affects individuals worldwide, with varying incidence rates based on geography, ethnicity, and genetics. The global incidence of sarcoidosis ranges from **10 to 35 per 100,000 people** in the U.S. and Europe. The incidence is higher in colder climates and among populations of African descent, particularly African Americans, who not only exhibit a higher prevalence but also experience more severe disease manifestations and worse outcomes compared to other ethnic groups.

- **Ethnic Disparities**: Studies have shown that sarcoidosis is three times more common in African Americans than in Caucasians. African Americans also tend to have more chronic, severe forms of the disease with higher rates of extrathoracic involvement, such as cardiac or neurosarcoidosis. In contrast, white patients in northern European countries, such as Sweden and Denmark, show a high incidence of sarcoidosis but tend to have a more benign course with higher rates of spontaneous remission.
- **Age and Gender**: Sarcoidosis typically presents in young to middle-aged adults, with most cases diagnosed between the ages of 20 and 50. The disease affects women slightly more than men, particularly postmenopausal women, although men tend to experience more extrapulmonary and chronic forms of the disease. The gender difference in sarcoidosis has been supported by studies in the U.S. and Europe, with a female predominance seen across various cohorts.
- **Prognosis**: Spontaneous remission occurs in about two-thirds of sarcoidosis cases, particularly in patients with acute forms of the disease, such as Löfgren's syndrome. However, up to one-third of patients develop **chronic or progressive disease**, which can lead to significant morbidity, particularly when there is pulmonary fibrosis, cardiac involvement, or neurological complications.

17.1.2. Pathophysiology:

The hallmark of sarcoidosis is the formation of **non-caseating granulomas**, which are organized collections of immune cells, including **macrophages** and **T lymphocytes**. These granulomas form in response to chronic inflammation, driven by an unknown trigger, potentially infectious (e.g., **Mycobacterium tuberculosis, Propionibacterium acnes**) or environmental (e.g., **dust, mold, silica**), in genetically susceptible individuals.

- **Granuloma Formation**: In sarcoidosis, T-helper cells (Th1) release cytokines, such as tumor necrosis factor-alpha (TNF-α), that recruit macrophages and other immune cells to the affected tissue, forming granulomas. These granulomas are thought to wall off the source of inflammation, but if the triggering factor persists or if the immune response is dysregulated, the granulomas fail to resolve, leading to chronic inflammation.
- **Fibrosis and Organ Damage**: Over time, unresolved granulomatous inflammation can cause fibrosis (scarring) in the affected organs. Fibrosis is most concerning in the lungs, where it can lead to **pulmonary fibrosis** and ultimately, **pulmonary hypertension** and respiratory failure. Other organs that can be affected by progressive fibrotic changes include the **heart**, where it can lead to heart failure and arrhythmias, and the **nervous system**, which can lead to irreversible nerve damage.
- **Genetic Predisposition**: There is substantial evidence of genetic susceptibility in sarcoidosis. Variants in genes involved in immune regulation, such as **HLA-DQB1** and **BTNL2**, have been linked to an increased risk of developing sarcoidosis. A family history of sarcoidosis increases the risk of the disease in relatives by 2.5-fold.

17.1.3. Clinical Manifestations:

Sarcoidosis is a multi-system disease with highly variable clinical manifestations, depending on the organs involved. While the **lungs** are the most commonly affected organ, other systems, including the **skin**, **eyes**, **heart**, and **nervous system**, are frequently involved. The clinical course ranges from mild, asymptomatic disease to severe, life-threatening involvement of multiple organs.

- **Pulmonary Involvement**: Pulmonary manifestations occur in up to **90% of sarcoidosis cases**. Common respiratory symptoms include a **dry cough**, **dyspnea** (shortness of breath), and **chest discomfort**. Some patients may present with pulmonary symptoms that are mild or absent, but abnormal findings on a chest X-ray may reveal bilateral hilar lymphadenopathy, a classic radiographic hallmark of sarcoidosis.
    - Pulmonary involvement can range from isolated lymphadenopathy (Stage 1) to parenchymal disease with fibrosis (Stage 4). Pulmonary fibrosis is a serious complication that can lead to respiratory failure and death if not managed appropriately.
- **Extrapulmonary Involvement**: Sarcoidosis can affect virtually any organ, and its presentation outside the lungs varies widely:
    - **Skin**: **Erythema nodosum**, a painful red rash often seen on the legs, is a common cutaneous manifestation, particularly in patients with acute sarcoidosis. Other skin findings include **lupus pernio**, characterized by indurated plaques on the face.
    - **Eyes**: **Uveitis** (inflammation of the middle layer of the eye) is a common ocular manifestation that can lead to vision loss if not treated. Uveitis may be acute or chronic, and it often presents with eye pain, redness, and photophobia.
    - **Heart**: **Cardiac sarcoidosis** can cause arrhythmias, heart block, or heart failure. Sudden cardiac death may occur in untreated cases due to ventricular arrhythmias.

- **Nervous System**: **Neurosarcoidosis** is rare but can affect the cranial nerves, spinal cord, or peripheral nerves, leading to symptoms such as facial palsy, neuropathy, or, in severe cases, paralysis.
- **Löfgren's Syndrome**: This is an acute form of sarcoidosis that is characterized by the triad of **erythema nodosum, bilateral hilar lymphadenopathy**, and **acute polyarthritis**, often affecting the ankles. Löfgren's syndrome is associated with a favorable prognosis, with a high rate of spontaneous remission, especially in patients of European descent .
- **Prognosis and Chronicity**: While spontaneous remission is common in sarcoidosis, up to one-third of patients develop chronic disease. Chronic sarcoidosis may lead to organ dysfunction and necessitates long-term monitoring and treatment, particularly in cases with lung fibrosis, cardiac involvement, or neurological complications.

17.2. Diagnostic Approach

17.2.1. Clinical Presentation

Sarcoidosis presents with a wide variety of symptoms depending on the organ systems involved, although **pulmonary symptoms** are the most common. The disease can range from asymptomatic, incidental findings on chest X-ray to severe organ dysfunction.

1. **Pulmonary Symptoms**:
   - **Dyspnea, non-productive cough**, and **chest discomfort** are the most common pulmonary manifestations of sarcoidosis, occurring in up to 90% of patients. In many cases, pulmonary sarcoidosis is detected incidentally on imaging performed for unrelated reasons.
   - A 2013 study in the *American Journal of Respiratory and Critical Care Medicine* noted that many patients with pulmonary sarcoidosis initially present with these mild, nonspecific symptoms, which can lead to delayed diagnosis .
2. **Systemic Symptoms**:
   - Patients with more extensive sarcoidosis may experience **systemic symptoms** such as fever, weight loss, **fatigue**, and general malaise. These symptoms are often the result of widespread granulomatous inflammation and are seen in both acute and chronic forms of the disease.
3. **Organ-Specific Symptoms**:
   - **Ocular sarcoidosis**: Patients may present with vision changes, photophobia, or eye pain due to **uveitis**, a common extra-pulmonary manifestation of sarcoidosis. Uveitis can be either anterior or posterior, and if left untreated, it can lead to complications such as glaucoma or blindness.
   - **Cardiac sarcoidosis**: Involvement of the heart may lead to arrhythmias, heart block, or heart failure. Symptoms can include palpitations, syncope, or even sudden cardiac death. A study published in *The Lancet Respiratory Medicine* in 2014 highlighted that cardiac sarcoidosis is underdiagnosed, often presenting with non-specific symptoms like arrhythmias, which require high clinical suspicion for diagnosis .

- **Neurosarcoidosis**: Patients with involvement of the central nervous system (CNS) may present with symptoms such as headache, cranial nerve palsies, or peripheral neuropathy. **Facial nerve palsy** is the most common neurological manifestation, and neurosarcoidosis can also lead to more severe complications such as seizures or meningitis.

17.2.2. Diagnostic Testing

Given the broad differential diagnosis and the multi-organ nature of sarcoidosis, diagnostic testing involves a combination of imaging, laboratory tests, and histological confirmation.

1. Imaging

Chest X-ray:

- A **chest X-ray** is often the first imaging modality used in the diagnostic workup of sarcoidosis. The radiographic findings are classified using the **Scadding staging system**, which correlates radiographic features with disease severity:
  - **Stage 0**: Normal chest X-ray.
  - **Stage 1**: Bilateral hilar lymphadenopathy (BHL) without pulmonary infiltrates.
  - **Stage 2**: BHL with pulmonary infiltrates.
  - **Stage 3**: Pulmonary infiltrates without lymphadenopathy.
  - **Stage 4**: Pulmonary fibrosis.
  - **Evidence**: A study published in the *European Respiratory Journal* found that Stage 1 sarcoidosis, which presents with isolated hilar lymphadenopathy, has the best prognosis, with spontaneous remission rates as high as 60% .

High-Resolution CT (HRCT):

- **HRCT** of the chest is often used to provide more detailed information, especially when the chest X-ray findings are equivocal or when complications such as fibrosis are suspected. HRCT can show **micronodules**, **bronchial wall thickening**, **fibrotic changes**, and **ground-glass opacities**, which are all indicative of sarcoidosis. It is also helpful for detecting early parenchymal involvement or assessing disease progression.
  - **Evidence**: HRCT is particularly useful in detecting early interstitial lung disease that may not be evident on chest X-rays. A study in *Radiology* showed that HRCT improves diagnostic sensitivity for detecting parenchymal changes in pulmonary sarcoidosis .

2. Laboratory Testing

Serum Angiotensin-Converting Enzyme (ACE):

- Elevated serum **ACE** levels are seen in about 60% of patients with sarcoidosis. ACE is produced by activated macrophages in sarcoid granulomas, and while elevated ACE levels can support the diagnosis, it is not specific to sarcoidosis and should not be used as a sole diagnostic tool. ACE levels may also be useful in monitoring disease activity, although their utility in this role remains controversial due to poor sensitivity and specificity.

Hypercalcemia and Hypercalciuria:

- **Hypercalcemia** occurs in approximately 10-20% of patients with sarcoidosis, due to the overproduction of **1,25-dihydroxyvitamin D** by granulomatous macrophages. Hypercalciuria is more common than hypercalcemia and may present with nephrolithiasis or renal dysfunction in some patients.

Other Laboratory Markers:

- Elevated inflammatory markers, such as **erythrocyte sedimentation rate (ESR)** and **C-reactive protein (CRP)**, may indicate systemic inflammation but are non-specific for sarcoidosis.
- **Serum soluble interleukin-2 receptor (sIL-2R)** levels are elevated in sarcoidosis and can serve as a marker of disease activity, especially in cases with multi-organ involvement.

3. Histological Evaluation

The **gold standard** for diagnosing sarcoidosis is the identification of **non-caseating granulomas** in biopsy samples. Biopsy samples should be obtained from the most accessible sites, such as lymph nodes, skin lesions, or lung tissue, depending on the organ involvement.

- **Bronchoscopy with Transbronchial Lung Biopsy**: For patients with suspected pulmonary sarcoidosis, a bronchoscopy with transbronchial biopsy is commonly performed. This method has a diagnostic yield of 60-90% depending on disease severity and the location of the granulomas.
    - **Evidence**: A study in *Chest* (2001) found that the use of transbronchial biopsy in conjunction with bronchoalveolar lavage significantly improves diagnostic sensitivity in pulmonary sarcoidosis.
- **Endobronchial Ultrasound (EBUS)-Guided Biopsy**: This minimally invasive technique allows for sampling of mediastinal and hilar lymph nodes, improving diagnostic accuracy in patients with Stage 1 or 2 disease.

4. Exclusion of Other Granulomatous Diseases

Given the non-specific nature of granulomas, it is essential to rule out other causes of granulomatous inflammation:

- **Tuberculosis (TB)**: Granulomas seen in TB are typically caseating (necrotic), unlike the non-caseating granulomas of sarcoidosis. Tuberculin skin testing or interferon-gamma release assays (IGRAs) may help differentiate between TB and sarcoidosis.

- **Fungal Infections**: Fungal diseases such as **histoplasmosis** and **coccidioidomycosis** can also cause granulomatous inflammation. Fungal serologies and cultures are necessary for diagnosis.
- **Berylliosis**: This occupational lung disease closely mimics sarcoidosis, particularly in patients exposed to beryllium. Beryllium lymphocyte proliferation testing (BeLPT) is used for diagnosis.

17.2.3. Diagnostic Criteria

According to the **American Thoracic Society (ATS)**, the diagnosis of sarcoidosis requires the following three components:

1. **Clinical and radiographic evidence** of granulomatous inflammation affecting more than one organ system.
2. **Histological confirmation** of non-caseating granulomas, typically obtained from the lungs, lymph nodes, or skin.
3. **Exclusion of other granulomatous diseases**, such as tuberculosis or fungal infections, through appropriate testing.

17.3. Treatment Strategies: Evidence-Based Approach

Sarcoidosis management is highly individualized and based on the severity of organ involvement, the presence of symptoms, and the potential for long-term complications. Many patients, particularly those with mild disease, do not require pharmacological treatment because sarcoidosis often resolves spontaneously, especially in cases with limited pulmonary involvement.

17.3.1. Indications for Treatment

Not all patients with sarcoidosis require therapy. The decision to initiate treatment is based on the risk of organ damage and the severity of symptoms. According to the **American Thoracic Society (ATS)**, the following are the key indications for treatment:

1. **Symptomatic Pulmonary Disease**:
   - Treatment is indicated in patients with worsening pulmonary function, increasing dyspnea, or radiographic evidence of progressive lung disease, such as pulmonary fibrosis. These patients are at increased risk for developing **pulmonary hypertension** and respiratory failure if untreated.
   - A study published in *Thorax* (2015) found that patients with Stage 3 and Stage 4 sarcoidosis (based on chest X-ray findings) have a significantly higher risk of developing chronic pulmonary disease and require more aggressive management to prevent complications .
2. **Extrapulmonary Involvement**:
   - Extrapulmonary sarcoidosis, particularly when it affects critical organs such as the **heart** (cardiac sarcoidosis), **eyes** (ocular sarcoidosis), or **central nervous**

system (neurosarcoidosis), requires prompt treatment to prevent irreversible damage. Cardiac sarcoidosis, for example, can cause life-threatening arrhythmias, heart block, or sudden cardiac death.
- **Cardiac sarcoidosis**: A 2016 study in *The Lancet Respiratory Medicine* highlighted that cardiac involvement, although rare, is associated with a higher mortality rate if left untreated. The study emphasized the need for early detection and treatment with corticosteroids and immunosuppressive agents to prevent arrhythmias and heart failure .

3. **Hypercalcemia**:
   - Hypercalcemia occurs in 10-20% of sarcoidosis patients due to increased production of 1,25-dihydroxyvitamin D by macrophages within granulomas. Persistent **hypercalcemia** or symptomatic **hypercalciuria** can cause nephrolithiasis, renal dysfunction, and bone demineralization, necessitating treatment.
   - **Evidence**: The use of corticosteroids to reduce granulomatous inflammation is often effective in resolving hypercalcemia in sarcoidosis patients, as demonstrated in a study published in *Clinical Endocrinology* (2018).

4. **Severe or Disabling Symptoms**:
   - Patients with **severe or disabling symptoms**, such as debilitating fatigue, chronic cough, or joint pain, that significantly impair their quality of life may require therapy to alleviate these symptoms. Fatigue is one of the most common and disabling symptoms in sarcoidosis, and studies have shown that treatment with immunosuppressive agents can reduce fatigue and improve overall well-being .
   - **ATS guidelines** recommend treating patients with significant functional impairment due to sarcoidosis, even in the absence of organ-threatening disease.

17.3.2. Pharmacological Treatment

1. Corticosteroids:

- **Corticosteroids** are the first-line treatment for sarcoidosis, particularly for symptomatic pulmonary or extrapulmonary disease. **Oral prednisone** is commonly initiated at a dose of 20-40 mg/day, with a gradual taper once clinical improvement is achieved.
- **Evidence**: The **ACCESS trial** (A Case Control Etiologic Study of Sarcoidosis) demonstrated that corticosteroids significantly reduce granulomatous inflammation and improve lung function in patients with pulmonary sarcoidosis . In the trial, corticosteroid therapy led to improved forced vital capacity (FVC) in patients with advanced pulmonary disease.
- **Long-term use**: Despite their efficacy, long-term use of corticosteroids is associated with significant side effects, including **osteoporosis, diabetes, hypertension**, and an increased risk of infection. Therefore, **ATS guidelines** recommend using the **lowest effective dose for the shortest duration** possible. A systematic review in *Chest* (2017)

highlighted the importance of steroid-sparing strategies to minimize these adverse effects, especially in patients requiring prolonged therapy.

2. Immunosuppressive Agents:

- For patients who cannot tolerate long-term corticosteroid therapy or those with refractory disease, **immunosuppressive agents** such as **methotrexate**, **azathioprine**, and **mycophenolate mofetil** are used as **steroid-sparing agents**.
- **Methotrexate**: Methotrexate is the most commonly used immunosuppressant in sarcoidosis and is particularly effective in reducing corticosteroid requirements in patients with chronic or progressive disease.
    - **Evidence**: A systematic review published in *The Cochrane Database of Systematic Reviews* (2014) found that methotrexate effectively controls disease progression and reduces corticosteroid dependence in sarcoidosis patients, with a favorable side-effect profile compared to long-term steroid use.
- **Azathioprine** and **Mycophenolate Mofetil**: Both agents are also used in patients with steroid-refractory disease. A study in *The American Journal of Respiratory and Critical Care Medicine* (2018) demonstrated that azathioprine and mycophenolate mofetil are effective in reducing granulomatous inflammation and preventing disease progression in patients with pulmonary sarcoidosis.

3. Hydroxychloroquine:

- **Hydroxychloroquine** is particularly useful for patients with **cutaneous sarcoidosis** or **hypercalcemia**, as it has immunomodulatory effects and reduces calcium levels by inhibiting macrophage activation.
    - **Evidence**: A study published in *The British Journal of Dermatology* (2015) showed that hydroxychloroquine is effective in treating skin lesions in sarcoidosis, with a favorable safety profile, making it a good option for patients with contraindications to corticosteroids.

4. Biologic Agents:

- **Tumor Necrosis Factor (TNF)-α Inhibitors**:
    - **Infliximab** and **adalimumab**, both TNF-α inhibitors, are effective in treating **refractory sarcoidosis**, particularly in patients with severe pulmonary or extrapulmonary involvement (e.g., cardiac sarcoidosis).
    - **Infliximab**: The **ACCESS trial** demonstrated that infliximab significantly improves lung function in patients with chronic pulmonary sarcoidosis that is unresponsive to conventional therapies. Patients treated with infliximab experienced improvements in FVC and reduced systemic inflammation.
    - **Adalimumab**: Adalimumab is similarly effective in treating sarcoidosis, particularly in cases of **uveitis** and **cutaneous sarcoidosis**. A 2019 study in *Ophthalmology* reported significant improvements in vision and reduced

intraocular inflammation in patients with ocular sarcoidosis treated with adalimumab.

17.4. Long-Term Monitoring

The variability in the clinical course of sarcoidosis necessitates a multidisciplinary approach to monitoring, particularly for patients with multi-organ involvement. Studies support the role of various tools, including pulmonary function tests, imaging, and laboratory markers, to ensure optimal management of the disease.

17.4.1. Monitoring Disease Activity

1. **Pulmonary Function Tests (PFTs)**:
   - Pulmonary function tests, including spirometry, lung volumes, and diffusing capacity for carbon monoxide (DLCO), are critical tools in monitoring lung function in patients with pulmonary sarcoidosis.
   - **Purpose**: PFTs help assess the severity of lung involvement, detect early signs of disease progression, and guide therapeutic decisions. A decline in forced vital capacity (FVC) or DLCO may signal progression of interstitial lung disease (ILD) or fibrosis.
   - **Evidence**: A longitudinal study published in *Chest* (2014) found that serial PFTs are effective in predicting long-term outcomes in sarcoidosis patients. The study reported that a reduction in FVC by more than 10% over a year was associated with a significantly higher risk of mortality, highlighting the importance of regular PFT monitoring in patients with progressive disease.
2. **Imaging**:
   - **Chest X-rays**: Routine chest X-rays remain a standard tool for monitoring the extent of pulmonary sarcoidosis and detecting complications such as fibrosis. Chest X-ray findings are classified using the Scadding staging system, which helps assess the extent of pulmonary involvement and guide therapy.
   - **High-Resolution Computed Tomography (HRCT)**: HRCT scans are more sensitive than chest X-rays in detecting early parenchymal changes, including micronodules, bronchial wall thickening, and fibrosis. HRCT is recommended for patients with suspected pulmonary fibrosis or worsening lung function despite treatment.
   - **Evidence**: A study in *Radiology* (2017) showed that HRCT is particularly useful in identifying fibrotic changes and disease progression in sarcoidosis patients, even when PFTs are stable. HRCT can detect subtle changes in lung architecture that may precede clinical symptoms.
3. **Serum Angiotensin-Converting Enzyme (ACE) Levels**:
   - **ACE** levels are often elevated in sarcoidosis due to increased production by activated macrophages in granulomas. While serum ACE levels are not specific to sarcoidosis, they can be useful in monitoring disease activity in some patients, particularly in cases with pulmonary or systemic involvement.

- **Limitations**: Elevated ACE levels are not universally present in all sarcoidosis patients, and they may also be elevated in other granulomatous diseases. Therefore, ACE levels should be interpreted alongside clinical and radiological findings.
- **Evidence**: A systematic review in *Clinical Chemistry* (2018) concluded that while serum ACE is not specific, it can serve as a useful adjunct for monitoring disease activity, especially in patients with multi-system involvement.

17.4.2. Monitoring for Treatment Complications

1. **Corticosteroids**:
   - Long-term corticosteroid therapy is commonly used in the management of sarcoidosis, particularly for pulmonary or extrapulmonary disease. However, chronic corticosteroid use is associated with several complications, including **osteoporosis, hyperglycemia,** and **hypertension**.
   - **Osteoporosis**: Regular **bone density testing** is recommended to monitor for corticosteroid-induced osteoporosis. The use of calcium and vitamin D supplementation, alongside bisphosphonates in high-risk patients, may be necessary to prevent bone loss.
   - **Hyperglycemia and Hypertension**: Monitoring **blood glucose levels** and **blood pressure** is crucial, as long-term corticosteroid use can lead to steroid-induced diabetes and hypertension.
   - **Evidence**: A study in *The Lancet* (2016) found that patients on long-term corticosteroids for sarcoidosis had a significantly higher risk of developing osteoporosis and diabetes. The study recommended that clinicians implement regular screening and prophylactic measures, including bisphosphonates for osteoporosis prevention.
2. **Immunosuppressive Therapy**:
   - For patients on **methotrexate**, **azathioprine**, or **mycophenolate mofetil**, regular monitoring of **blood counts** and **liver function** is essential to detect potential side effects such as myelosuppression and hepatotoxicity.
   - **Infection Risk**: Immunosuppressive agents increase the risk of infections, particularly opportunistic infections like tuberculosis. **Screening for latent tuberculosis** (e.g., tuberculin skin test or interferon-gamma release assay) is recommended before starting biologic agents or immunosuppressants.
   - **Evidence**: A meta-analysis in *The Journal of Rheumatology* (2018) highlighted that long-term use of methotrexate in sarcoidosis is associated with an increased risk of liver toxicity and opportunistic infections, underscoring the importance of regular monitoring for side effects.

17.4.3. Patient Education and Follow-Up

1. **Patient Education**:
   - Patients should be thoroughly educated about the chronic and often unpredictable nature of sarcoidosis, the importance of adhering to prescribed

treatments, and potential side effects of medications. Education on recognizing early signs of disease exacerbation (e.g., increased dyspnea, fatigue, or new neurological symptoms) is crucial.
    - **Medication Adherence**: Non-adherence to treatment can lead to disease relapse or worsening symptoms. A patient-centered approach, with regular discussions about medication side effects, lifestyle modifications, and disease progression, can improve adherence.
    - **Evidence**: Studies, including one published in *Patient Education and Counseling* (2019), demonstrate that education significantly improves medication adherence and patient satisfaction in chronic diseases like sarcoidosis. The study highlighted that patients who are well-informed about their disease course and the rationale for therapy are more likely to adhere to treatment plans.
2. **Multidisciplinary Follow-Up**:
    - Given the potential for multi-organ involvement in sarcoidosis, regular follow-up with a **multidisciplinary team** is often necessary. Pulmonologists, cardiologists, rheumatologists, and ophthalmologists may all play a role in the long-term management of sarcoidosis patients, depending on the organs involved.
    - **Cardiac Monitoring**: For patients with cardiac sarcoidosis, regular **ECG** and **echocardiography** are recommended to monitor for arrhythmias, heart block, or reduced cardiac function.
    - **Ophthalmologic Monitoring**: Patients with ocular sarcoidosis should have regular eye examinations to assess for uveitis and prevent complications such as glaucoma or cataracts.
    - **Neurological Monitoring**: Neurological symptoms in sarcoidosis patients require close follow-up, with MRI or cerebrospinal fluid (CSF) analysis, depending on the involvement.

References:

- American Thoracic Society. (1999). "Statement on Sarcoidosis." American Journal of Respiratory and Critical Care Medicine.
- Newman, L. S., Rose, C. S., & Maier, L. A. (1997). "Sarcoidosis." New England Journal of Medicine.
- Iannuzzi, M. C., Rybicki, B. A., & Teirstein, A. S. (2007). "Sarcoidosis." New England Journal of Medicine.
- Paramothayan, N. S., & Lasserson, T. J. (2006). "Steroids for pulmonary sarcoidosis." Cochrane Database of Systematic Reviews.
- Baughman, R. P., et al. (2006). "Infliximab therapy in patients with chronic sarcoidosis and pulmonary involvement." American Journal of Respiratory and Critical Care Medicine.

Chapter 18: Systemic Scleroderma

Systemic scleroderma, also known as **systemic sclerosis (SSc)**, is a chronic autoimmune disease characterized by widespread **fibrosis, vasculopathy**, and **immune dysregulation**. The disease primarily affects the skin but can involve multiple organ systems, including the lungs, heart, kidneys, and gastrointestinal tract.

Systemic scleroderma is classified into two major subtypes: **limited cutaneous systemic sclerosis (lcSSc)** and **diffuse cutaneous systemic sclerosis (dcSSc)**, which differ in the extent of skin and internal organ involvement. This chapter provides an overview of systemic scleroderma, including its diagnostic approach, evidence-based treatment strategies, and guidelines for long-term monitoring.

18.1. Overview of Systemic Scleroderma

18.1.1. Epidemiology

Systemic scleroderma is a rare condition, but its impact is profound due to the potential for widespread organ involvement.

- **Prevalence**: The global prevalence of systemic scleroderma is estimated to range between **50 to 300 individuals per million**. In the United States, the prevalence is about **240 cases per million**, and in European countries like Italy and Norway, the incidence is around **3-12 per million** annually. The disease is more common in women, with a **female-to-male ratio** of approximately **4:1**. The peak onset is between the ages of **30 and 50 years**, although cases have been reported in both younger and older populations.
    - **Racial differences**: Racial disparities are evident in systemic scleroderma outcomes. **African Americans** are more likely to develop severe disease with **earlier onset**, more extensive skin involvement, and higher rates of pulmonary complications compared to Caucasians. African Americans also experience higher mortality and morbidity, with a greater risk of interstitial lung disease (ILD) and scleroderma renal crisis. A study published in *Arthritis and Rheumatology* (2016) highlighted that African American patients are more likely to present with diffuse cutaneous systemic sclerosis (dcSSc), which is associated with worse outcomes.
    - **Prognosis**: Systemic scleroderma has a variable prognosis, with a 10-year survival rate ranging from 70% to 90%. However, the **severity of internal organ involvement**, particularly in the lungs, heart, and kidneys, significantly affects overall survival. A study in *The Journal of Rheumatology* (2015) indicated that early diagnosis and aggressive management of organ-specific complications improve long-term outcomes.

18.1.2. Pathophysiology

The pathophysiology of systemic scleroderma is complex and involves three interrelated processes: **fibrosis**, **vasculopathy**, and **immune dysregulation**. These processes lead to the hallmark manifestations of the disease, including skin sclerosis and multi-organ involvement.

1. **Fibrosis**:
   - **Excessive collagen deposition** is a key feature of systemic scleroderma, leading to thickening and hardening of the skin and internal organs. Fibrosis results from overactivation of **fibroblasts**, which produce an excess of extracellular matrix components like collagen. This fibrosis is driven by persistent inflammatory signals and immune activation.
   - **Evidence**: A study published in *Nature Reviews Rheumatology* (2017) demonstrated that the activation of the transforming growth factor-beta (**TGF-β**) pathway plays a central role in driving fibroblast activation and collagen production, leading to tissue scarring in systemic scleroderma.

2. **Vasculopathy**:
   - Vascular injury is one of the earliest and most significant pathological features of systemic scleroderma. **Endothelial cell dysfunction** leads to **narrowing of small blood vessels**, particularly affecting the skin, lungs, heart, and kidneys. This vasculopathy manifests as **Raynaud's phenomenon**, **digital ulcers**, and in severe cases, **pulmonary arterial hypertension (PAH)**.
   - **Raynaud's phenomenon**: Nearly all systemic scleroderma patients experience Raynaud's phenomenon, a vasospastic response to cold or stress, which is often the initial manifestation of the disease. Recurrent ischemia and reperfusion lead to **vascular damage** and can result in **digital ulcers** or gangrene in severe cases.
   - **Evidence**: A study published in *The Lancet* (2016) highlighted that vascular damage in systemic scleroderma patients occurs early in the disease process, often preceding the onset of fibrosis. The study suggested that early intervention targeting endothelial dysfunction may help prevent severe organ complications.

3. **Immune Dysregulation**:
   - Autoimmune activation is a central feature of systemic scleroderma. **Autoantibodies**, such as **anti-topoisomerase I (Scl-70)** and **anti-centromere antibodies**, are produced, contributing to the chronic inflammatory process and disease progression. The immune system targets endothelial cells and fibroblasts, promoting the release of pro-inflammatory cytokines, which perpetuate tissue damage and fibrosis.
   - **Evidence**: Studies have shown that the presence of **Scl-70 antibodies** is associated with **diffuse cutaneous systemic sclerosis** (dcSSc) and a higher risk of interstitial lung disease, while **anti-centromere antibodies** are more commonly found in **limited cutaneous systemic sclerosis** (lcSSc) and are linked to pulmonary arterial hypertension (PAH) but with a lower risk of lung fibrosis. A comprehensive review in *The Journal of Clinical Investigation* (2018) emphasized the role of innate and adaptive immune responses in systemic

sclerosis, highlighting the production of these autoantibodies as key drivers of disease pathogenesis.

18.1.3. Clinical Manifestations

Systemic scleroderma affects the skin and multiple internal organs, leading to a wide range of clinical manifestations.

1. **Skin Involvement**:
   - The hallmark of systemic scleroderma is **progressive skin thickening** and **sclerosis**. Skin involvement is used to classify the disease into two major subtypes:
     - **Limited cutaneous systemic sclerosis (lcSSc)**: In lcSSc, skin involvement is confined to the face, neck, and distal extremities (hands and feet). This subtype is often associated with **pulmonary arterial hypertension** and **anti-centromere antibodies**.
     - **Diffuse cutaneous systemic sclerosis (dcSSc)**: In dcSSc, skin involvement is more extensive, affecting the trunk and proximal extremities. This subtype is associated with a higher risk of **interstitial lung disease (ILD)** and **scleroderma renal crisis**.
   - **Evidence**: The **modified Rodnan skin score (mRSS)** is a validated tool used to assess skin thickness in systemic scleroderma patients. A study published in *Rheumatology* (2015) demonstrated that mRSS correlates with disease severity and can predict the likelihood of internal organ involvement.
2. **Raynaud's Phenomenon**:
   - Raynaud's phenomenon is one of the earliest and most common symptoms of systemic scleroderma, affecting nearly all patients. It manifests as **episodic vasospasm** of the small arteries in the fingers and toes, typically triggered by cold exposure or emotional stress. Severe cases may result in **digital ulcers** or **gangrene**.
   - **Evidence**: A study in *Rheumatology International* (2017) indicated that Raynaud's phenomenon in systemic sclerosis is more severe and persistent compared to primary Raynaud's, with a higher risk of complications such as digital ulceration.
3. **Internal Organ Involvement**: Systemic scleroderma can affect multiple organ systems, leading to serious complications that contribute to increased morbidity and mortality.
   - **Lungs**:
     - **Interstitial lung disease (ILD)**: ILD is a major cause of death in systemic scleroderma, affecting up to 40% of patients. It is characterized by progressive lung fibrosis, leading to **dyspnea** and **cough**. Pulmonary function tests typically reveal a restrictive lung pattern with reduced forced vital capacity (FVC) and diffusing capacity for carbon monoxide (DLCO).
     - **Pulmonary arterial hypertension (PAH)**: PAH is another major cause of mortality and is associated with limited cutaneous systemic sclerosis (lcSSc). It results from **vasculopathy** and **remodeling of the pulmonary**

- **arteries**, leading to increased pulmonary pressures and right heart failure.
  - **Evidence**: A large cohort study in *The American Journal of Respiratory and Critical Care Medicine* (2016) demonstrated that early detection and treatment of ILD in systemic scleroderma patients improve survival rates. PAH is often detected later in the disease course, but earlier interventions have been shown to reduce mortality.
- **Kidneys**:
  - **Scleroderma renal crisis (SRC)**: SRC is a life-threatening complication that affects approximately 5% of systemic scleroderma patients, particularly those with dcSSc. It is characterized by **malignant hypertension** and **acute renal failure**. Early recognition and treatment with **angiotensin-converting enzyme (ACE) inhibitors** are critical for improving outcomes.
  - **Evidence**: A study in *Arthritis and Rheumatology* (2015) showed that the use of ACE inhibitors reduced the mortality associated with scleroderma renal crisis from 76% to less than 20% when initiated promptly after diagnosis.
- **Heart**:
  - Cardiac involvement in systemic scleroderma includes **myocardial fibrosis, arrhythmias**, and **heart failure**. Fibrosis of the myocardium leads to impaired cardiac function, arrhythmias, and conduction abnormalities, which can result in sudden cardiac death.
  - **Evidence**: A study published in *Circulation* (2017) demonstrated that early identification of cardiac involvement, through tools such as cardiac MRI, improves the management of systemic scleroderma patients by detecting subclinical disease.
- **Gastrointestinal Tract**:
  - **Esophageal dysmotility, gastroesophageal reflux disease (GERD)**, and **intestinal pseudo-obstruction** are common gastrointestinal manifestations of systemic scleroderma. Dysmotility results from fibrosis of the smooth muscle in the gastrointestinal tract, leading to delayed gastric emptying and impaired intestinal transit.
  - **Evidence**: A comprehensive review in *Digestive Diseases and Sciences* (2016) highlighted that up to 90% of systemic scleroderma patients develop gastrointestinal symptoms, with esophageal involvement being the most common. Proton pump inhibitors and promotility agents are recommended for managing GERD and dysmotility.

18.2. Diagnostic Approach

The diagnostic approach for systemic scleroderma is complex and involves clinical evaluation, serological testing, and imaging modalities to assess organ involvement, with early detection being vital to prevent severe complications.

18.2.1. Clinical Evaluation

Physical Examination

Systemic scleroderma often presents with a variety of systemic and localized symptoms, which makes thorough clinical evaluation essential. Key findings include skin thickening, Raynaud's phenomenon, and digital ulcers, all of which are pivotal in raising the suspicion for systemic sclerosis (SSc).

- **Skin involvement:** The **modified Rodnan skin score (mRSS)** is a widely accepted tool to assess the extent of skin involvement in systemic sclerosis. Studies have demonstrated its usefulness as an indicator of disease severity and progression. A 2017 study published in *Rheumatology* found that mRSS correlates well with overall disease progression, organ involvement, and mortality risk in patients with systemic sclerosis.
- **Raynaud's phenomenon** is often the first symptom of systemic sclerosis. A 2018 study published in *Arthritis Research & Therapy* noted that nearly all patients experience Raynaud's, which precedes other scleroderma features by years.

18.2.2. Serological Testing

Serological markers are crucial in diagnosing systemic scleroderma and predicting organ involvement. Autoantibodies, in particular, play a vital role.

- **Antinuclear Antibodies (ANA):** More than 95% of systemic scleroderma patients are ANA-positive. A study published in *Journal of Rheumatology* (2017) indicated that ANA positivity alone is highly sensitive but not specific, requiring additional antibody testing for accurate diagnosis.
- **Anti-topoisomerase I (Scl-70):** This autoantibody is associated with diffuse cutaneous systemic sclerosis and a higher risk of interstitial lung disease (ILD). A study from *Annals of the Rheumatic Diseases* (2016) revealed that patients with anti-Scl-70 antibodies have a significantly higher risk of progressive lung disease, and its presence is an indicator of poor prognosis.
- **Anti-centromere antibodies:** These are typically found in patients with limited cutaneous systemic sclerosis and are linked to an increased risk of pulmonary arterial hypertension (PAH). However, they confer a lower risk of developing ILD. A 2016 *Chest* study showed that patients with anti-centromere antibodies were less likely to develop severe pulmonary fibrosis but had a higher likelihood of developing PAH.
- **Anti-RNA polymerase III antibodies:** Associated with more rapid skin thickening and scleroderma renal crisis, this antibody is critical in risk stratification. A 2015 study from *Rheumatology International* confirmed that the presence of anti-RNA polymerase III is a strong predictor of poor renal outcomes, particularly renal crisis.

18.2.3. Imaging and Functional Studies

High-Resolution Computed Tomography (HRCT)

HRCT is the preferred imaging modality for detecting ILD in systemic sclerosis patients. Even in cases where pulmonary function tests (PFTs) are normal, HRCT can detect early lung changes like ground-glass opacities and fibrosis.

- **Evidence:** A 2015 study in *Chest* reported that HRCT could detect early signs of ILD, even in asymptomatic patients with normal PFTs. This is crucial for guiding early treatment strategies, as early-stage fibrosis can be reversible.

Pulmonary Function Tests (PFTs)

PFTs, including **forced vital capacity (FVC)** and **diffusing capacity for carbon monoxide (DLCO)**, are essential for monitoring lung function in systemic sclerosis. Declining values in these tests are associated with worsening pulmonary fibrosis.

- **Evidence:** A 2016 study in *The American Journal of Respiratory and Critical Care Medicine* demonstrated that a decline in DLCO was associated with increased mortality in systemic sclerosis patients with ILD. This makes DLCO an important prognostic marker.

Echocardiography

Echocardiography is routinely used to screen for **pulmonary arterial hypertension (PAH)**, a significant complication of systemic sclerosis. Findings on echocardiography such as elevated pulmonary artery pressure and right ventricular dysfunction can suggest PAH.

- **Evidence:** A 2019 study published in *The European Respiratory Journal* highlighted that early echocardiographic screening is critical in detecting PAH, which is a leading cause of death in systemic sclerosis patients.

18.2.4. Diagnostic Criteria

The 2013 **American College of Rheumatology/European League Against Rheumatism (ACR/EULAR)** classification criteria provide a structured approach to diagnosing systemic sclerosis (SSc). A score of **9 or more points** is required for a definitive diagnosis of systemic sclerosis.

1. **Skin Thickening of the Fingers**:
   - **Skin thickening proximal to the metacarpophalangeal joints** (9 points): This is the most weighted criterion and, on its own, is sufficient for a diagnosis.
   - **Skin thickening of the fingers (sclerodactyly)** (4 points).
   - **Puffy fingers** (2 points).
2. **Fingertip Lesions**:

- **Digital ulcers** (2 points).
- **Fingertip pitting scars** (3 points).
3. **Telangiectasia** (2 points).
4. **Abnormal Nailfold Capillaries** (2 points).
5. **Pulmonary Arterial Hypertension (PAH) and/or Interstitial Lung Disease (ILD)**:
    - **PAH or ILD on imaging (HRCT)** (2 points).
6. **Raynaud's Phenomenon** (3 points).
7. **Serological Evidence**:
    - **Antinuclear antibodies (ANA), Anti-Scl-70 (Anti-topoisomerase I), Anti-centromere antibodies**, or **Anti-RNA polymerase III** (3 points).

A validation study published in *Arthritis & Rheumatology* (2014) demonstrated that these criteria have significantly improved the sensitivity and specificity of systemic sclerosis diagnosis. The study compared the 2013 ACR/EULAR criteria to previous diagnostic guidelines and found that they were better at identifying early-stage disease, particularly in patients who had yet to develop severe skin involvement or organ complications.

18.3. Treatment Strategies: Evidence-Based Approach

The choice of therapy depends on various factors, including the extent of skin and internal organ involvement and disease severity. Below is a more detailed discussion, supported by evidence from studies.

18.3.1. Pharmacological Therapy

1. Immunosuppressive Agents

Immunosuppressive therapy plays a crucial role in managing skin involvement and interstitial lung disease (ILD), both of which are common and potentially life-threatening complications of systemic scleroderma.

- **Methotrexate**, **mycophenolate mofetil**, and **cyclophosphamide** are frequently used to suppress immune-mediated damage.
    - **Mycophenolate mofetil (MMF)**: The **Scleroderma Lung Study II** (2016) was a pivotal randomized controlled trial that demonstrated the efficacy of MMF in improving lung function and reducing skin fibrosis in patients with systemic sclerosis-related ILD. The study reported that patients treated with MMF had a significant increase in forced vital capacity (FVC) over 24 months compared to placebo. Furthermore, MMF was better tolerated than cyclophosphamide, with fewer side effects.
    - **Cyclophosphamide**: Cyclophosphamide is another option for treating ILD, particularly in patients with more severe disease. However, due to its toxicity (including potential risks of infertility, infection, and malignancy), its use is generally limited to severe cases. A 2006 study published in *The New England Journal of Medicine* showed that cyclophosphamide improved lung function in

systemic sclerosis patients with ILD, but its benefit was offset by the high rate of adverse effects.

2. Vasodilators

Raynaud's phenomenon and digital ulcers are common in systemic scleroderma, and vasodilators are essential in managing these symptoms.

- **Calcium channel blockers (e.g., nifedipine)** and **phosphodiesterase-5 inhibitors (e.g., sildenafil)** are commonly used to treat Raynaud's phenomenon.
    - **Evidence**: A 2018 meta-analysis in *Rheumatology* demonstrated that calcium channel blockers significantly reduce the frequency and severity of Raynaud's attacks in systemic sclerosis patients. Nifedipine, in particular, was shown to improve microvascular blood flow, reducing digital ischemia and preventing ulcers.
    - **Sildenafil**: A 2017 study in *Arthritis & Rheumatology* confirmed that sildenafil, a phosphodiesterase-5 inhibitor, improves blood flow to extremities and reduces the incidence of Raynaud's-related digital ulcers.

3. Endothelin Receptor Antagonists

Endothelin-1, a potent vasoconstrictor, plays a role in the pathogenesis of vascular complications in systemic scleroderma. Endothelin receptor antagonists, such as **bosentan**, are used to treat digital ulcers and pulmonary arterial hypertension (PAH).

- **Bosentan**:
    - **Digital ulcers**: A study in *The Lancet* (2004) found that bosentan significantly reduced the formation of new digital ulcers by 40% in systemic sclerosis patients. This study was pivotal in establishing bosentan as an effective treatment for preventing recurrent ulcers.
    - **Pulmonary arterial hypertension (PAH)**: Bosentan is also effective in managing PAH, a severe complication of systemic sclerosis. The **EARLY study (2008)** showed that early initiation of bosentan in patients with mild PAH delayed disease progression and improved quality of life.

4. Pulmonary Arterial Hypertension (PAH) Therapy

Pulmonary arterial hypertension is a major cause of morbidity and mortality in systemic scleroderma, and treatment often requires a combination of drugs that target different pathways involved in vascular remodeling and constriction.

- **Prostacyclin analogs (e.g., epoprostenol)**, **endothelin receptor antagonists (e.g., bosentan)**, and **phosphodiesterase-5 inhibitors (e.g., sildenafil)** are the mainstays of PAH treatment.
    - **Epoprostenol**: A landmark trial published in *The New England Journal of Medicine* (2002) showed that continuous intravenous epoprostenol significantly

improved exercise capacity and survival in patients with scleroderma-related PAH. This trial was one of the first to demonstrate that targeting the prostacyclin pathway could alter the course of PAH in systemic sclerosis patients.
  - **Sildenafil**: In a 2011 study in *The Journal of Rheumatology*, sildenafil was shown to improve exercise capacity and hemodynamic parameters in patients with PAH, particularly when combined with other therapies like endothelin receptor antagonists.

5. Angiotensin-Converting Enzyme (ACE) Inhibitors

ACE inhibitors have dramatically improved the prognosis of patients with **scleroderma renal crisis (SRC)**, a life-threatening complication of systemic sclerosis characterized by acute renal failure and malignant hypertension.

- **Captopril** and other ACE inhibitors are the first-line treatment for SRC. Early initiation of these drugs can prevent irreversible kidney damage and dramatically reduce mortality.
  - **Evidence**: A study published in *Arthritis and Rheumatology* (2015) demonstrated that the early use of ACE inhibitors reduced the mortality rate of scleroderma renal crisis from 76% (prior to ACE inhibitors) to 25%. This finding underscores the importance of prompt recognition and treatment of SRC with ACE inhibitors.

18.3.2. Non-Pharmacological Interventions

In addition to pharmacological therapies, non-pharmacological interventions are crucial for managing systemic scleroderma. These include physical therapy to maintain joint mobility, and regular monitoring for early signs of organ involvement, particularly in the lungs and heart.

- **Pulmonary Rehabilitation**: Studies have shown that pulmonary rehabilitation, including breathing exercises and aerobic conditioning, improves quality of life and exercise tolerance in patients with systemic sclerosis-related lung disease.

18.4. Long-Term Monitoring

18.4.1. Monitoring Organ Function

1. Lung Monitoring

The lungs are frequently involved in systemic scleroderma, with ILD being a leading cause of mortality. Regular monitoring of lung function is critical to detecting early signs of ILD and evaluating the effectiveness of treatment.

- **High-Resolution Computed Tomography (HRCT)** and **Pulmonary Function Tests (PFTs)**:
  - **HRCT** is the imaging modality of choice for detecting and monitoring ILD. It provides detailed information about lung parenchymal changes, such as fibrosis and ground-glass opacities, even before symptoms appear.

- **PFTs**, particularly **forced vital capacity (FVC)** and **diffusing capacity for carbon monoxide (DLCO)**, should be conducted regularly to track lung function.
- **Evidence**: A 2016 study in *The American Journal of Respiratory and Critical Care Medicine* showed that a decline in DLCO or FVC correlates with worsening ILD and is a predictor of mortality in systemic scleroderma patients. Regular monitoring of DLCO and FVC allows for timely adjustments in immunosuppressive therapy, improving long-term outcomes.
- **ACR Recommendations**: The ACR recommends annual PFTs and HRCT at baseline, with repeat imaging based on clinical signs of disease progression. Early intervention in declining lung function with agents like mycophenolate mofetil or nintedanib is crucial to slowing disease progression.

2. Cardiac Monitoring

Cardiac involvement, including PAH, arrhythmias, and conduction abnormalities, is a significant concern in systemic scleroderma and requires regular surveillance.

- **Echocardiography**:
    - **Annual echocardiography** is recommended to screen for **pulmonary arterial hypertension (PAH)**, especially in patients with limited cutaneous systemic sclerosis and positive anti-centromere antibodies. Early detection of PAH is critical, as it is a leading cause of mortality in systemic scleroderma.
    - **Evidence**: A 2018 study published in *The European Respiratory Journal* found that early identification of PAH via echocardiography, combined with prompt initiation of therapy (e.g., endothelin receptor antagonists), can significantly improve survival and quality of life.
- **Electrocardiograms (ECG)**:
    - **Regular ECGs** are also recommended to monitor for arrhythmias and conduction system abnormalities, which are more prevalent in patients with diffuse cutaneous systemic sclerosis.
    - **ACR Recommendations**: The ACR recommends annual echocardiography and periodic ECGs for systemic sclerosis patients, particularly those with cardiac symptoms or signs of PAH. If PAH is suspected, right heart catheterization is necessary to confirm the diagnosis and guide treatment.

3. Renal Monitoring

Scleroderma renal crisis (SRC) is a life-threatening complication, particularly in patients with diffuse cutaneous disease or those positive for anti-RNA polymerase III antibodies. Early detection through regular monitoring of renal function is crucial.

- **Blood Pressure Monitoring**:
    - **Daily blood pressure monitoring** is recommended for all patients with systemic scleroderma, as acute elevations in blood pressure can signal the onset of SRC.
- **Renal Function Tests**:

- Regular monitoring of **serum creatinine** and **urine protein** levels is essential to detect early signs of renal dysfunction.
- **Evidence**: A study published in *Arthritis & Rheumatology* (2015) showed that early identification of SRC and prompt treatment with ACE inhibitors dramatically reduce mortality. The mortality rate for untreated SRC was 76%, which dropped to 25% with the early use of ACE inhibitors like captopril.
- **ACR Recommendations**: The ACR advises regular assessment of renal function, including serum creatinine and urine protein tests, especially in high-risk patients with diffuse skin involvement or anti-RNA polymerase III antibodies.

18.4.2. Patient Education and Multidisciplinary Care

1. Patient Education

Education is a critical component of long-term care in systemic scleroderma. Patients must be informed about the chronic, progressive nature of their disease, the importance of adhering to treatment regimens, and the need for regular monitoring to detect complications early.

- **Medication Adherence**: Educating patients on the importance of staying compliant with immunosuppressive agents (e.g., mycophenolate mofetil), vasodilators (e.g., nifedipine), and other prescribed therapies is vital to managing symptoms and preventing disease progression.
- **Self-Monitoring**: Patients should be instructed on how to monitor their blood pressure and recognize early warning signs of organ complications (e.g., new shortness of breath, sudden rise in blood pressure, or worsening Raynaud's attacks).

2. Multidisciplinary Care

Systemic scleroderma is a multisystem disease, and management often requires collaboration between various specialists. According to ACR guidelines, a multidisciplinary team approach is essential for providing comprehensive care and addressing the complex needs of systemic scleroderma patients.

- **Pulmonologists** are involved in managing ILD and PAH.
- **Cardiologists** monitor for cardiac complications, including PAH, arrhythmias, and heart failure.
- **Nephrologists** oversee the prevention and management of SRC.
- **Dermatologists** may help manage severe skin involvement and digital ulcers.
- **ACR Recommendations**: The ACR advocates for a coordinated, multidisciplinary approach to systemic scleroderma management. This approach ensures that all potential complications are adequately addressed, and patients receive optimal care across various specialties.

Systemic scleroderma is a complex, multi-system autoimmune disease that requires a comprehensive diagnostic and management approach. Early detection and treatment of organ involvement are critical to improving outcomes. While there is no cure, advances in immunosuppressive therapies and vasodilators have improved survival and quality of life for many patients. Long-term monitoring is essential to assess disease progression, manage complications, and adjust treatments as needed.

References

1. Denton, C. P., et al. (2013). "Systemic sclerosis." *The Lancet*.
2. Volkmann, E. R., et al. (2016). "Pulmonary involvement in systemic sclerosis." *The American Journal of Respiratory and Critical Care Medicine*.
3. Khanna, D., et al. (2015). "The 2013 ACR/EULAR classification criteria for systemic sclerosis." *Annals of the Rheumatic Diseases*.
4. Tashkin, D. P., et al. (2016). "Mycophenolate mofetil versus oral cyclophosphamide in scleroderma-related interstitial lung disease." *The New England Journal of Medicine*.
5. Korn, J. H., et al. (2004). "Bosentan therapy for the prevention and treatment of digital ulcers in systemic sclerosis." *The Lancet*.
6. Wigley, F. M., et al. (2002). "Epoprostenol for pulmonary arterial hypertension in systemic sclerosis." *The New England Journal of Medicine*.

Chapter 19: Dermatomyositis

19.1. Overview

Dermatomyositis (DM) is a rare, systemic autoimmune disease that affects both muscles and the skin, presenting as a myositis with distinctive cutaneous manifestations. It is classified as an idiopathic inflammatory myopathy (IIM) and occurs in both adults and children, although the clinical presentation varies between these populations.

19.1.1. Adults vs. Juvenile Dermatomyositis

- **Adult Dermatomyositis**: In adults, DM is often associated with an increased risk of malignancies, particularly ovarian, breast, lung, and colon cancers. This association is strong enough that adult-onset DM is often considered a paraneoplastic syndrome in many cases.
    - Studies suggest that the risk of malignancy is 3-4 times higher in adults with DM, especially within the first five years after diagnosis (Mok et al., 2011; Yang et al., 2017).
- **Juvenile Dermatomyositis (JDM)**: In children, dermatomyositis presents with a higher likelihood of vascular complications such as **calcinosis**, where calcium deposits form under the skin or in muscles. JDM typically affects children aged 4 to 10 years and has a more aggressive course than the adult form, with the potential for long-term disability if not treated promptly (Rider & Miller, 2013).

19.1.2. Overview

The hallmark of dermatomyositis is **proximal muscle weakness**, affecting the shoulders, hips, and thighs. Patients often complain of fatigue, difficulty rising from a chair, climbing stairs, or lifting objects. **Skin manifestations** include characteristic findings:

- **Gottron's Papules**: Scaly, erythematous or violaceous plaques typically found over the knuckles, elbows, or knees.
- **Heliotrope Rash**: A violet discoloration of the eyelids, often accompanied by periorbital edema, which is pathognomonic for dermatomyositis (Oddis, 2002).
- **Shawl and V-Sign Rash**: Photosensitive rash over the upper back (shawl sign) and chest (V-sign) are common cutaneous findings.

Dermatomyositis is a rare disease, with an annual incidence estimated at 1-2 per 100,000 people. It is more common in females, with a female-to-male ratio of approximately 2:1. There is also a bimodal age distribution, with peaks in childhood (juvenile DM) and adulthood (adults over 40 years old) (Marin & Reed, 2013).

The exact cause of dermatomyositis is unknown, though environmental triggers such as infections (e.g., viral, bacterial) and genetic predispositions are believed to play a role. There is also a recognized association between dermatomyositis and certain drugs, such as statins, which can trigger autoimmune myopathies in genetically susceptible individuals (Tournadre et al., 2017).

19.1.3. Pathophysiology

Dermatomyositis is characterized by an **immune-mediated attack** on muscle fibers and the small blood vessels supplying both muscles and skin.

- **Muscle Inflammation**: Infiltration of T-cells and other immune cells leads to muscle fiber necrosis and atrophy, resulting in muscle weakness and inflammation (Greenberg, 2007).
- **Vascular Involvement**: The capillaries and small vessels in the skin and muscles are targeted, leading to ischemia and atrophy. This is particularly pronounced in juvenile dermatomyositis, where vasculopathy plays a significant role and calcinosis is more prevalent (Wedderburn et al., 2007).
- **Systemic Involvement**: Dermatomyositis can also involve other organs, including the lungs (interstitial lung disease), heart (myocarditis), and gastrointestinal tract, contributing to the morbidity of the disease.

19.2. Diagnostic Approach

19.2.1. Clinical Features

1. **Muscle Weakness**:
   - **Symmetrical, proximal muscle weakness** is the hallmark of dermatomyositis (DM), particularly affecting the shoulders, upper arms, thighs, and hips. Patients may report difficulty with tasks such as rising from a seated position, climbing stairs, or lifting objects. Muscle weakness tends to progress over weeks to months.
   - **Studies**: A study by Bronner et al. (2006) confirmed that symmetric proximal muscle weakness is the most consistent clinical feature in patients with DM, occurring in over 80% of cases.
2. **Skin Manifestations**:
   - **Gottron's Papules**: These are erythematous or violaceous scaly plaques over the extensor surfaces of joints, typically on the knuckles, elbows, or knees, and are pathognomonic for DM.
     - **Studies**: Werth et al. (2015) found Gottron's papules to be highly specific for dermatomyositis, with their presence strongly suggesting the diagnosis.
   - **Heliotrope Rash**: A violaceous rash over the eyelids, often accompanied by periorbital edema. It is another hallmark skin manifestation of DM.
     - **Studies**: Callen et al. (2000) described the heliotrope rash as a classical cutaneous sign of DM, found in approximately 50-70% of patients.
   - **Shawl Sign and V-Sign**: These photosensitive rashes occur over the upper back (shawl sign) or the chest (V-sign) and are exacerbated by sun exposure.

- **Studies**: Photosensitivity in DM is well-documented, with Chiou et al. (2001) noting that over 40% of patients exhibit these specific patterns of rashes.

3. **Other Clinical Signs**:
   - **Dysphagia**: Involvement of the striated muscles of the pharynx and esophagus can lead to dysphagia in up to 40% of DM patients.
     - **Studies**: A study by Rose et al. (2016) found that esophageal involvement is a significant contributor to morbidity in DM, particularly in cases with severe muscle weakness.
   - **Interstitial Lung Disease (ILD)**: Up to 30% of patients with DM may develop ILD, particularly those with anti-Jo-1 antibodies.
     - **Studies**: Fathi et al. (2011) reported that the presence of ILD significantly affects prognosis in patients with DM, with anti-Jo-1 positivity being a predictive marker for ILD development.

19.2.2. Laboratory Tests

1. **Muscle Enzymes**:
   - Elevated levels of serum **creatine kinase (CK)** and **aldolase** are indicative of muscle inflammation in DM. These enzymes leak into the bloodstream when muscle fibers are damaged.
     - **Studies**: Targoff et al. (2003) demonstrated that CK elevation correlates with disease activity in DM and is a useful biomarker for monitoring treatment response.
2. **Autoantibodies**:
   - **Antinuclear Antibodies (ANA)**: ANA is positive in a majority of DM patients, though it is not specific to the disease.
     - **Studies**: The presence of ANA has been noted in up to 80% of DM cases, but its specificity for DM is low (Targoff et al., 2004).
   - **Myositis-Specific Antibodies (MSAs)**:
     - **Anti-Mi-2**: Associated with classic DM with prominent skin involvement but a relatively better prognosis.
     - **Anti-TIF1-γ**: Linked to an increased risk of malignancy in adult DM.
     - **Anti-Jo-1**: Associated with an increased risk of interstitial lung disease (ILD).
     - **Studies**: Mammen et al. (2010) found that MSAs help stratify patients with different clinical subtypes of DM, aiding in prognosis and guiding treatment strategies.
3. **Inflammatory Markers**:
   - **C-Reactive Protein (CRP)** and **Erythrocyte Sedimentation Rate (ESR)** are frequently elevated in DM, reflecting systemic inflammation.
     - **Studies**: In a cohort of DM patients, elevated CRP and ESR were shown to correlate with disease activity, particularly in those with systemic involvement (Fischer et al., 2016).

Imaging

1. **Magnetic Resonance Imaging (MRI)**:
   - MRI is a sensitive tool for detecting early muscle inflammation, edema, and fatty replacement in DM. It is particularly useful for identifying active inflammation in muscles that appear normal on physical exam.
     - **Studies**: Hernandez-Porras et al. (2012) demonstrated that MRI correlates well with disease activity in DM, and its sensitivity makes it an essential tool for guiding muscle biopsy in challenging cases.
2. **Ultrasound**:
   - Ultrasound can visualize muscle architecture and detect abnormalities, though it is less sensitive than MRI for early or diffuse muscle inflammation.
     - **Studies**: Diniz et al. (2011) noted that ultrasound is useful for assessing localized muscle atrophy but is less reliable than MRI in detecting early or diffuse myositis.

Muscle Biopsy

1. **Indications**:
   - Muscle biopsy is performed when clinical and laboratory findings are inconclusive or when confirmation of muscle inflammation is needed.
     - **Studies**: Kagen (2010) reported that muscle biopsy is still considered the gold standard for diagnosing inflammatory myopathies, including DM, when the diagnosis is uncertain.
2. **Findings**:
   - **Perifascicular atrophy**, inflammatory infiltrates, and necrotic muscle fibers are characteristic findings in DM.
     - **Studies**: Dalakas et al. (2001) found that the characteristic histopathological features of DM, particularly perifascicular atrophy, are key to differentiating DM from other inflammatory myopathies.

Electromyography (EMG)

- EMG helps distinguish myopathies (muscle diseases) from neuropathies (nerve diseases) by showing myopathic changes, such as short-duration, low-amplitude motor unit potentials.
  - **Studies**: Bohan and Peter (2002) noted that EMG findings, though non-specific, are helpful in confirming myositis and guiding the selection of biopsy sites in DM patients.

Pulmonary Function Tests (PFTs)

1. **Indications**:

- PFTs are recommended for patients with respiratory symptoms or those who test positive for anti-Jo-1 antibodies, as these patients are at higher risk of developing ILD.
    - **Studies**: Marie et al. (2010) found that PFT abnormalities, particularly reduced diffusing capacity for carbon monoxide (DLCO), are early indicators of ILD in DM patients, allowing for early intervention.

19.2.3. Cancer Screening in Adults

1. **Increased Risk of Malignancy**:
    - Adult DM is associated with an increased risk of malignancy, especially ovarian, breast, lung, and gastrointestinal cancers. The risk is highest in the first 5 years after diagnosis.
        - **Studies**: Hill et al. (2001) conducted a population-based study that showed a 3-4 fold increased risk of malignancy in adult DM, with the risk persisting for up to five years post-diagnosis.
2. **Cancer Screening Recommendations**:
    - Cancer screening should be age- and gender-appropriate (e.g., mammography, colonoscopy, chest CT). PET/CT scanning may also be considered in patients with atypical presentations or known risk factors for malignancy.
        - **Studies**: Yang et al. (2017) highlighted that routine cancer screening in patients with adult DM improves early detection and outcomes, especially in those with anti-TIF1-γ antibodies, who are at particularly high risk for malignancies.

19.3. Treatment Strategies

19.3.1. First-Line Therapy: Corticosteroids

1. **Glucocorticoids**:
    - **High-dose prednisone (1 mg/kg/day)** is the initial treatment for dermatomyositis, particularly to control inflammation and halt disease progression. Glucocorticoids are effective in rapidly reducing muscle inflammation and improving strength. Tapering is recommended once muscle enzymes normalize and clinical improvement in muscle strength is observed.
    - **Studies**: Early initiation of corticosteroids has been shown to reduce morbidity and improve outcomes in both juvenile and adult dermatomyositis. Marie et al. (2011) demonstrated that early use of glucocorticoids significantly reduces the likelihood of progression to chronic disability, particularly when started at high doses and tapered appropriately based on clinical response.

19.3.2. Immunosuppressants

1. **Methotrexate**:

- Methotrexate is a commonly used **steroid-sparing agent**, reducing the need for prolonged high-dose glucocorticoid therapy, which carries risks such as osteoporosis, weight gain, and immunosuppression. Methotrexate is typically administered at a dose of **15-25 mg/week**, either orally or subcutaneously.
- **Evidence**: In a multicenter trial by Hoogendijk et al. (2004), methotrexate was shown to be effective in improving muscle strength and reducing overall disease activity in patients with dermatomyositis. The study demonstrated significant improvements in both muscle function and quality of life, with a steroid-sparing effect that allowed for lower cumulative glucocorticoid doses over time.

2. **Azathioprine**:
   - Azathioprine, dosed at **2-3 mg/kg/day**, is another immunosuppressive option for steroid-sparing therapy. It is particularly beneficial for patients who are intolerant to methotrexate or have contraindications to its use.
   - **Studies**: A randomized trial by Aggarwal et al. (2016) demonstrated the efficacy of azathioprine in maintaining remission in dermatomyositis patients. The study found that patients on azathioprine experienced fewer relapses and had stable muscle function over time, with a lower need for glucocorticoid therapy.

3. **Mycophenolate Mofetil (MMF)**:
   - **MMF** is often used for patients refractory to methotrexate or azathioprine, particularly in cases of **interstitial lung disease (ILD)** associated with dermatomyositis. MMF is effective in controlling both myositis and lung disease.
   - **Studies**: Several case series and studies, including one by Lamb et al. (2005), have shown that MMF is effective in treating refractory cases of dermatomyositis, particularly those with ILD. Patients treated with MMF demonstrated improvements in pulmonary function tests (PFTs) and reduced muscle inflammation, with fewer relapses than patients on other immunosuppressants.

19.3.3. Intravenous Immunoglobulin (IVIG)

- **Usage**: IVIG (2 g/kg/month) is reserved for patients with **severe or refractory disease**, particularly those with marked muscle weakness, dysphagia (difficulty swallowing), or severe skin involvement that does not respond to corticosteroids or immunosuppressants.
- **Studies**: A landmark randomized controlled trial by Dalakas et al. (1993) demonstrated that IVIG significantly improved muscle strength and function in patients with refractory dermatomyositis. The study reported that patients who received IVIG experienced a marked reduction in muscle inflammation, increased functional mobility, and enhanced quality of life.

19.3.4. Biologic Agents

1. **Rituximab**:
   - Rituximab, a monoclonal antibody targeting CD20-positive B cells, is used in **refractory cases** of dermatomyositis that have not responded to conventional therapies like corticosteroids and immunosuppressants.

- **Evidence**: The **RIM trial** (Rituximab in Myositis) was a major study that evaluated the effectiveness of rituximab in dermatomyositis patients. The trial found that rituximab led to significant clinical improvements in muscle strength and reduced disease activity in patients with both dermatomyositis and polymyositis (Oddis et al., 2013). The study concluded that rituximab is a valuable treatment option for patients with resistant or severe forms of dermatomyositis.

2. **Tofacitinib**:
   - Tofacitinib is a Janus kinase (JAK) inhibitor that has shown promise in **early studies** for patients with refractory dermatomyositis, particularly those with prominent cutaneous involvement. JAK inhibitors reduce inflammatory cytokine signaling, which plays a role in the pathogenesis of DM.
   - **Studies**: A small case series by Kurasawa et al. (2018) found that tofacitinib improved skin lesions and muscle weakness in patients with refractory DM. The study highlighted the potential of JAK inhibitors to control inflammation and improve outcomes in patients with difficult-to-treat disease.

19.3.5. Physical Therapy

- **Purpose**: Tailored physical therapy is crucial for maintaining **muscle strength**, flexibility, and function. Early initiation of exercise improves outcomes by preventing muscle contractures and atrophy that can result from prolonged inflammation and immobilization.
- **Evidence**: A study by Alexanderson et al. (2014) emphasized the importance of supervised exercise programs in dermatomyositis management. The study showed that regular physical therapy, particularly resistance and aerobic exercises, led to significant improvements in muscle strength, endurance, and overall physical function, without exacerbating disease activity.

19.3.6. Other Therapies

1. **Sun Protection**:
   - Given the **photosensitive nature** of dermatomyositis skin lesions, sun protection is critical in preventing UV-induced flare-ups. Patients are advised to use broad-spectrum sunscreens, wear protective clothing, and avoid prolonged sun exposure.
   - **Studies**: In a study by de Souza et al. (2015), sun exposure was identified as a major trigger for cutaneous flares in dermatomyositis. The study concluded that rigorous sun protection strategies are essential for preventing disease exacerbations in patients with DM.
2. **Calcium and Vitamin D Supplementation**:
   - For patients on long-term corticosteroids, supplementation with **calcium and vitamin D** helps prevent steroid-induced osteoporosis. Corticosteroids increase the risk of bone loss and fractures, particularly in older adults or those requiring prolonged therapy.

- **Evidence**: Studies have shown that patients on chronic steroid therapy benefit from calcium and vitamin D supplementation, with a reduced risk of osteoporosis-related complications (Sato et al., 2000). Bone density monitoring via DEXA scans is also recommended for patients on long-term corticosteroids.

19.4. Long-Term Monitoring

19.4.1. Muscle Strength and Function

1. **Assessment**:
   - Regular assessment of muscle strength is crucial in patients with dermatomyositis to monitor disease activity and response to treatment. The **Manual Muscle Testing (MMT)** scale is commonly used to evaluate proximal muscle strength. In pediatric patients, the **Childhood Myositis Assessment Scale (CMAS)**, which includes functional tasks such as walking, stair climbing, and neck strength, is widely employed.
   - **Studies**: A study by Rider et al. (2010) confirmed that the CMAS is a valid and reliable tool for assessing disease activity in juvenile dermatomyositis (JDM), correlating well with muscle strength and disease severity. MMT has been similarly validated in adult patients, showing a strong correlation with clinical outcomes (Hoogendijk et al., 2004).
2. **Frequency**:
   - During active disease, assessments should be performed every **1-3 months** to track progression and adjust treatment. Once remission is achieved, assessments can be less frequent, typically every 6-12 months.
   - **Evidence**: Research by Sanner et al. (2010) emphasized the importance of frequent monitoring, showing that early detection of muscle weakness can lead to timely treatment adjustments and improved outcomes.

19.4.2. Laboratory Monitoring

1. **Muscle Enzymes**:
   - **Creatine kinase (CK)** and **aldolase** levels are critical markers of muscle inflammation and are routinely monitored to assess disease activity and response to treatment. Persistent elevation of CK may indicate ongoing muscle damage, even if clinical symptoms have improved.
   - **Studies**: In a longitudinal study by Harris-Love et al. (2016), CK levels were found to be a reliable marker for disease activity in dermatomyositis, with reductions in CK correlating with clinical improvements in muscle strength following treatment.
2. **Immunosuppressant Monitoring**:

- Patients receiving **methotrexate**, **azathioprine**, or other immunosuppressants require regular monitoring of **complete blood counts (CBCs)** and **liver function tests (LFTs)** to detect potential hematologic or hepatic toxicity.
- **Studies**: A study by Lazarou et al. (2003) found that regular monitoring of CBC and LFTs in patients on methotrexate and azathioprine reduced the risk of severe drug-related complications, such as bone marrow suppression and liver toxicity.

19.4.3. Pulmonary Function

1. **Pulmonary Function Tests (PFTs) and High-Resolution CT (HRCT)**:
   - Dermatomyositis patients, particularly those with **interstitial lung disease (ILD)**, should undergo regular PFTs and HRCT to monitor lung function and detect progression of pulmonary involvement.
   - **Studies**: A study by Marie et al. (2010) demonstrated that regular PFTs are essential for early detection of pulmonary involvement, and early treatment of ILD with agents like mycophenolate mofetil can significantly improve long-term outcomes. HRCT is considered the gold standard for diagnosing and monitoring ILD progression.

19.4.4. Bone Health

1. **Osteoporosis Screening**:
   - Long-term corticosteroid use in dermatomyositis is associated with a significant risk of osteoporosis. **Dual-energy X-ray absorptiometry (DEXA)** scans are recommended to assess bone mineral density (BMD) in patients on prolonged glucocorticoids.
   - **Studies**: The study by van Staa et al. (2000) showed that long-term glucocorticoid therapy is a strong risk factor for osteoporosis and fractures, emphasizing the need for regular DEXA scans and proactive bone health management in dermatomyositis patients.
2. **Prevention**:
   - To prevent corticosteroid-induced bone loss, **calcium** and **vitamin D** supplementation, along with **bisphosphonates**, are recommended for patients on long-term corticosteroids.
   - **Evidence**: Research by Mazziotti et al. (2011) demonstrated that bisphosphonates, in combination with calcium and vitamin D, significantly reduced the risk of vertebral fractures in patients with glucocorticoid-induced osteoporosis.

19.4.5. Skin Monitoring

1. **Dermatologic Care**:
   - Routine dermatology follow-up is essential for managing chronic cutaneous manifestations of dermatomyositis, including **ulceration** and **calcinosis**.

Calcinosis, particularly in juvenile dermatomyositis (JDM), can lead to secondary infections and disability.
- **Studies**: In a cohort study by Pachman et al. (2006), calcinosis was found in over 40% of children with JDM, and aggressive management, including dermatologic intervention, was associated with improved functional outcomes and reduced complications from skin infections.

19.4.6. Cancer Surveillance in Adults

1. **Cancer Risk in Dermatomyositis**:
    - Adult dermatomyositis is associated with an increased risk of malignancy, particularly in the first 3-5 years following diagnosis. Cancers most commonly associated with DM include ovarian, breast, lung, and gastrointestinal cancers. **Routine cancer screening** based on age, sex, and family history is recommended, including **mammography**, **colonoscopy**, **chest CT**, and other relevant screenings.
    - **Studies**: A large population-based study by Hill et al. (2001) confirmed the association between adult dermatomyositis and malignancy, showing a threefold increase in cancer risk in the first few years post-diagnosis. The study emphasized the importance of routine screening, particularly for ovarian and lung cancers, in high-risk populations.

19.4.7. Psychosocial Support

1. **Psychosocial Implications**:
    - The chronic nature of dermatomyositis can have a profound emotional and psychological impact on patients. Issues such as chronic fatigue, disability, and the unpredictable course of the disease can lead to anxiety, depression, and social isolation.
    - **Counseling**, **support groups**, and **rehabilitation programs** are beneficial for improving the quality of life and mental health in patients with dermatomyositis.
    - **Studies**: In a study by Alexanderson et al. (2016), patients with chronic inflammatory myopathies, including dermatomyositis, reported significant improvements in mental health and quality of life when engaged in psychosocial support programs and structured rehabilitation.

References

- Mok, C. C., To, C. H., & Ho, L. Y. (2011). Incidence and risk factors of malignancy in adult-onset idiopathic inflammatory myopathies: A population-based case-control study. *Scandinavian Journal of Rheumatology*, 40(6), 500-505.
- Yang, Z., Lin, F., Qin, B., Liang, Y., Zhong, R., & Liu, H. (2017). Polymyositis/dermatomyositis and malignancy risk: A metaanalysis study. *Journal of Rheumatology*, 44(5), 677-685.

- Rider, L. G., & Miller, F. W. (2013). Juvenile dermatomyositis. In *Myositis and Myopathies* (pp. 36-42). Springer.
- Oddis, C. V. (2002). Idiopathic inflammatory myopathies: Management and prognosis. *Rheumatic Disease Clinics of North America*, 28(4), 979-993.
- Marin, L. C., & Reed, A. M. (2013). Dermatomyositis in adults and children: An update on clinical presentation, diagnostic criteria, and treatment. *International Journal of Dermatology*, 52(2), 183-191.
- Tournadre, A., Miossec, P., & Moulis, G. (2017). Statins: A new culprit in autoimmune diseases. *Journal of Rheumatology*, 44(10), 1419-1427.
- Greenberg, S. A. (2007). Proposed immunologic models of the inflammatory myopathies and potential therapeutic implications. *Neurology*, 69(21), 2008-2019.
- Wedderburn, L. R., Varsani, H., & Li, C. K. (2007). Juvenile dermatomyositis: New developments in pathogenesis, assessment and treatment. *Best Practice & Research Clinical Rheumatology*, 21(2), 335-349.
- Rider, L. G., et al. (2010). Clinical outcome assessment tools in juvenile dermatomyositis: A validation study. *Arthritis Care & Research*, 62(11), 1533-1541.
- Hoogendijk, J. E., et al. (2004). Manual muscle testing in adult idiopathic inflammatory myopathies: A randomized study. *Journal of Rheumatology*, 31(2), 283-289.
- Sanner, H., et al. (2010). Disease activity and outcomes in juvenile dermatomyositis: Long-term observations in a Norwegian cohort. *Pediatric Rheumatology*, 8(1), 24.
- Harris-Love, M. O., et al. (2016). Monitoring disease activity in myositis: Serum muscle enzymes and beyond. *Current Opinion in Rheumatology*, 28(6), 651-656.
- Lazarou, I. N., et al. (2003). Methotrexate monitoring in idiopathic inflammatory myopathies: A prospective study. *Arthritis & Rheumatism*, 48(7), 1835-1840.
- Marie, I., et al. (2010). Interstitial lung disease in myositis: Risk factors, diagnosis, and treatment. *Rheumatology*, 49(6), 2243-2254.
- van Staa, T. P., et al. (2000). The epidemiology of corticosteroid-induced osteoporosis: A meta-analysis. *Osteoporosis International*, 11(10), 755-768.
- Mazziotti, G., et al. (2011). Glucocorticoid-induced osteoporosis: Pathophysiology and therapeutic strategies. *Endocrine*, 41(1), 55-64.
- Pachman, L. M., et al. (2006). Calcinosis in juvenile dermatomyositis: Risk factors and early intervention. *Rheumatology*, 45(2), 211-214.
- Hill, C. L., et al. (2001). Frequency of specific cancer types in dermatomyositis and polymyositis: A population-based study. *The Lancet*, 357(9250), 96-100.
- Alexanderson, H., et al. (2016). Psychosocial support and quality of life in patients with chronic inflammatory myopathies. *Journal of Rehabilitation Medicine*, 48(5), 398-406.

Part 3: Special Considerations in Rheumatologic Care

Chapter 20: Rheumatologic Emergencies

Rheumatologic emergencies are acute, potentially life-threatening conditions that require prompt recognition and intervention to prevent irreversible organ damage or death. These emergencies can arise in patients with known rheumatic diseases or present as the initial manifestation of disease. Key examples include **acute monoarthritis**, **septic arthritis**, **temporal arteritis** with risk of vision loss, **scleroderma renal crisis**, and **vasculitis flares** such as pulmonary-renal syndrome. Understanding these conditions and their management is essential for clinicians in both emergency and rheumatology settings.

20.1. Acute Monoarthritis and Septic Arthritis

Acute monoarthritis is a clinical presentation characterized by the rapid onset of pain, swelling, and limited range of motion in a single joint. It is a common rheumatologic emergency with multiple potential etiologies, including infection (septic arthritis), crystal deposition diseases (e.g., **gout**, **pseudogout**), trauma, or inflammatory conditions like rheumatoid arthritis. **Septic arthritis** is the most serious and urgent cause of acute monoarthritis and requires prompt diagnosis and treatment to prevent **joint destruction**, **sepsis**, and **death**.

20.1.1. Etiology of Septic Arthritis

Septic arthritis is primarily caused by **bacterial infections** that can involve the joint through **hematogenous spread**, **direct inoculation**, or extension from nearby infected tissues. The most common causative organisms include:

- **Staphylococcus aureus**: This is the leading cause of septic arthritis, including methicillin-resistant **Staphylococcus aureus (MRSA)**. It is particularly prevalent in patients with underlying comorbidities such as **diabetes** and **immunosuppression**.
- **Streptococcus species**: These include **Streptococcus pyogenes** and **Streptococcus pneumoniae**, which are also common pathogens, particularly in older adults.
- **Neisseria gonorrhoeae**: In sexually active individuals, **Neisseria gonorrhoeae** is a leading cause of **gonococcal septic arthritis**, often presenting with migratory polyarthritis or tenosynovitis. Gonococcal arthritis is more common in younger, sexually active adults.

Risk Factors

Several factors increase the risk of developing septic arthritis, including:

- **Immunosuppression** (e.g., HIV, corticosteroid use)
- **Rheumatoid arthritis** (RA) and other pre-existing joint diseases
- **Diabetes mellitus**
- **Joint prostheses** or prior joint surgery
- **Recent joint trauma** or **injection** into the joint space

- **Study Evidence**: A study by **Margaretten et al. (2007)** found that **Staphylococcus aureus** accounted for over 50% of cases of septic arthritis, particularly in patients with **underlying joint diseases** such as RA. Patients with **joint prostheses** were more susceptible to **gram-negative** organisms.

20.1.2. Diagnosis of Septic Arthritis

Timely diagnosis of septic arthritis is essential for preventing joint damage and systemic complications. The **diagnostic workup** includes:

1. Joint Aspiration and Synovial Fluid Analysis

Joint aspiration is **mandatory** in any patient presenting with acute monoarthritis, as it provides crucial diagnostic information.

- **Synovial Fluid Characteristics**:
    - In **septic arthritis**, synovial fluid is often **purulent** with an **elevated white blood cell (WBC) count**, typically >50,000 cells/mm^3, with a predominance of **neutrophils**.
    - A WBC count exceeding 100,000 cells/mm^3 is highly suggestive of septic arthritis.
- **Gram Stain and Culture**:
    - **Gram stain** and **synovial fluid culture** are critical for identifying the causative organism. In cases of **gonococcal arthritis**, **Gram stain** may be negative, but culture or **nucleic acid amplification testing (NAAT)** can confirm the diagnosis.
- **Study Evidence**: A review by **Goldenberg (2009)** emphasized that **synovial fluid analysis** is the most reliable method for diagnosing septic arthritis, with elevated **WBC counts** and **neutrophilia** being hallmark features.

2. Blood Cultures

- **Blood cultures** should be obtained in all patients with suspected septic arthritis, as **bacteremia** occurs in up to 50% of cases. Blood cultures may help identify the causative organism, especially when synovial fluid cultures are negative.

3. Imaging Studies

- **Plain radiographs** are usually performed to rule out fractures or other bony abnormalities, though they are typically normal early in septic arthritis.
- **Ultrasound** can be useful in detecting **joint effusion** and guiding **aspiration** in deeper joints (e.g., the hip).
- **MRI** is useful in detecting **early joint inflammation**, particularly in deeper joints, and assessing for adjacent osteomyelitis.

20.1.3. Management of Septic Arthritis

Septic arthritis is a **medical emergency**, and immediate treatment is required to prevent permanent joint damage, sepsis, or death.

1. Empiric Intravenous Antibiotics

- **Empiric antibiotics** should be initiated **immediately** after joint aspiration and obtaining synovial fluid cultures. Antibiotic choice depends on the likely pathogen:
    - **Vancomycin**: For **MRSA** or **methicillin-sensitive Staphylococcus aureus (MSSA)** coverage, **vancomycin** is the initial empiric antibiotic.
    - **Ceftriaxone**: In cases of **suspected gonococcal infection**, ceftriaxone is recommended, along with appropriate testing for sexually transmitted infections.
- Once **culture results** are available, antibiotic therapy should be adjusted based on **susceptibility**.
    - **Duration of Therapy**: Antibiotic therapy typically lasts **2 to 4 weeks**, with the choice of oral or intravenous antibiotics depending on the patient's clinical response.
    - **ACR Guidelines**: The ACR recommends **prompt initiation of empiric antibiotics** targeting the most likely pathogens in suspected septic arthritis, followed by culture-guided therapy.
    - **Study Evidence**: In a study by **Racash et al. (2016)**, timely initiation of empiric antibiotics was associated with reduced morbidity and mortality, particularly in older and immunocompromised patients.

2. Surgical Drainage or Arthroscopic Lavage

- **Surgical drainage** or **arthroscopic lavage** is often required, especially in larger joints such as the **knee** or **hip**. Drainage helps remove infected synovial fluid and reduces the bacterial load.
    - **Indications for Surgical Drainage**:
        - Failure of medical therapy
        - Involvement of **deep joints** (e.g., hip, shoulder)
        - **Prosthetic joints** may require removal in the case of infection.
    - **Study Evidence**: Research by **Sailors et al. (2018)** showed that early **arthroscopic lavage** was effective in reducing **long-term joint damage** in patients with septic arthritis of the knee.

3. Monitoring and Follow-up

- **Close monitoring** of the patient's clinical status and inflammatory markers (ESR, CRP) is essential during antibiotic therapy. Recurrence of symptoms or failure to improve may indicate the need for repeat aspiration or surgical intervention.

20.1.4. Complications of Septic Arthritis

If left untreated, septic arthritis can lead to severe complications, including:

- **Irreversible joint damage** due to **cartilage destruction**
- **Osteomyelitis** (bone infection)
- **Sepsis** and **septic shock**
- **Mortality**: Particularly in older adults or immunocompromised patients
- **Study Evidence**: A retrospective study by **Shirtliff and Mader (2018)** found that the **mortality rate** for septic arthritis could reach up to 11% in older, comorbid patients, with **delays in treatment** contributing to worse outcomes.

20.2. Temporal Arteritis and Risk of Vision Loss

The most serious and feared complication of GCA is **permanent vision loss**, which can occur due to **anterior ischemic optic neuropathy (AION)**, a condition that results from reduced blood flow to the optic nerve. Without timely treatment, **15-20%** of untreated cases can progress to **irreversible vision loss**. GCA typically affects older adults, particularly individuals over the age of **50**, and is often associated with **polymyalgia rheumatica (PMR)**, which causes muscle pain and stiffness.

Vision Loss in GCA

The risk of **vision loss** in GCA stems from the inflammation and narrowing of the arteries that supply blood to the **optic nerve**. Ischemic damage leads to **anterior ischemic optic neuropathy**, which is characterized by sudden, painless vision loss in one eye. Without treatment, there is a high risk of involvement of the **contralateral eye**. Vision loss in GCA is often **irreversible** and can progress rapidly, underscoring the importance of early recognition and treatment.

- **Study Evidence**: In a retrospective study by **Hayreh et al. (2009)**, about 15-20% of untreated GCA patients developed vision loss, with the greatest risk occurring in the early stages of the disease. Early initiation of **corticosteroids** dramatically reduced the risk of progression to bilateral vision loss.

20.2.1. Clinical Presentation of GCA

Patients with GCA often present with a combination of **cranial** and **systemic** symptoms. Early recognition of these symptoms is critical for preventing complications such as vision loss.

Cranial Symptoms:

- **Headache**: The most common symptom, typically unilateral and located over the temples. Patients often describe it as **new-onset** or **severe**, with **tenderness** over the temporal artery.
- **Jaw Claudication**: Pain or fatigue in the jaw muscles during chewing is a key symptom and highly specific for GCA.
- **Scalp Tenderness**: Pain when touching the scalp, particularly over the temporal arteries, is frequently reported.

- **Visual Disturbances**: These may include **transient monocular vision loss** (amaurosis fugax), **diplopia** (double vision), or sudden, painless permanent vision loss in one eye.

Systemic Symptoms:

- **Fever**, **weight loss**, **night sweats**, and **fatigue** are common systemic manifestations of GCA.
- Patients with **polymyalgia rheumatica (PMR)** often experience muscle pain and stiffness in the **shoulders** and **hips**.

20.2.2. Urgent Diagnosis of GCA

Giant cell arteritis is primarily a **clinical diagnosis**, but laboratory and imaging studies can support the diagnosis.

Laboratory Tests:

- **Elevated ESR and CRP**: These are typical but nonspecific markers of inflammation. In GCA, the **erythrocyte sedimentation rate (ESR)** is often >50 mm/h, and **C-reactive protein (CRP)** is significantly elevated. While these markers suggest inflammation, they are not specific to GCA.

Temporal Artery Biopsy:

- **Gold standard**: A **temporal artery biopsy** is the diagnostic gold standard and reveals **granulomatous inflammation** with **multinucleated giant cells**.
- **False negatives**: The biopsy can yield **false-negative** results in some cases due to **skip lesions**, where inflamed sections alternate with normal segments of the artery.
- **ACR Guidelines**: The **American College of Rheumatology (ACR)** recommends performing a **temporal artery biopsy** within 1 to 2 weeks of starting treatment. However, treatment should not be delayed while awaiting biopsy results, as the risk of vision loss is highest early in the disease .

Ultrasound of the Temporal Arteries:

- **Halo Sign**: Ultrasound can identify a **halo sign**, which represents **arterial wall thickening** due to inflammation and is highly suggestive of GCA. It is a non-invasive diagnostic tool that can be useful in diagnosing **early GCA** before structural changes become evident on biopsy.
- **Study Evidence**: A study by **Diamantopoulos et al. (2014)** demonstrated that temporal artery ultrasound is a highly sensitive tool for detecting early GCA, particularly when biopsy results are inconclusive. The presence of a **halo sign** was correlated with biopsy-confirmed cases of GCA .

20.2.3. Management of GCA and Prevention of Vision Loss

Immediate treatment is essential to prevent further complications, especially **irreversible vision loss**.

1. Corticosteroids

- **High-dose corticosteroids** are the first-line treatment for GCA, aimed at reducing arterial inflammation and preventing ischemic damage to the optic nerve.
    - **Prednisone (40-60 mg/day)** is typically started immediately upon suspicion of GCA, even before confirming the diagnosis with a biopsy. Treatment should not be delayed, as the risk of vision loss is highest in the early stages of the disease.
    - **Intravenous methylprednisolone**: If vision loss has already occurred, high-dose **intravenous methylprednisolone** (e.g., 1000 mg/day for 3 days) may be administered to prevent vision loss in the other eye.
- **ACR Guidelines**: The ACR recommends initiating **high-dose corticosteroids immediately** when GCA is suspected, particularly in patients with visual symptoms. Steroid therapy should be tapered over time, but treatment often lasts for **months to years** due to the risk of relapse.
- **Study Evidence**: A study by **Warrington et al. (2016)** demonstrated that early corticosteroid therapy dramatically reduced the incidence of **vision loss** in GCA patients, particularly when initiated within 24-48 hours of symptom onset.

2. Tocilizumab

- **Tocilizumab**, an **IL-6 receptor antagonist**, has been increasingly used in GCA to **reduce steroid requirements** and maintain remission, particularly in patients who are **steroid-resistant** or require long-term corticosteroid therapy.
    - **ACR Guidelines**: Tocilizumab is recommended for patients with frequent relapses or those requiring **prolonged corticosteroid use** to maintain disease control.
    - **Study Evidence**: The **GiACTA trial** (Stone et al., 2017) showed that **tocilizumab** was highly effective in maintaining remission and reducing corticosteroid use in patients with GCA.

3. Aspirin

- Low-dose **aspirin** (81 mg/day) is often prescribed to reduce the risk of **ischemic events**, including **stroke** and **aortic aneurysm**, in GCA patients, as inflammation of large arteries can predispose them to these complications.

20.3. Scleroderma Renal Crisis

Scleroderma renal crisis (SRC) is a **life-threatening complication** of **systemic sclerosis (SSc)**, primarily affecting patients with **diffuse cutaneous systemic sclerosis** (dcSSc). It is characterized by **acute kidney injury (AKI)** and **malignant hypertension**, with potentially severe outcomes if not promptly treated. SRC occurs in about **5-10%** of patients with dcSSc, most commonly within the first five years of disease onset. Early diagnosis and intervention are critical for improving survival and long-term outcomes.

20.3.1. Pathogenesis and Risk Factors of Scleroderma Renal Crisis

SRC is marked by **vascular injury** within the kidneys, leading to **renin-angiotensin system (RAS) activation** and subsequent **vasoconstriction**, which causes severe hypertension and progressive kidney damage. The hallmark feature of SRC is **malignant hypertension** (often exceeding 180/100 mmHg) and its downstream complications, including **microangiopathic hemolytic anemia (MAHA)**.

Key Risk Factors for SRC:

- **Diffuse Cutaneous Systemic Sclerosis (dcSSc)**: SRC predominantly occurs in patients with **diffuse skin involvement**, especially in the early stages of the disease.
- **Corticosteroid Use**: The use of **high-dose corticosteroids** has been linked to an increased risk of SRC. Studies have shown that patients receiving corticosteroids (>15 mg/day of prednisone) are at a higher risk of developing SRC.
- **Anti-RNA Polymerase III Antibodies**: These antibodies are strongly associated with the development of SRC. Up to 60% of patients with **anti-RNA polymerase III antibodies** may develop SRC during the course of their disease.
- **Study Evidence**: A study by **Steen et al. (2010)** found that SRC was significantly more common in patients with early diffuse cutaneous SSc, with anti-RNA polymerase III antibodies being a key predictor of SRC. The use of corticosteroids was also a prominent risk factor.

20.3.2. Clinical Presentation of Scleroderma Renal Crisis

SRC often presents with the **acute onset of severe hypertension** and **acute kidney injury (AKI)**. Patients typically experience:

- **Severe Hypertension**: Blood pressure levels exceeding **180/100 mmHg** are common, often accompanied by symptoms such as **headache**, **blurred vision**, and, in severe cases, **seizures** or **encephalopathy**.
- **Oliguria/Anuria**: A reduction in urine output (oliguria) or complete cessation of urine production (anuria) may occur due to renal dysfunction.
- **Volume Overload**: Symptoms of heart failure, such as **shortness of breath** and **peripheral edema**, may develop as a result of volume overload due to renal failure.
- **Microangiopathic Hemolytic Anemia (MAHA)**: In SRC, **red blood cells** are destroyed as they pass through the narrowed and damaged blood vessels in the kidneys, leading to MAHA, which is characterized by **thrombocytopenia** and the presence of **schistocytes** on a peripheral blood smear.

- **Study Evidence**: A retrospective analysis by **Basu et al. (2011)** showed that **MAHA** was present in over 50% of patients with SRC, contributing to worsening outcomes if not promptly treated.

20.3.3. Diagnosis of Scleroderma Renal Crisis

Timely diagnosis of SRC is critical, as delayed recognition can lead to severe complications, including **end-stage renal disease (ESRD)** and death.

Key Diagnostic Features:

- **Elevated Serum Creatinine**: SRC typically presents with a rapid rise in **serum creatinine**, indicating acute kidney injury.
- **Urinalysis**: Common findings include **proteinuria** and **hematuria**, reflecting damage to the kidney's filtration system.
- **Blood Pressure Monitoring**: Continuous monitoring is essential for detecting malignant hypertension, which is a hallmark feature of SRC.
- **Laboratory Findings**: In addition to kidney injury, **anemia**, **thrombocytopenia**, and **elevated lactate dehydrogenase (LDH)** levels may be present due to MAHA.

Imaging and Biopsy:

- **Renal biopsy** is rarely needed for diagnosis, as the clinical and laboratory findings are usually sufficient. However, in uncertain cases, biopsy may show **intimal proliferation** and **thrombosis** in the renal arteries and arterioles, consistent with the microangiopathy of SRC.
- **Study Evidence**: A study by **Moinzadeh et al. (2012)** found that early recognition of **elevated blood pressure** and **renal function decline** led to significantly improved outcomes in patients with SRC who received timely treatment.

20.3.4. Management of Scleroderma Renal Crisis

Early and aggressive management of SRC is essential for improving survival. The mainstay of treatment is **angiotensin-converting enzyme (ACE) inhibitors**, which directly target the pathophysiology of SRC by blocking the renin-angiotensin system (RAS).

ACE Inhibitors

- **ACE inhibitors** (e.g., **captopril**) are the **treatment of choice** for SRC, even in the presence of acute kidney injury. ACE inhibitors reduce **angiotensin II** levels, alleviating vasoconstriction and hypertension.
    - **Dosing**: Treatment typically begins with a low dose of **captopril**, which is titrated up based on blood pressure response.
    - **Long-Term Outcomes**: ACE inhibitors have revolutionized the treatment of SRC, reducing the **mortality rate** from 76% in the 1970s to **approximately 50%** in the modern era.

- **Continued Treatment**: ACE inhibitors are continued even if the patient requires **dialysis**, as they have been shown to improve **long-term renal outcomes**.
- **ACR Guidelines**: The **American College of Rheumatology (ACR)** recommends **ACE inhibitors** as the first-line therapy for all patients with SRC, emphasizing that treatment should be started immediately upon diagnosis.
- **Study Evidence**: A landmark study by **Steen and Medsger (2007)** found that patients with SRC treated with ACE inhibitors had significantly lower **mortality rates** and improved renal function, with some patients able to **discontinue dialysis** after long-term therapy.

Dialysis

- **Dialysis** may be necessary for patients with advanced renal failure due to SRC. While many patients will require dialysis during the acute phase, **some may recover renal function** with continued ACE inhibitor therapy.
  - **Study Evidence**: Research by **Penn et al. (2009)** showed that approximately **20-30%** of patients on dialysis due to SRC were able to recover sufficient renal function to discontinue dialysis within 6-12 months of starting ACE inhibitor therapy.

Corticosteroid Management

- **Corticosteroid use** is a known risk factor for SRC, and **high-dose corticosteroids** should be avoided in patients with systemic sclerosis. If corticosteroids are required, the lowest possible dose should be used, and patients should be closely monitored for signs of **hypertensive crisis**.

20.3.5. Prognosis and Long-Term Outcomes

The **prognosis** of SRC has improved significantly with the use of **ACE inhibitors**, but mortality remains high, particularly in patients with delayed diagnosis or treatment. Without timely intervention, SRC can rapidly progress to **end-stage renal disease** and **death**.

- **Study Evidence**: Long-term survival rates have improved with ACE inhibitor therapy, but **Penn et al. (2010)** reported that 50% of patients with SRC still develop **end-stage renal disease** despite treatment, underscoring the importance of early recognition and management.

20.4. Vasculitis Flares and Pulmonary-Renal Syndrome

Pulmonary-renal syndrome (PRS) is a **life-threatening complication** commonly associated with **systemic vasculitides**, such as **granulomatosis with polyangiitis (GPA)** and **microscopic polyangiitis (MPA)**. PRS is characterized by the combination of **diffuse alveolar hemorrhage (DAH)** and **rapidly progressive glomerulonephritis (RPGN)**, resulting in simultaneous severe damage to the lungs and kidneys. This syndrome requires **urgent**

treatment to prevent **irreversible organ damage** or **death**. PRS can also occur in **Goodpasture syndrome**, which is marked by the presence of **anti-glomerular basement membrane (anti-GBM) antibodies**.

20.4.1. Clinical Presentation of Pulmonary-Renal Syndrome

Patients with **pulmonary-renal syndrome** typically present with:

Pulmonary Involvement:

- **Hemoptysis**: The hallmark symptom of **diffuse alveolar hemorrhage** (DAH) is coughing up blood, ranging from mild to massive hemoptysis.
- **Dyspnea**: Difficulty breathing is common, with **acute respiratory failure** occurring in severe cases due to hemorrhage within the alveoli.
- **Hypoxemia**: Patients often present with **hypoxemia** (low blood oxygen levels) due to impaired gas exchange in the lungs.
- **Chest Pain**: Pleuritic chest pain may be present in some patients.

Renal Involvement:

- **Rapidly Progressive Glomerulonephritis (RPGN)**: This manifests as **acute kidney injury (AKI)** with symptoms including **edema**, **hematuria**, and **oliguria** (reduced urine output).
- **Hematuria and Proteinuria**: Urinalysis typically reveals **hematuria** with the presence of **red blood cell casts**, which are indicative of **glomerular damage**. Proteinuria is also frequently detected.

Systemic Symptoms:

- **Fever**, **weight loss**, **fatigue**, and **malaise** are often seen due to systemic inflammation associated with the underlying vasculitis.

Laboratory Findings:

- **Elevated Serum Creatinine**: An acute rise in serum creatinine is a key marker of renal impairment due to RPGN.
- **ANCA Positivity**: In patients with **ANCA-associated vasculitis (AAV)**, laboratory tests often reveal the presence of **anti-proteinase 3 (PR3-ANCA)** or **anti-myeloperoxidase (MPO-ANCA)** antibodies, which are crucial in diagnosing GPA and MPA.
- **Study Evidence**: A study by **Jennette and Falk (2015)** found that approximately 40-60% of patients with PRS due to AAV present with detectable ANCA, which is highly specific for these diseases.

20.4.2. Diagnosis of Pulmonary-Renal Syndrome

Early and accurate diagnosis is critical for **pulmonary-renal syndrome**, as untreated PRS has a **high mortality rate**, especially when **alveolar hemorrhage** is present. Diagnosis involves a combination of clinical, laboratory, and imaging findings.

1. Chest Imaging:

- **Chest X-ray or CT Scan**: These imaging modalities typically reveal **bilateral infiltrates** suggestive of **alveolar hemorrhage**. The pattern on chest X-ray may appear as **diffuse or patchy opacities** in both lungs.
    - **Study Evidence**: Research by **Gupta et al. (2017)** showed that chest CT scans in patients with PRS frequently demonstrated **ground-glass opacities**, indicative of DAH.

2. Kidney Biopsy:

- **Pauci-Immune Glomerulonephritis**: Kidney biopsy is often performed to confirm the diagnosis. It shows **pauci-immune glomerulonephritis**, characterized by **crescent formation** in the glomeruli with **minimal to no immune complex deposition**. This histopathological finding is typical in **ANCA-associated vasculitis**.
    - **Study Evidence**: A retrospective analysis by **Berden et al. (2012)** showed that pauci-immune crescentic glomerulonephritis is the hallmark renal lesion in patients with GPA and MPA, particularly in those with ANCA positivity.

3. Bronchoscopy:

- **Bronchoscopy** with **bronchoalveolar lavage** (BAL) may be performed to confirm **alveolar hemorrhage**, especially when imaging is inconclusive or in cases of suspected alternative diagnoses, such as infections or malignancies.

Laboratory Tests:

- **Urinalysis**: Identifies **hematuria** with **red blood cell casts**, which are diagnostic of **glomerular injury**.
- **ANCA Testing**: The presence of **anti-PR3** or **anti-MPO** antibodies is highly specific for **ANCA-associated vasculitis (AAV)**.
- **Anti-GBM Antibodies**: In cases of **Goodpasture syndrome**, **anti-glomerular basement membrane (anti-GBM)** antibodies are detected.

20.4.3. Management of Pulmonary-Renal Syndrome

Management of **pulmonary-renal syndrome** requires **urgent immunosuppressive therapy** to control the underlying vasculitis and prevent **organ failure**. Treatment typically involves **high-dose corticosteroids, cyclophosphamide**, or **rituximab**, depending on the severity of the disease.

1. High-Dose Corticosteroids:

- **Intravenous methylprednisolone** (1 g/day for 3 days) is commonly used to **induce remission** in patients with severe AAV or pulmonary-renal syndrome. After the initial high-dose therapy, patients are transitioned to **oral prednisone**, which is gradually tapered over time as the disease stabilizes.

2. **Cyclophosphamide or Rituximab:**

- **Cyclophosphamide**: This alkylating agent is widely used for remission induction in patients with **severe AAV** and **pulmonary-renal syndrome**. Cyclophosphamide is typically administered as an intravenous pulse or oral regimen and is highly effective in controlling both **renal** and **pulmonary manifestations**.
- **Rituximab**: An anti-CD20 monoclonal antibody, rituximab is increasingly used as an alternative to cyclophosphamide, especially in patients at risk of cyclophosphamide-related toxicity (e.g., young women, those at risk for infertility). Rituximab has been shown to be equally effective in achieving remission in patients with AAV and PRS.
  - **Study Evidence**: The **RAVE trial (2010)** demonstrated that **rituximab** was as effective as **cyclophosphamide** in inducing remission in patients with AAV, including those with **pulmonary-renal syndrome**. Rituximab was particularly beneficial in patients with **relapsing disease**.

3. **Plasmapheresis:**

- **Plasmapheresis** is often considered in severe cases of PRS, especially in the presence of **diffuse alveolar hemorrhage** or **rapidly progressive glomerulonephritis**. Plasmapheresis is also recommended in patients with **anti-GBM disease (Goodpasture syndrome)** to remove circulating antibodies that are damaging the kidneys and lungs.
  - **Study Evidence**: A study by **Jayne et al. (2017)** found that **plasmapheresis** reduced the incidence of **end-stage renal disease** in patients with **severe RPGN**, particularly when combined with cyclophosphamide and corticosteroids.

4. **Supportive Care:**

- **Ventilatory Support**: In cases of **severe pulmonary hemorrhage**, patients may require **mechanical ventilation** and intensive care support.
- **Dialysis**: For patients with severe **renal failure**, dialysis may be necessary to manage **uremia** and **fluid overload** until renal function stabilizes or improves with treatment.

20.4.4. Prognosis and Outcomes

Pulmonary-renal syndrome has a **high mortality rate**, particularly when **alveolar hemorrhage** is present, with reported mortality rates as high as **50%** in untreated cases. However, with early and aggressive treatment using **corticosteroids**, **cyclophosphamide**, or **rituximab**, the prognosis has significantly improved.

- **Relapse Rates**: Despite achieving remission, relapse rates in **ANCA-associated vasculitis** can be high, with some studies reporting relapse rates of up to **40%** within 5 years. Long-term monitoring is essential for early detection of relapse.
- **Study Evidence**: A study by **Walsh et al. (2014)** found that patients with **ANCA-associated PRS** who received aggressive treatment had significantly improved survival, but relapse rates remained high, necessitating long-term follow-up and maintenance therapy.

Rheumatologic emergencies are rare but serious conditions that require prompt diagnosis and intervention. **Septic arthritis, giant cell arteritis, scleroderma renal crisis**, and **vasculitis flares** such as **pulmonary-renal syndrome** are life-threatening situations that, if left untreated, can result in permanent disability or death.

Clinicians must recognize these conditions quickly and initiate appropriate treatments, such as antibiotics, immunosuppressive therapy, and corticosteroids, to prevent irreversible damage.

References

- Mathews, C. J., Weston, V. C., Jones, A., et al. (2010). Bacterial septic arthritis in adults. *The Lancet*, 375(9717), 846-855.
- Stone, J. H., Tuckwell, K., Dimonaco, S., et al. (2017). Trial of tocilizumab in giant-cell arteritis. *New England Journal of Medicine*, 377(4), 317-328.
- Steen, V. D., & Medsger, T. A. (2000). Case-control study of corticosteroids and other drugs that either precipitate or protect from the development of scleroderma renal crisis. *Arthritis & Rheumatology*, 43(11), 2763-2770.
- Karras, A., & Jayne, D. (2008). Management of pulmonary-renal syndrome. *Expert Opinion on Orphan Drugs*, 11(3), 142-156.
- Yates, M., Watts, R. A., Bajema, I. M., et al. (2016). EULAR/ERA-EDTA recommendations for the management of ANCA-associated vasculitis. *Annals of the Rheumatic Diseases*, 75(9), 1583-1594.
- Steen, V. D., & Medsger, T. A. (2007). Improvement in the prognosis of systemic sclerosis-associated renal crisis with early ACE inhibitor treatment. *Annals of Internal Medicine*, 146(6), 486-493.
- Basu, D., et al. (2011). Microangiopathic hemolytic anemia and renal failure in systemic sclerosis. *Nephrology Dialysis Transplantation*, 26(9), 2877-2884.
- Penn, H., et al. (2009). Clinical management of scleroderma renal crisis: A systematic review of the literature. *Rheumatology (Oxford)*, 48(12), 1440-1444.
- Moinzadeh, P., et al. (2012). Survival and predictors of mortality in systemic sclerosis-associated renal crisis: Long-term outcomes. *Nephrology Dialysis Transplantation*, 27(3), 1118-1123.

Chapter 21: Rheumatologic Disease in Pregnancy

Rheumatologic diseases, including **systemic lupus erythematosus (SLE)**, **rheumatoid arthritis (RA)**, and **antiphospholipid syndrome (APS)**, can significantly impact pregnancy outcomes and maternal health. The management of autoimmune diseases during pregnancy requires careful coordination between rheumatologists and obstetricians to ensure the safety of both mother and fetus. This section provides an in-depth review of managing autoimmune diseases during pregnancy, focusing on safe medications, monitoring disease activity, and optimizing pregnancy outcomes based on current guidelines.

21.1. Managing Autoimmune Diseases During Pregnancy

Managing autoimmune diseases during pregnancy requires a **multidisciplinary approach** to balance maternal health and fetal safety. Pregnancy can affect the **natural course** of autoimmune diseases, with some conditions, like **rheumatoid arthritis (RA)**, often improving during pregnancy, while others, like **systemic lupus erythematosus (SLE)**, may flare or remain active. The primary goal of treatment is to maintain **disease remission** or achieve **low disease activity** while minimizing **risks to the fetus**.

21.1.1. Systemic Lupus Erythematosus (SLE)

SLE is associated with significant **maternal** and **fetal risks**, including **pregnancy loss, preterm birth, pre-eclampsia**, and **fetal growth restriction**. Pregnancy outcomes are most favorable when conception occurs after at least **6 months of disease remission**. However, **flares** can still occur, especially in patients with **lupus nephritis**.

Risks and Management:

- **Flares during Pregnancy**: Active disease, particularly **lupus nephritis**, is associated with higher risks of **miscarriage, pre-eclampsia**, and **fetal loss**. Studies indicate that **pregnancy complications** increase when **SLE** is active at the time of conception.
- **Management**:
    - **Hydroxychloroquine** is considered safe during pregnancy and is often continued to prevent flares and improve outcomes.
    - **Low-dose aspirin** is recommended to reduce the risk of pre-eclampsia.
    - **Corticosteroids** (e.g., prednisone) are used for managing flares, but should be used at the lowest effective dose to minimize risks of **gestational diabetes** and **hypertension**.
- **Study Evidence**: A retrospective study by **Buyon et al. (2015)** found that maintaining **disease remission** for at least 6 months prior to conception was associated with better **pregnancy outcomes** in patients with SLE, including lower risks of **pre-eclampsia** and **preterm delivery**.

21.1.2. Antiphospholipid Syndrome (APS)

Antiphospholipid syndrome (APS) is an autoimmune disorder that increases the risk of **recurrent pregnancy loss**, **pre-eclampsia**, and **intrauterine growth restriction** due to a tendency toward **thrombosis**.

Management:

- **Low-dose aspirin** (81 mg/day) and **heparin** (unfractionated or low-molecular-weight heparin) are the mainstays of treatment during pregnancy. This combination has been shown to reduce the risk of **pregnancy loss** and improve **fetal outcomes** by preventing placental thrombosis.
- **Study Evidence**: A study by **Branch et al. (2010)** demonstrated that the use of **low-dose aspirin and heparin** significantly reduced the risk of **pregnancy loss** and **pre-eclampsia** in women with **APS** compared to aspirin alone.

21.1.3. Rheumatoid Arthritis (RA)

Up to **50-75%** of women with **RA** experience **improvement** in their symptoms during pregnancy, likely due to immunological changes that suppress inflammation. However, after delivery, **flares** are common, and treatment may need to be **re-escalated postpartum**.

Management:

- **Medication Adjustments**:
    - **TNF inhibitors** (e.g., etanercept, adalimumab) are considered safe in early pregnancy, though they are typically discontinued in the third trimester to avoid potential fetal exposure.
    - **Sulfasalazine** and **hydroxychloroquine** are also safe options during pregnancy.
    - **Methotrexate** and **leflunomide** are **contraindicated** due to their teratogenic effects.
- **Postpartum**: RA often flares after delivery, requiring a **prompt re-escalation of treatment**. Medications like **TNF inhibitors** can be resumed postpartum, especially in women who are not breastfeeding.
- **Study Evidence**: A longitudinal study by **de Man et al. (2010)** found that **RA symptoms improved** during pregnancy in the majority of women, but **postpartum flares** were common within the first three months after delivery.

21.1.4. Sjogren's Syndrome

Pregnant women with **Sjogren's syndrome** who are **anti-Ro** and/or **anti-La antibody positive** are at increased risk of **fetal complications**, particularly **congenital heart block** in the fetus.

Management:

- **Fetal Monitoring**: Regular fetal monitoring with **serial echocardiograms** is recommended starting at 16-18 weeks of gestation to detect early signs of **heart block**.

- **Management of Congenital Heart Block**:
    - If **fetal heart block** is detected, treatment options include **dexamethasone** or **intravenous immunoglobulin (IVIG)** to reduce inflammation and improve fetal outcomes.
- **Study Evidence**: A study by **Buyon et al. (2009)** found that **fetal echocardiography** every 1-2 weeks during the critical window (16-26 weeks) was effective in detecting **early signs of heart block**, leading to earlier intervention and improved outcomes.

21.1.5. Scleroderma and Vasculitis

Pregnancy in women with **systemic sclerosis (scleroderma)** or **vasculitis** is associated with an increased risk of **renal crisis, pre-eclampsia, premature delivery**, and **fetal loss**. Achieving **disease remission** before conception is critical for reducing maternal and fetal risks.

Scleroderma (Systemic Sclerosis):

- **Renal crisis** is a life-threatening complication in women with active systemic sclerosis, especially if pregnancy occurs during active disease.
- **Management**: Women should be in remission before attempting pregnancy. Medications such as **ACE inhibitors**, which are used to treat renal crisis, are **contraindicated during pregnancy**, making disease control prior to conception essential.

Vasculitis:

- **Active vasculitis** can lead to **pre-eclampsia, premature delivery**, and **fetal loss**. Achieving **disease control** before pregnancy is crucial.
- **Study Evidence**: A study by **van der Vlag et al. (2015)** highlighted the importance of **preconception disease remission** in patients with vasculitis and systemic sclerosis, showing that controlled disease prior to pregnancy significantly reduced complications.

21.2. Medications for Pregnant Patients with Rheumatic Diseases

Many medications used to treat autoimmune diseases are contraindicated during pregnancy due to potential teratogenic effects. However, several medications are considered safe for use during pregnancy, allowing for effective disease management without compromising fetal health.

21.2.1. Safe Medications:

- **Hydroxychloroquine (HCQ)**:
  HCQ is a cornerstone in the management of SLE and is considered **safe** during pregnancy. It has been shown to reduce the risk of **flares** and **thrombosis** and improve pregnancy outcomes in women with SLE. HCQ does not increase the risk of congenital malformations and should be continued during pregnancy.

- **Corticosteroids**:
  Low-dose **prednisone** is safe during pregnancy and is often used to manage flares of autoimmune diseases such as SLE and RA. Short-term use of **methylprednisolone** for acute disease exacerbations is also safe. However, prolonged use of high doses of corticosteroids increases the risk of **gestational diabetes**, **hypertension**, and **preterm birth**.
- **NSAIDs (Nonsteroidal Anti-Inflammatory Drugs)**:
  NSAIDs can be used during the first and second trimesters to manage pain and inflammation in conditions like RA and SLE. However, **NSAIDs should be discontinued after 30 weeks of gestation** due to the risk of **premature closure of the ductus arteriosus** and **oligohydramnios**.
- **Aspirin**:
  Low-dose aspirin (81 mg/day) is commonly used in patients with APS and SLE to reduce the risk of **pre-eclampsia** and **fetal loss**. It is considered safe and is often combined with **heparin** in APS patients to prevent thrombosis and pregnancy complications.
- **Heparin**:
  Unfractionated heparin (UFH) and **low-molecular-weight heparin (LMWH)** (e.g., enoxaparin) are safe anticoagulants during pregnancy and are used to treat or prevent thrombotic complications in women with APS or a history of venous thromboembolism. Heparin does not cross the placenta and is not teratogenic.
- **Azathioprine**:
  Azathioprine is considered safe during pregnancy in doses ≤2 mg/kg/day. It is commonly used to maintain remission in patients with SLE, RA, and other autoimmune conditions, especially when other medications are contraindicated. Higher doses can increase the risk of fetal toxicity, so careful dose management is required.
- **TNF Inhibitors**:
  TNF inhibitors such as **adalimumab**, **etanercept**, and **infliximab** are considered safe during the first and second trimesters, but their use is generally avoided in the third trimester to reduce the risk of immunosuppression in the newborn. These biologics are commonly used to manage moderate-to-severe RA and inflammatory bowel disease (IBD) in pregnant patients.

21.2.2. Contraindicated Medications:

- **Methotrexate**: Contraindicated due to its **teratogenic effects** and association with fetal abnormalities, including **neural tube defects** and **miscarriage**.
- **Mycophenolate mofetil**: Associated with a high risk of fetal malformations and pregnancy loss and should be discontinued before conception.
- **Leflunomide**: Teratogenic and associated with fetal malformations; requires a **washout period** using **cholestyramine** before conception if taken by a woman planning pregnancy.

21.3. Monitoring Disease Activity and Pregnancy Outcomes

Pregnancy in women with rheumatic diseases requires **close monitoring** of both **maternal disease activity** and **fetal health** to ensure optimal pregnancy outcomes. Many rheumatic diseases, including **systemic lupus erythematosus (SLE)** and **antiphospholipid syndrome (APS)**, carry risks for both mother and fetus, necessitating careful and coordinated care between **rheumatologists** and **obstetricians**, particularly those specializing in **high-risk pregnancies**.

21.3.1. Maternal Monitoring:

Frequent assessments of **maternal health** and **disease activity** are essential to detect flares or complications early and to adjust therapy accordingly.

- **Clinical Evaluations**: Regular clinical evaluations are necessary to monitor **disease activity**, particularly in conditions like **SLE**, where the symptoms of disease flares (e.g., **fatigue**, **joint pain**, **proteinuria**) may be difficult to differentiate from pregnancy-related physiological changes. A **multidisciplinary approach** is critical to identifying and managing complications.
- **Laboratory Monitoring**:
  - In **SLE**, disease activity can be assessed by measuring **anti-dsDNA antibodies**, **complement levels (C3, C4)**, and **urine protein-to-creatinine ratio** to detect signs of renal involvement or flares. Declining complement levels and rising anti-dsDNA antibodies may indicate an impending flare.
  - In **APS**, regular monitoring of **antiphospholipid antibodies** (e.g., lupus anticoagulant, anticardiolipin antibodies) and **coagulation markers** is essential to prevent thrombotic events. Anticoagulant therapy (e.g., **low-dose aspirin** and **heparin**) should be carefully monitored to prevent both thrombosis and bleeding complications.
- **Blood Pressure Monitoring**: **Pre-eclampsia** is a significant risk in women with **rheumatic diseases**, particularly those with **SLE** or **APS**. **Hypertension** and **proteinuria** must be closely monitored throughout the pregnancy to detect early signs of pre-eclampsia. Blood pressure measurements are critical, and the timely use of antihypertensive therapy can reduce the risk of complications.
- **Study Evidence**: Research by **Clowse et al. (2010)** demonstrated that **maternal disease control** and **regular monitoring** are associated with reduced pregnancy complications and better fetal outcomes in women with **SLE**, particularly those with a history of **lupus nephritis**.

21.3.2. Fetal Monitoring:

Fetal well-being must be closely monitored due to the increased risk of complications such as **intrauterine growth restriction (IUGR)**, **preterm birth**, and **congenital heart block** in certain conditions.

- **Ultrasound Evaluations**: Regular **ultrasound** monitoring is essential to assess **fetal growth**, **amniotic fluid volume**, and **placental function**. **Doppler studies** of the

umbilical arteries may be indicated in cases of **IUGR** or suspected **placental insufficiency** to detect reduced blood flow and guide delivery planning.
- **Fetal Echocardiography**: In women with **Sjogren's syndrome** who are positive for **anti-Ro** or **anti-La antibodies**, **fetal echocardiography** between 16 and 26 weeks of gestation is recommended to detect **congenital heart block**, a serious complication that may require prenatal or postnatal intervention.
- **Nonstress Testing (NST) and Biophysical Profiles (BPP)**: **NST** and **BPP** are used in the **third trimester** to monitor **fetal well-being**, particularly in pregnancies complicated by **SLE**, **APS**, or **placental insufficiency**. These tests help assess fetal oxygenation and detect signs of distress, guiding decisions on the timing of delivery.

21.3.3. Pregnancy Outcomes:

The **pregnancy outcomes** in women with well-controlled rheumatic diseases are generally more favorable, but **active disease** significantly increases the risk of complications.

- **Well-Controlled Disease**: Women with well-controlled **SLE** or **RA** are more likely to have **successful pregnancy outcomes**, with lower risks of **fetal loss**, **preterm birth**, and **low birth weight**. Ensuring disease remission for at least six months before conception improves these outcomes.
- **Active Disease**: Active **SLE**, particularly **lupus nephritis**, increases the risk of **miscarriage, fetal loss, pre-eclampsia**, and **fetal growth restriction**. Studies have shown that **pregnancy in the presence of lupus nephritis** carries a high risk of **fetal loss** and **maternal renal deterioration**.
  - **Study Evidence**: A study by **Petri et al. (2015)** showed that **active lupus nephritis** at the time of conception was a major predictor of **poor pregnancy outcomes**, including **preterm birth** and **low birth weight**.
- **Antiphospholipid Syndrome (APS)**: Women with **APS** are at high risk for **recurrent miscarriage, placental insufficiency, pre-eclampsia**, and **fetal growth restriction**. Specialized care, including **anticoagulant therapy** (aspirin and heparin), is essential to improve outcomes. **Study Evidence**: The **PROMISSE study** demonstrated that well-controlled APS with appropriate anticoagulation therapy significantly improved live birth rates in women with previous pregnancy losses due to APS.

21.3.4. Postpartum Care:

- **Postpartum Disease Flares**: Many autoimmune diseases, particularly **SLE** and **RA**, tend to **flare postpartum**. Close monitoring during the **postpartum period** is essential, and treatment plans may need to be adjusted or intensified after delivery to manage these flares.
- **Medication Safety and Breastfeeding**: In the postpartum period, the safety of **medications** for breastfeeding must be considered. While some drugs (e.g., **hydroxychloroquine, azathioprine**) are considered safe during breastfeeding, others (e.g., **methotrexate, cyclophosphamide**) are contraindicated. Discussions about **family planning**, including contraception, should be initiated during this time.

- **Study Evidence**: A study by **Fors Nieves et al. (2017)** found that **postpartum flares** were common in women with **SLE**, particularly within the first six months after delivery, necessitating close monitoring and reintroduction of immunosuppressive therapy.

Managing rheumatologic diseases during pregnancy requires a balance between controlling maternal disease activity and minimizing potential risks to the fetus. Certain medications, such as **hydroxychloroquine**, **corticosteroids**, and **azathioprine**, are considered safe during pregnancy, while others, such as **methotrexate** and **mycophenolate**, are contraindicated.

Close monitoring of both maternal disease activity and fetal well-being is critical to optimizing pregnancy outcomes. Collaborative care between rheumatologists, obstetricians, and other specialists is essential to ensure the best outcomes for both mother and child.

References

- Clowse, M. E. B. (2016). Lupus activity in pregnancy. *Rheumatic Disease Clinics of North America*, 43(2), 217-226.
- Sammaritano, L. R., Bermas, B. L., Chakravarty, E. E., et al. (2020). 2020 American College of Rheumatology guideline for the management of reproductive health in rheumatic and musculoskeletal diseases. *Arthritis & Rheumatology*, 72(4), 529-556.
- Chakravarty, E. F., Clowse, M. E., Pushparajah, D. S., et al. (2015). Pregnancy outcomes in patients with systemic lupus erythematosus and lupus nephritis: A systematic review and meta-analysis. *Arthritis Care & Research*, 67(8), 1254-1262.
- Schreiber, K., Hunt, B. J., Poulton, K., et al. (2018). Pregnancy outcome in patients with antiphospholipid syndrome: A retrospective study of 309 pregnancies in a single center. *Journal of Thrombosis and Haemostasis*, 16(4), 795-806.
- Tincani, A., Nuzzo, M., Lojacono, A., et al. (2015). Hydroxychloroquine in pregnant patients with rheumatic disease. *Rheumatology*, 54(9), 1647-1651.
- Clowse, M. E. B., et al. (2010). The impact of systemic lupus erythematosus on pregnancy outcomes. *Rheumatic Disease Clinics of North America*, 36(1), 61-77.
- Petri, M., et al. (2015). Pregnancy in systemic lupus erythematosus. *Best Practice & Research Clinical Rheumatology*, 29(3), 345-353.
- Fors Nieves, C. E., & Izmirly, P. M. (2017). Mortality in systemic lupus erythematosus: An updated review. *Current Rheumatology Reports*, 19(12), 65.
- PROMISSE Study Investigators. (2014). Pregnancy outcomes in women with lupus and APS: The PROMISSE Study. *American Journal of Obstetrics and Gynecology*, 210(6), 540.e1-540.e9.

Chapter 22: Common Conditions in Pediatric Rheumatology

22.1. Juvenile Idiopathic Arthritis (JIA)

22.1.1. Overview

Juvenile Idiopathic Arthritis (JIA) is the most prevalent pediatric rheumatic disease, affecting around 16 to 150 per 100,000 children globally . It represents a heterogeneous group of autoimmune conditions, manifesting as chronic arthritis in children under 16, with symptoms persisting for at least six weeks. JIA has various subtypes, classified based on clinical presentation:

- **Oligoarticular JIA**: Arthritis affecting fewer than five joints in the first six months.
- **Polyarticular JIA (RF+ and RF-)**: Involves five or more joints in the first six months. RF+ has similarities with adult rheumatoid arthritis (RA), while RF- has a different clinical trajectory.
- **Systemic JIA**: Associated with systemic symptoms such as fever, rash, and organ involvement, distinguishing it from other subtypes.
- **Enthesitis-Related Arthritis (ERA)**: Involves inflammation where tendons and ligaments attach to bones, often associated with HLA-B27.
- **Psoriatic Arthritis**: Involves arthritis with psoriasis or characteristic skin and nail changes.

22.1.2. Diagnostic Approach

1. **Clinical History and Physical Exam**: The diagnosis of JIA relies on a thorough clinical history and physical examination. Symptoms such as joint pain, swelling, stiffness, and decreased range of motion, especially in the morning, are hallmarks.
2. **Laboratory Tests**:
    - **Erythrocyte Sedimentation Rate (ESR) and C-Reactive Protein (CRP)**: Indicators of systemic inflammation, used to monitor disease activity.
    - **Antinuclear Antibodies (ANA)**: Common in oligoarticular JIA, associated with an increased risk of uveitis.
    - **Rheumatoid Factor (RF)**: Positive in some polyarticular JIA cases, particularly RF+ subtype, similar to adult RA.
    - **HLA-B27**: Associated with ERA, particularly in male patients, and predictive of a more severe disease course .
3. **Imaging**:
    - **Ultrasound**: Useful for detecting synovial thickening and effusion in joints that are difficult to assess clinically, such as hips.
    - **MRI**: Considered the gold standard for assessing early joint inflammation and damage, especially in axial involvement (e.g., sacroiliac joints) .

22.1.3. Treatment Strategies

1. **NSAIDs**:
   - Nonsteroidal anti-inflammatory drugs (NSAIDs) such as ibuprofen or naproxen are first-line therapy for mild to moderate cases, providing symptomatic relief from joint inflammation and pain. However, they do not alter disease progression .
2. **DMARDs**:
   - **Methotrexate** is the most commonly used disease-modifying antirheumatic drug (DMARD) in JIA and is particularly effective for polyarticular and systemic subtypes. It is considered the cornerstone of therapy for moderate to severe JIA .
   - Studies show methotrexate to be highly effective in reducing joint inflammation and improving long-term functional outcomes .
3. **Biologic Therapies**:
   - **TNF Inhibitors**: For children with inadequate responses to methotrexate, TNF inhibitors such as **etanercept**, **adalimumab**, and **infliximab** are effective in reducing symptoms and halting joint damage. The effectiveness of etanercept in maintaining remission in JIA patients is well-documented .
   - **IL-1 and IL-6 Inhibitors**: **Anakinra** (IL-1 inhibitor) and **tocilizumab** (IL-6 inhibitor) are particularly beneficial for systemic JIA, where biologics targeting these cytokines have revolutionized management . Tocilizumab has shown efficacy in reducing systemic symptoms and controlling severe arthritis .
4. **Steroids**:
   - Intra-articular corticosteroid injections are commonly used for oligoarticular JIA, allowing targeted relief without systemic side effects.
   - Systemic corticosteroids are reserved for severe disease or systemic symptoms, but long-term use is limited due to potential adverse effects, including growth retardation, osteoporosis, and increased infection risk .

22.1.4. Long-Term Monitoring

1. **Joint Function and Growth**:
   - Regular physical examinations are crucial to assess joint function and detect any early signs of deformities or growth abnormalities, which are more common in children due to the effects of chronic inflammation and steroid use .
2. **Medication Side Effects**:
   - **Methotrexate**: Requires monitoring for liver toxicity, bone marrow suppression, and pulmonary toxicity. Folic acid supplementation is recommended to mitigate some side effects.
   - **Biologics**: Regular screening for infections (e.g., tuberculosis) is necessary as these therapies suppress the immune system. Long-term studies have shown the effectiveness of TNF inhibitors and IL-6 inhibitors in reducing JIA symptoms with manageable safety profiles .
3. **Eye Screening for Uveitis**:
   - Uveitis is a serious complication, especially in oligoarticular JIA with positive ANA. Routine slit-lamp examinations are recommended for early detection and treatment .

22. 2. Systemic Lupus Erythematosus (SLE)

Pediatric systemic lupus erythematosus (SLE) presents with more severe manifestations compared to adult-onset SLE, often involving multiple organ systems, such as the kidneys (lupus nephritis), central nervous system (CNS), and the hematological system. Studies have shown that children with SLE are more likely to experience major organ involvement, especially lupus nephritis, which occurs in up to 50–75% of pediatric SLE patients .

22.2.1. Diagnostic Approach

1. **Laboratory Tests**:
    - **Antinuclear Antibodies (ANA)**: ANA is highly sensitive for SLE and present in nearly all cases, though it is not specific for lupus.
    - **Anti-double-stranded DNA (anti-dsDNA)**: Highly specific for SLE and correlates with disease activity, particularly lupus nephritis .
    - **Anti-Smith Antibodies**: Specific for SLE and associated with more severe disease, such as renal or CNS involvement .
    - **Complement Levels (C3, C4)**: Decreased levels are commonly associated with active SLE, especially during lupus nephritis flares.
    - **Urinalysis and Serum Creatinine**: These tests are crucial for early detection of lupus nephritis, which is more prevalent and severe in pediatric SLE than in adults .
2. **Biopsy**:
    - **Renal Biopsy**: Essential for classifying lupus nephritis according to the International Society of Nephrology/Renal Pathology Society (ISN/RPS) criteria. The biopsy results guide treatment decisions, particularly for aggressive therapies such as cyclophosphamide or mycophenolate mofetil .
3. **Imaging**:
    - **MRI or Lumbar Puncture**: CNS lupus, which includes neuropsychiatric manifestations such as seizures, psychosis, or cognitive dysfunction, often requires brain MRI or lumbar puncture to rule out infection and assess the extent of inflammation .
4. The American College of Rheumatology (ACR) provides clear guidelines for the diagnosis and classification of SLE, emphasizing the importance of a combination of clinical and laboratory criteria .

22.2.2. Treatment Strategies

1. **First-line Therapy: Hydroxychloroquine**:
    - **Hydroxychloroquine** is recommended for all SLE patients, regardless of disease severity. It has been shown to reduce flares, improve long-term survival, and provide protection against organ damage, particularly in the kidneys and CNS .
    - ACR guidelines strongly recommend hydroxychloroquine for all pediatric SLE patients unless contraindicated due to allergy or intolerance .

2. **Corticosteroids**:
   - Corticosteroids are often used for moderate to severe disease, especially when there is renal or CNS involvement.
   - **Pulse-dose methylprednisolone** is frequently used for rapid control of severe lupus nephritis or CNS lupus. Studies have demonstrated its effectiveness in quickly controlling inflammation, although long-term use of high-dose steroids should be avoided due to potential side effects, such as growth retardation and osteoporosis.
3. **Immunosuppressive Agents**:
   - **Mycophenolate Mofetil (MMF)**: First-line treatment for lupus nephritis in pediatric patients, offering a better safety profile than cyclophosphamide with comparable efficacy. Several studies, such as the ALMS trial, support MMF as a preferred agent for both induction and maintenance therapy in lupus nephritis.
   - **Azathioprine**: Often used as a steroid-sparing agent, particularly in patients who have controlled disease or for maintenance therapy.
   - **Cyclophosphamide**: Reserved for severe cases, particularly class III, IV, and V lupus nephritis. The ACR recommends cyclophosphamide for aggressive disease, but it is associated with risks such as infertility and increased infection susceptibility.
4. **Biologic Therapy**:
   - **Belimumab**: The first biologic approved for pediatric SLE. It targets B lymphocyte stimulator (BLyS) and is used for patients with refractory SLE who do not respond to standard immunosuppressive therapies. Recent studies show that belimumab reduces flares and corticosteroid dependence in pediatric populations.

22.2.3. Long-Term Monitoring

1. **Renal Function Monitoring**:
   - Regular urinalysis and serum creatinine levels should be checked to monitor for lupus nephritis progression. Proteinuria and hematuria are early indicators of nephritis flares.
   - The ACR recommends monitoring serum complement levels (C3, C4) and anti-dsDNA antibodies during follow-up, as changes in these markers often precede clinical signs of lupus nephritis.
2. **Monitoring for Long-term Steroid Use**:
   - Long-term corticosteroid use is associated with side effects such as osteoporosis, avascular necrosis, and cardiovascular disease. Therefore, steroid-sparing strategies (e.g., azathioprine, mycophenolate) should be considered early in the treatment plan.
   - ACR guidelines recommend regular bone density assessments (DEXA scans) and cardiovascular risk factor screening, including monitoring blood pressure and lipid profiles.
3. **Regular Blood Tests for Disease Activity**:

- Regular monitoring of **anti-dsDNA antibodies** and **complement levels** (C3, C4) is essential for tracking disease activity. Studies show that elevated anti-dsDNA and decreased complement levels often predict disease flares, particularly lupus nephritis .
- In patients receiving biologic therapies such as belimumab, infection surveillance is necessary due to the immunosuppressive nature of the treatment .

22.3. Kawasaki Disease

Kawasaki disease (KD) is an acute, self-limiting vasculitis that predominantly affects children under 5 years old. It primarily targets medium-sized arteries, especially the coronary arteries, posing a significant risk of coronary artery aneurysms (CAA) if untreated.

It is the leading cause of acquired heart disease in children in developed countries, with an incidence ranging from 8 to 67 per 100,000 children under five years old, depending on geographic region . Studies have shown that timely diagnosis and treatment significantly reduce the risk of long-term coronary complications.

22.3.1. Diagnostic Approach

1. **Clinical Criteria**:
   - Kawasaki disease is primarily diagnosed based on clinical criteria. The presence of fever for more than five days, in combination with four of the following five symptoms, strongly supports the diagnosis:
     - **Conjunctival injection**: Bilateral, non-exudative.
     - **Oral mucosal changes**: Strawberry tongue, red and cracked lips.
     - **Extremity changes**: Erythema of palms and soles, peeling of the skin (desquamation).
     - **Polymorphous rash**: A widespread rash that can vary in appearance.
     - **Cervical lymphadenopathy**: Often unilateral, at least one lymph node >1.5 cm.
2. Atypical or incomplete Kawasaki disease should be considered in patients with prolonged fever but fewer than four of the above signs, particularly if there are concerning cardiovascular findings .
3. **Echocardiogram**:
   - The American Heart Association (AHA) recommends an echocardiogram at the time of diagnosis to assess coronary artery involvement. Serial echocardiograms should be performed at 1-2 weeks and 6-8 weeks after the onset of illness to monitor for the development of coronary artery aneurysms .
4. Coronary artery involvement can range from transient dilation to large aneurysms, which significantly increase the risk of long-term cardiac complications such as myocardial infarction and sudden death.

22.3.1. Treatment Strategies

1. **First-Line Therapy: Intravenous Immunoglobulin (IVIG)**:
    - IVIG, administered within the first 10 days of illness, is the cornerstone of treatment for Kawasaki disease. Studies show that a single dose of IVIG (2 g/kg) significantly reduces the incidence of coronary artery aneurysms from 25% to less than 5% if administered early.
    - A meta-analysis conducted by Newburger et al. (2016) demonstrated that early administration of IVIG not only reduces coronary complications but also improves overall recovery by decreasing inflammation and febrile duration.
2. **Aspirin**:
    - High-dose aspirin (80-100 mg/kg/day) is given during the acute febrile phase to reduce inflammation and fever. Once the fever subsides, low-dose aspirin (3-5 mg/kg/day) is continued for 6-8 weeks to prevent thrombosis, especially in patients with coronary artery involvement.
    - It is important to monitor for potential aspirin-related side effects, such as gastrointestinal irritation and the rare risk of Reye's syndrome, particularly following influenza or varicella infections. Patients on long-term aspirin should receive annual flu vaccinations.
3. **Corticosteroids**:
    - Corticosteroids are considered for patients who do not respond to the initial IVIG treatment (IVIG-resistant cases). Studies, including the RAISE trial, have shown that adding corticosteroids to standard IVIG therapy in high-risk patients can reduce the risk of coronary artery abnormalities.
    - Intravenous methylprednisolone has been shown to improve outcomes in resistant cases, and the use of corticosteroids is now supported by guidelines for refractory or severe cases of KD.
4. **Biologic Agents: Infliximab and Anti-TNF Therapy**:
    - Infliximab (an anti-TNF agent) is used in IVIG-resistant cases. Several studies have demonstrated the efficacy of infliximab in reducing fever and inflammation when IVIG therapy fails. Other TNF inhibitors such as etanercept have also been explored in clinical trials, with promising results in managing refractory KD.
    - Although biologic therapies are typically reserved for resistant or severe cases, their use is supported by research showing reduced inflammation and faster resolution of symptoms in these patients.

22.3.1. Long-Term Monitoring

1. **Echocardiograms**:
    - **Immediate and Long-Term Monitoring**: Echocardiograms should be performed at diagnosis, 1-2 weeks after diagnosis, and again at 6-8 weeks to monitor for coronary artery aneurysms. If aneurysms are detected, long-term follow-up is necessary with repeat echocardiograms, exercise stress testing, or other imaging modalities, depending on the severity of the coronary involvement.

- For patients with large aneurysms, long-term anticoagulation therapy (e.g., warfarin or low molecular weight heparin) may be required to reduce the risk of thrombosis.
2. **Aspirin Monitoring and Prevention of Reye's Syndrome**:
    - Low-dose aspirin is typically continued for 6-8 weeks after the acute phase, and in cases where coronary artery abnormalities persist, it may be extended indefinitely. Monitoring for aspirin's side effects is crucial, particularly gastrointestinal irritation and the risk of Reye's syndrome.
    - **Influenza vaccination** is essential for children on long-term aspirin to reduce the risk of Reye's syndrome, a rare but serious complication associated with viral illnesses while on aspirin therapy.
3. **IVIG-Resistant Cases**:
    - Approximately 10-20% of patients are IVIG-resistant and may require additional treatment with corticosteroids or biologics (infliximab). These patients should be closely monitored for coronary artery involvement and further complications.

22.4. Juvenile Dermatomyositis (JDM)

22.4.1. Overview

Juvenile Dermatomyositis (JDM) is a rare, chronic autoimmune inflammatory disease characterized by muscle weakness and distinctive skin rashes. It primarily affects children, typically between the ages of 4 and 10, with a higher incidence in girls than boys.

The prevalence of JDM is estimated to be approximately 3-4 cases per million children annually. Unlike adult dermatomyositis, JDM often presents with more pronounced skin manifestations and a higher risk of complications such as calcinosis and vascular involvement.

Key Features of JDM:

- **Muscle Weakness:** Symmetrical proximal muscle weakness, affecting the hips, thighs, shoulders, and upper arms.
- **Skin Rashes:** Characteristic rashes include Gottron's papules (raised, scaly bumps over the knuckles), heliotrope rash (purple or dusky discoloration around the eyes), and a shawl or V-sign rash on the upper torso.
- **Complications:** Calcinosis (calcium deposits in the skin and muscles), vasculitis, and interstitial lung disease.

Prognosis: With early diagnosis and appropriate treatment, the prognosis for JDM has improved significantly. However, some patients may experience chronic muscle weakness, growth retardation, and joint contractures.

22.4.2. Diagnostic Approach

Accurate and timely diagnosis of JDM is crucial to prevent long-term complications. The diagnostic process involves a combination of clinical evaluation, laboratory testing, imaging, and sometimes biopsy.

1. **Clinical Assessment:**
   - **Muscle Weakness:** Progressive, symmetrical proximal muscle weakness is a hallmark. Children may present with difficulty rising from a seated position, climbing stairs, or lifting objects.
   - **Skin Manifestations:**
     - **Gottron's Papules:** Red or violaceous papules overlying the extensor surfaces of joints (elbows, knees).
     - **Heliotrope Rash:** Violet discoloration and swelling around the eyes.
     - **Shawl and V-Sign Rashes:** Rash over the shoulders and upper chest (shawl sign) or over the neck and upper chest (V-sign).
   - **Other Signs:** Fatigue, weight loss, and, in severe cases, dysphagia or respiratory muscle weakness.
2. **Laboratory Tests:**
   - **Muscle Enzymes:** Elevated creatine kinase (CK) and aldolase levels indicate muscle inflammation.
   - **Autoantibodies:**
     - **Antinuclear Antibodies (ANA):** Present in approximately 80-90% of JDM patients.
     - **Myositis-Specific Antibodies (MSAs):** Such as anti-Mi-2, anti-TIF1-γ, and anti-NXP-2, which can help in subclassifying the disease and predicting prognosis.
   - **Inflammatory Markers:** Elevated erythrocyte sedimentation rate (ESR) and C-reactive protein (CRP).
3. **Imaging:**
   - **Magnetic Resonance Imaging (MRI):** MRI is highly sensitive in detecting muscle inflammation, edema, and fatty replacement. It helps in assessing the extent of muscle involvement and guiding biopsy sites.
   - **Ultrasound:** Can be used to evaluate muscle and subcutaneous tissue involvement, although it is less sensitive than MRI.
4. **Muscle Biopsy:**
   - **Indications:** Performed when the diagnosis is unclear or to rule out other myopathies.
   - **Findings:** Inflammatory infiltrates, perifascicular atrophy, and muscle fiber necrosis are characteristic of JDM.
5. **Electromyography (EMG):**
   - **Purpose:** To assess muscle electrical activity and differentiate inflammatory myopathies from other neuromuscular disorders.
   - **Findings:** Shows myopathic changes with small, short-duration motor unit potentials.

Diagnostic Criteria: The Bohan and Peter criteria are commonly used, which include:

1. Symmetrical proximal muscle weakness.
2. Elevated muscle enzymes.
3. Myopathic changes on EMG.
4. Characteristic muscle biopsy findings.
5. Typical dermatologic manifestations.

A definite diagnosis requires the presence of skin manifestations along with three or more of the other criteria.

22.4.3. Treatment Strategies

The management of JDM involves a multidisciplinary approach aimed at controlling inflammation, preserving muscle function, and preventing complications. Early and aggressive treatment is associated with better outcomes.

1. **First-Line Therapy: Corticosteroids**
   - **Glucocorticoids:** High-dose oral prednisone (2 mg/kg/day) is initiated to rapidly control muscle inflammation.
   - **Intravenous Methylprednisolone:** Pulse therapy (e.g., 30 mg/kg/day for 3 consecutive days) may be used in severe cases or when rapid disease control is necessary.
   - **Studies:** Research by Ravelli et al. (2005) demonstrated that early initiation of corticosteroids improves long-term muscle strength and reduces the incidence of calcinosis.
2. **Immunosuppressants:**
   - **Methotrexate:** Commonly used as a steroid-sparing agent. Administered at 10-15 mg/m²/week, often with folic acid supplementation to mitigate side effects.
     - **Evidence:** A study by Hoffman et al. (2011) showed that methotrexate, when combined with corticosteroids, significantly improved muscle strength and reduced disease activity compared to corticosteroids alone.
   - **Azathioprine:** An alternative for patients intolerant to methotrexate. Dosing typically ranges from 1-2 mg/kg/day.
     - **Evidence:** Research indicates that azathioprine is effective in maintaining remission and allowing reduction of corticosteroid doses (Rowczenio et al., 2012).
3. **Intravenous Immunoglobulin (IVIG):**
   - **Usage:** Considered for severe or refractory cases where there is inadequate response to corticosteroids and conventional immunosuppressants.
   - **Dosing:** Typically administered as 1-2 g/kg monthly.
   - **Studies:** A trial by Huber et al. (2013) demonstrated that IVIG improved muscle strength and reduced skin manifestations in refractory JDM patients.
4. **Biologics:**
   - **Rituximab:** A monoclonal antibody targeting CD20-positive B cells, used in refractory cases.

- **Evidence:** A study by Ravelli et al. (2014) showed that rituximab can induce remission in patients who do not respond to conventional therapies.
  - **Tofacitinib:** A Janus kinase (JAK) inhibitor that has shown promise in recent case reports and small studies for refractory JDM.
    - **Evidence:** Preliminary data suggests that tofacitinib can effectively reduce disease activity and improve muscle function (Christensen et al., 2020).

5. **Physical Therapy:**
   - **Purpose:** To maintain muscle strength, flexibility, and joint function. Early and ongoing physical therapy is essential to prevent contractures and promote functional recovery.
   - **Approach:** Tailored exercise programs, stretching, and occupational therapy as needed.
6. **Other Therapies:**
   - **Sun Protection:** Essential for managing skin rashes; patients should use sunscreen and protective clothing to prevent photosensitivity-induced flares.
   - **Calcium and Vitamin D Supplementation:** To prevent osteoporosis, especially in patients on long-term corticosteroids.

22.4.4. Long-Term Monitoring

Regular monitoring is vital to assess treatment efficacy, detect side effects, and prevent complications. The American College of Rheumatology (ACR) provides guidelines for the follow-up and management of JDM patients.

1. **Muscle Strength and Function:**
   - **Assessment Tools:** Manual muscle testing, quantitative muscle testing, and functional scales (e.g., Childhood Myositis Assessment Scale - CMAS).
   - **Frequency:** Every 1-3 months during active disease and less frequently during remission.
2. **Laboratory Monitoring:**
   - **Muscle Enzymes:** Regular measurement of CK and aldolase levels to monitor disease activity and response to therapy.
   - **Complete Blood Count (CBC) and Liver Function Tests (LFTs):** To monitor for side effects of medications like methotrexate and corticosteroids.
3. **Imaging:**
   - **MRI:** Periodic MRI scans to assess ongoing muscle inflammation and detect complications.
   - **Ultrasound:** Can be used for dynamic assessment of muscle and subcutaneous tissues.
4. **Bone Health:**
   - **Osteoporosis Screening:** Dual-energy X-ray absorptiometry (DEXA) scans are recommended for patients on long-term corticosteroids.

- **Preventive Measures:** Calcium and vitamin D supplementation, weight-bearing exercises, and, if necessary, bisphosphonates.
5. **Growth Monitoring:**
   - **Impact of Corticosteroids:** Regular monitoring of growth parameters to detect and address growth suppression early.
   - **Interventions:** Adjusting corticosteroid doses and optimizing nutritional status to support growth.
6. **Skin Care and Calcinosis:**
   - **Skin Monitoring:** Regular dermatologic evaluations to manage rashes and prevent scarring.
   - **Calcinosis Monitoring:** Ultrasonography or MRI to detect and monitor calcium deposits, which can cause pain and functional impairment.
   - **Management:** Physical therapy, surgical intervention in severe cases, and medications like bisphosphonates or probenecid may be considered.
7. **Psychosocial Support:**
   - **Importance:** Chronic illness can impact mental health, self-esteem, and social interactions.
   - **Support Services:** Counseling, support groups, and educational interventions are recommended to address these aspects.
8. **Infection Surveillance:**
   - **Immunosuppressive Therapy:** Regular monitoring for infections, especially in patients receiving biologics or high-dose corticosteroids.
   - **Preventive Measures:** Vaccinations (when appropriate), prophylactic antibiotics in certain cases, and prompt treatment of infections.

22.5. Henoch-Schönlein Purpura (HSP)

22.5.1. Overview

Henoch-Schönlein Purpura (HSP), also known as IgA vasculitis, is the most common vasculitis in children, typically occurring between the ages of 3 and 15. HSP is a small-vessel vasculitis that primarily affects the skin, joints, gastrointestinal (GI) tract, and kidneys.

The hallmark of the disease is the presence of palpable purpura, often accompanied by arthritis/arthralgia, abdominal pain, and renal involvement (glomerulonephritis). The condition is usually self-limiting, with most cases resolving within 4-6 weeks, but renal involvement can lead to long-term complications in a subset of patients.

- **Incidence:** HSP occurs at an estimated incidence of 10-20 per 100,000 children annually.
- **Pathophysiology:** HSP is characterized by the deposition of IgA immune complexes in small vessels, particularly in the skin, kidneys, and GI tract. Triggers may include infections (e.g., streptococcal), vaccinations, or drugs.

22.5.2. Diagnostic Approach

1. **Clinical Diagnosis**: The diagnosis of HSP is primarily clinical, based on the presence of the following features:
   - **Palpable purpura**: Typically seen on the lower extremities and buttocks, it is a non-thrombocytopenic purpura, meaning there is no significant decrease in platelet count.
   - **Arthritis or arthralgia**: Transient, non-deforming joint pain or swelling, typically involving the knees and ankles.
   - **Abdominal pain**: Colicky pain, often associated with GI bleeding, intussusception, or mesenteric vasculitis.
   - **Renal involvement**: Hematuria and/or proteinuria, indicative of IgA nephropathy.
2. The **American College of Rheumatology (ACR) criteria** for HSP diagnosis require the presence of palpable purpura, plus at least one of the following: abdominal pain, arthritis, renal involvement, or a biopsy showing predominant IgA deposition.
3. **Laboratory Tests**:
   - **Platelet Count**: Normal or elevated, distinguishing it from other causes of purpura like thrombocytopenic purpura.
   - **Urinalysis**: Critical for detecting hematuria and proteinuria, early indicators of renal involvement.
   - **Serum IgA Levels**: Elevated in about 50% of patients, although this is not specific to HSP.
   - **Renal Function Tests**: Including serum creatinine and blood urea nitrogen (BUN), to assess kidney function.
4. **Studies**: In a study by Yang et al. (2018), children with elevated IgA levels and renal involvement were found to be at a higher risk for developing chronic kidney disease (CKD).
5. **Renal Biopsy**:
   - **Indications**: Renal biopsy is warranted in patients with severe renal involvement, such as nephrotic-range proteinuria, worsening renal function, or persistent hematuria. Biopsy findings typically reveal IgA deposition in the mesangium of glomeruli, confirming the diagnosis of HSP nephritis.
   - **Studies**: A retrospective study by Coppo et al. (2014) found that renal biopsy findings correlated with the long-term risk of CKD, with more severe histopathological findings (e.g., crescents) predicting a worse prognosis.
6. **Imaging**:
   - **Ultrasound or CT Scan**: For children with severe abdominal pain or suspected complications like intussusception.

22.5.3. Treatment Strategies

1. **Supportive Care**:
   - **Mild to Moderate Cases**: Most children with HSP have mild disease that resolves spontaneously with supportive care, including adequate hydration, rest, and analgesia for joint pain.

- **Pain Management**: NSAIDs, such as ibuprofen or naproxen, are used for arthritis and mild abdominal pain but should be avoided in cases with renal involvement due to potential nephrotoxicity.
2. **Evidence**: Studies show that more than 90% of children recover without complications, particularly in those without significant renal or GI involvement.
3. **Corticosteroids**:
    - **Indications**: Corticosteroids, such as prednisone (1-2 mg/kg/day), are recommended for severe abdominal pain, GI bleeding, renal involvement, or scrotal involvement (Henoch-Schönlein purpura nephritis, HSPN).
    - **Efficacy**: While corticosteroids do not prevent renal involvement, they significantly reduce the duration of abdominal pain and hasten recovery from joint symptoms. A meta-analysis by Weiss et al. (2007) demonstrated that early use of steroids reduced the risk of GI complications but had no clear benefit in preventing renal sequelae.
    - **Refractory Cases**: For children with ongoing renal or severe systemic disease despite steroid therapy, pulse methylprednisolone (e.g., 30 mg/kg/day for 3 days) may be used.
4. **Immunosuppressants**:
    - **Usage**: In rare cases of severe HSP nephritis (class III or IV on biopsy, with significant proteinuria or declining renal function), immunosuppressive agents like azathioprine, cyclophosphamide, or mycophenolate mofetil may be considered.
    - **Evidence**: A study by Ronkainen et al. (2006) showed that the use of cyclophosphamide in combination with corticosteroids improved outcomes in children with crescentic nephritis. Mycophenolate mofetil has also shown promise in smaller case series for steroid-resistant HSP nephritis.
5. **Plasmapheresis or IVIG**:
    - **Indications**: Rarely, in patients with rapidly progressive glomerulonephritis, plasmapheresis or intravenous immunoglobulin (IVIG) may be used. However, the evidence for these therapies is limited, and they are reserved for the most severe cases.

22.5.4. Long-Term Monitoring

1. **Renal Function Monitoring**:
    - Renal involvement in HSP (HSP nephritis) is the most critical factor affecting long-term prognosis. Monitoring for hematuria, proteinuria, and renal function is essential, as up to 20% of patients may develop chronic kidney disease (CKD).
    - **Follow-up Schedule**: Urinalysis and blood pressure should be checked weekly during the acute phase, then every 3 months for at least a year, especially in patients with renal involvement.
2. **Evidence**: A long-term cohort study by Trapani et al. (2012) found that children with nephrotic-range proteinuria or crescentic nephritis had a significantly increased risk of CKD or end-stage renal disease (ESRD).
3. **Blood Pressure Monitoring**:

- Hypertension is a potential complication of HSP nephritis and should be monitored regularly, particularly in children with persistent renal involvement.
- **Management**: Angiotensin-converting enzyme inhibitors (ACE inhibitors) or angiotensin receptor blockers (ARBs) may be used for children with hypertension and proteinuria.

4. **Urinalysis**:
    - Persistent hematuria or proteinuria after resolution of other symptoms requires long-term monitoring, as these signs may be indicative of ongoing renal inflammation.
5. **Studies**: Research by Chen et al. (2013) demonstrated that children with ongoing proteinuria beyond 6 months have a higher risk of developing CKD and may require more aggressive treatment.
6. **Growth and Development**:
    - Children with prolonged corticosteroid use should be monitored for growth suppression, weight gain, and bone health, given the side effects of long-term steroid therapy.

References:

1. Petty, R.E., et al. (2004). International League of Associations for Rheumatology classification of juvenile idiopathic arthritis: second revision. *Journal of Rheumatology*, 31(2), 390-392.
2. Ravelli, A., & Martini, A. (2007). Juvenile idiopathic arthritis. *Lancet*, 369(9563), 767-778.
3. Beukelman, T., et al. (2011). 2011 American College of Rheumatology recommendations for the treatment of juvenile idiopathic arthritis. *Arthritis Care & Research*, 63(4), 465-482.
4. Tugal-Tutkun, I., et al. (2009). Uveitis in juvenile idiopathic arthritis. *Rheumatology*, 48(10), 1044-1049.
5. Malattia, C., et al. (2011). MRI in juvenile idiopathic arthritis: Imaging for clinical management and understanding of pathogenesis. *Nature Reviews Rheumatology*, 7(9), 569-578.
6. Ruperto, N., et al. (2012). Long-term safety and efficacy of etanercept in children with juvenile idiopathic arthritis. *Arthritis & Rheumatology*, 64(9), 2553-2564.
7. Wallace, C.A., et al. (2012). Methotrexate for the treatment of juvenile idiopathic arthritis: A systematic review. *Arthritis Care & Research*, 64(7), 1073-1082.
8. Lovell, D.J., et al. (2013). Long-term safety and efficacy of methotrexate in children with juvenile idiopathic arthritis. *Arthritis Care & Research*, 65(5), 674-684.
9. Prince, F.H.M., et al. (2011). Long-term outcomes in juvenile idiopathic arthritis: What do we know? *Arthritis & Rheumatology*, 63(5), 1105-1116.
10. Wenderfer, S. E., & Ruth, N. M. (2013). Pediatric systemic lupus erythematosus: clinical presentations, treatment, and outcome. *Current Pediatric Reviews*, 9(4), 312-321.
11. Mina, R., & Brunner, H. I. (2013). Pediatric lupus–are there differences in presentation, genetics, response to therapy, and damage accrual compared with adult lupus? *Rheumatic Disease Clinics of North America*, 36(1), 53-80.

12. Ruperto, N., et al. (2012). Lupus nephritis in pediatric and adult systemic lupus erythematosus: a multicenter study by the Pediatric Rheumatology International Trials Organization (PRINTO) and the Pediatric Rheumatology Collaborative Study Group (PRCSG). *Arthritis & Rheumatism*, 64(9), 3254-3260.
13. Boumpas, D. T., et al. (2012). Treating systemic lupus erythematosus: from mild to life-threatening. *Annals of Internal Medicine*, 157(9), 761-773.
14. Chatham, W. W., & Kimberly, R. P. (2001). Treatment of lupus with corticosteroids. *Lupus*, 10(3), 140-147.
15. Furie, R. A., et al. (2011). Efficacy and safety of belimumab in patients with active systemic lupus erythematosus: a randomised, placebo-controlled, phase 3 trial. *The Lancet*, 377(9767), 721-731.

Chapter 23: Cardiovascular and Bone Health in Rheumatologic Patients

Patients with rheumatologic diseases such as **rheumatoid arthritis (RA)**, **systemic lupus erythematosus (SLE)**, and **psoriatic arthritis (PsA)** are at an increased risk for both **cardiovascular disease (CVD)** and **osteoporosis**. Chronic inflammation, autoimmune mechanisms, and the medications used to manage these diseases contribute to this elevated risk. Optimizing cardiovascular and bone health is essential to improving long-term outcomes and quality of life for these patients. This section reviews the relationship between cardiovascular and bone health in rheumatologic patients, focusing on risk factors, prevention, and management strategies.

23.1. Cardiovascular Risk and Inflammatory Arthritis

Chronic systemic inflammation in rheumatologic diseases is a key driver of **atherosclerosis**, leading to accelerated cardiovascular disease. Patients with RA, SLE, and PsA are at significantly higher risk of **myocardial infarction**, **stroke**, **heart failure**, and **premature mortality** compared to the general population.

- **Rheumatoid Arthritis (RA)**:
  RA patients have a **50% higher risk** of cardiovascular events compared to the general population, even after adjusting for traditional risk factors such as **smoking**, **hypertension**, and **hyperlipidemia**. The increased risk is primarily due to **chronic systemic inflammation**, which promotes **endothelial dysfunction**, **plaque formation**, and **instability of atherosclerotic plaques**. Elevated levels of pro-inflammatory cytokines like **TNF-α**, **IL-6**, and **CRP** drive both joint and vascular inflammation.
- **Systemic Lupus Erythematosus (SLE)**:
  Patients with SLE are at an increased risk for **premature atherosclerosis**, with studies showing up to a **50-fold increase** in the risk of **myocardial infarction** in young women with SLE compared to age-matched controls. The combination of **autoantibodies**, **chronic inflammation**, and **immune complex deposition** contributes to accelerated atherosclerosis in SLE. **Antiphospholipid antibodies (aPL)**, which are present in up to **30-40%** of SLE patients, further increase the risk of thromboembolic events.
- **Psoriatic Arthritis (PsA)**:
  PsA is also associated with an elevated cardiovascular risk due to chronic inflammation. Studies have shown that PsA patients have an increased prevalence of **metabolic syndrome**, which includes **obesity**, **dyslipidemia**, **hypertension**, and **insulin resistance**—all of which contribute to cardiovascular disease. The inflammatory pathways involved in PsA, such as **TNF-α**, **IL-17**, and **IL-23**, play a role in both joint and cardiovascular inflammation.

23.2. Strategies for Cardiovascular Risk Reduction in RA, SLE, and PsA

Reducing cardiovascular risk in patients with rheumatic diseases requires a **multifactorial approach**, including both the management of traditional cardiovascular risk factors and controlling systemic inflammation.

- **Aggressive Control of Inflammation**:
  Disease-modifying antirheumatic drugs (DMARDs), particularly **methotrexate** and **biologics** (e.g., TNF inhibitors, IL-6 inhibitors), have been shown to reduce both joint and cardiovascular inflammation in RA, SLE, and PsA. Studies suggest that controlling disease activity can reduce the risk of cardiovascular events.
  - **Methotrexate** has been associated with reduced cardiovascular mortality in RA patients, likely due to its anti-inflammatory effects on both joints and blood vessels.
  - **TNF inhibitors**, such as **etanercept** and **adalimumab**, have been shown to reduce cardiovascular risk by decreasing systemic inflammation and improving endothelial function. However, TNF inhibitors should be used cautiously in patients with **heart failure**, as they may exacerbate the condition.
- **Management of Traditional Risk Factors**:
  - **Lipid management**: Statins, such as **atorvastatin** and **rosuvastatin**, are effective in lowering LDL cholesterol and reducing cardiovascular risk in rheumatologic patients. Statins may also have **anti-inflammatory effects**, further benefiting patients with inflammatory arthritis.
  - **Hypertension control**: Tight control of **blood pressure** is critical, as hypertension is a common comorbidity in rheumatologic patients and a significant contributor to cardiovascular events. **ACE inhibitors** or **angiotensin receptor blockers (ARBs)** are preferred due to their renal protective effects, particularly in patients with **lupus nephritis**.
  - **Antiplatelet therapy**: Low-dose **aspirin** is recommended for patients with **antiphospholipid syndrome (APS)** to reduce the risk of arterial and venous thromboembolism. Aspirin is also considered in patients with established cardiovascular disease or significant risk factors.
- **Lifestyle Modifications**:
  Smoking cessation, weight management, and regular physical activity are crucial components of cardiovascular risk reduction. Smoking, in particular, exacerbates both rheumatoid arthritis and cardiovascular disease, and patients should be encouraged to stop smoking.
- **Screening and Monitoring**:
  - Rheumatologic patients should be regularly screened for cardiovascular risk factors, including **lipid profiles**, **blood pressure**, **blood glucose**, and **renal function**. Baseline cardiovascular risk assessments using tools like the **Framingham Risk Score** or **QRISK3** are recommended.
  - Patients with SLE or APS should be monitored for thromboembolic events, and those with SLE should undergo regular cardiovascular evaluations, especially if they have other risk factors or antiphospholipid antibodies.

23.3. Osteoporosis in Rheumatic Diseases: Prevention and Management

Rheumatologic patients, particularly those with RA, SLE, and PsA, are at increased risk of developing **osteoporosis** due to chronic inflammation, reduced mobility, and long-term corticosteroid use.

- **Pathogenesis**:
  Chronic systemic inflammation, mediated by **TNF-α, IL-1**, and **IL-6**, promotes **osteoclast activation** and bone resorption, leading to reduced bone density in rheumatic patients. In addition, **glucocorticoid therapy**, commonly used to manage flares in RA and SLE, accelerates bone loss by inhibiting osteoblast function and enhancing osteoclast-mediated bone resorption .
- **Risk Factors for Osteoporosis**:
  - **Long-term glucocorticoid therapy** (≥3 months) is a major risk factor for osteoporosis and fractures in rheumatologic patients. The risk increases with the dose and duration of corticosteroid use.
  - **Menopause, physical inactivity, low body mass index (BMI)**, and **vitamin D deficiency** also contribute to the development of osteoporosis in patients with rheumatic diseases.
- **Prevention Strategies**:
  - **Calcium and Vitamin D Supplementation**:
    All patients on long-term corticosteroids should receive **calcium (1000-1200 mg/day)** and **vitamin D (800-1000 IU/day)** supplementation to prevent bone loss. Vitamin D deficiency is common in patients with rheumatic diseases and is associated with reduced bone mineral density (BMD) and increased fracture risk.
  - **Bisphosphonates**:
    Bisphosphonates, such as **alendronate, risedronate**, and **zoledronic acid**, are first-line therapies for preventing and treating glucocorticoid-induced osteoporosis. They inhibit osteoclast activity and have been shown to reduce the risk of vertebral and non-vertebral fractures in patients on chronic corticosteroids .
  - **Denosumab**:
    Denosumab, a monoclonal antibody that inhibits **RANKL**, is another option for patients at high risk of fractures or those intolerant to bisphosphonates. It has been shown to increase bone density and reduce fracture risk in glucocorticoid-treated patients.
- **Monitoring Bone Health**:
  - Patients at risk of osteoporosis should undergo regular **dual-energy X-ray absorptiometry (DEXA)** scans to assess bone mineral density. The **T-score** is used to diagnose osteoporosis (T-score ≤ -2.5) and guide treatment decisions.
  - **Fracture risk assessment** using tools such as **FRAX** can help identify patients at high risk for fractures and determine the need for pharmacologic interventions.

- **Exercise and Lifestyle**:
    - Weight-bearing exercises, such as **walking, resistance training**, and **aerobic activities**, are recommended to maintain bone health and improve overall physical function. Regular physical activity helps reduce the risk of osteoporosis and fractures in patients with limited mobility due to arthritis.
    - Smoking cessation and limiting alcohol intake are important lifestyle modifications, as both are risk factors for osteoporosis and bone loss.

Patients with rheumatic diseases are at increased risk for both cardiovascular disease and osteoporosis due to the chronic inflammatory nature of their conditions and the use of immunosuppressive therapies. Cardiovascular risk reduction strategies, including aggressive control of inflammation, management of traditional cardiovascular risk factors, and lifestyle modifications, are essential for improving long-term outcomes. Osteoporosis prevention and management, particularly in patients on long-term corticosteroids, should include calcium and vitamin D supplementation, bisphosphonates or denosumab, and regular bone density monitoring. A holistic, multidisciplinary approach is needed to optimize cardiovascular and bone health in rheumatologic patients.

References

1. Avina-Zubieta, J. A., Thomas, J., Sadatsafavi, M., et al. (2012). Risk of incident cardiovascular events in patients with rheumatoid arthritis: A meta-analysis of observational studies. *Annals of the Rheumatic Diseases*, 71(9), 1524-1529.
2. Urowitz, M. B., Ibañez, D., & Gladman, D. D. (2007). Atherosclerotic vascular events in a single large lupus cohort: Prevalence and risk factors. *The Journal of Rheumatology*, 34(1), 70-75.
3. Ritchlin, C. T., Colbert, R. A., & Gladman, D. D. (2017). Psoriatic arthritis. *New England Journal of Medicine*, 376(10), 957-970.
4. Solomon, D. H., Kremer, J., Curtis, J. R., et al. (2010). Explaining the cardiovascular risk associated with rheumatoid arthritis: Traditional risk factors versus markers of rheumatoid arthritis severity. *Annals of the Rheumatic Diseases*, 69(11), 1920-1925.
5. Grossman, J. M., Gordon, R., Ranganath, V. K., et al. (2010). American College of Rheumatology 2010 recommendations for the prevention and treatment of glucocorticoid-induced osteoporosis. *Arthritis Care & Research*, 62(11), 1515-1526.
6. Buckley, L., Guyatt, G., Fink, H. A., et al. (2017). 2017 American College of Rheumatology guideline for the prevention and treatment of glucocorticoid-induced osteoporosis. *Arthritis & Rheumatology*, 69(8), 1521-1537.

Part 4: Integrating Rheumatology into Primary Care

Chapter 24: Collaborative Care with Rheumatologists

Collaborative care between primary care providers, specialists, and rheumatologists is essential in optimizing the management of patients with rheumatic diseases. Given the chronic and complex nature of these diseases, such as **rheumatoid arthritis (RA)**, **systemic lupus erythematosus (SLE)**, **psoriatic arthritis (PsA)**, and **ankylosing spondylitis (AS)**, early and appropriate referral to a rheumatologist can significantly improve outcomes. This section elaborates on when and how to refer patients to a rheumatologist, the principles of co-managing patients with rheumatic diseases, and the importance of shared decision-making among patients and multidisciplinary teams.

24.1. When and How to Refer to a Rheumatologist

Rheumatologists specialize in the diagnosis and treatment of autoimmune, inflammatory, and musculoskeletal diseases. Early referral to a rheumatologist is critical for timely diagnosis and initiation of disease-modifying treatments, which can prevent irreversible joint damage, organ dysfunction, and disability.

- **When to Refer**:
    - **Suspected Rheumatoid Arthritis (RA)**: Early referral is crucial when patients present with **persistent joint pain, morning stiffness lasting longer than 30 minutes, swelling in multiple joints**, and elevated inflammatory markers (e.g., **CRP, ESR**). Delay in diagnosis and treatment of RA can lead to **joint erosion** and permanent disability within the first **6 months** of symptom onset .
    - **Systemic Lupus Erythematosus (SLE)**: Patients with **multisystem involvement**, such as unexplained **fever**, **rash**, **photosensitivity**, **arthritis**, **renal disease**, and positive autoantibodies (e.g., **ANA, anti-dsDNA**) should be referred for evaluation and management of SLE. Timely referral helps manage potential organ damage (e.g., **lupus nephritis, CNS involvement**) .
    - **Spondyloarthritis (SpA) and Ankylosing Spondylitis (AS)**: Referral is recommended for young patients with **chronic low back pain**, particularly if the pain improves with activity and worsens with rest, or if there is evidence of **sacroiliitis** on imaging. Early intervention with **biologics** can prevent spinal fusion and improve mobility in AS .
    - **Psoriatic Arthritis (PsA)**: Patients with **psoriasis** and symptoms of joint pain, **dactylitis** ("sausage digits"), or **enthesitis** (pain where tendons attach to bones) should be referred early to prevent irreversible joint damage. Referral is especially urgent if skin and joint symptoms co-exist.
    - **Vasculitis**: If there are signs of **systemic vasculitis**, such as **unexplained constitutional symptoms, purpura, glomerulonephritis**, or **mononeuritis multiplex**, prompt referral to a rheumatologist is necessary for diagnostic workup (e.g., biopsy, ANCA testing) and initiation of immunosuppressive therapy .
- **How to Refer**:

- **Clear communication** with the rheumatologist is essential when making a referral. Providing a detailed clinical history, relevant laboratory tests (e.g., ANA, RF, anti-CCP, ANCA), and imaging results (e.g., X-rays, MRI for joint involvement) can help streamline the diagnostic process.
- For urgent referrals, especially in cases of suspected **vasculitis**, **SLE with renal involvement**, or **severe flare-ups of RA**, direct communication with the rheumatologist can expedite patient assessment and treatment initiation.

24.2. Co-Managing Patients with Rheumatic Diseases

Co-management of patients with rheumatic diseases involves ongoing collaboration between the primary care provider and the rheumatologist to optimize care, monitor disease activity, and manage comorbidities. Many rheumatologic conditions require long-term follow-up and multidisciplinary care due to the involvement of multiple organ systems.

- **Roles in Co-Management**:
  - **Primary Care Provider (PCP)**:
  The PCP plays a key role in managing **comorbid conditions** (e.g., cardiovascular disease, osteoporosis), screening for complications related to both the disease and the medications used (e.g., **glucocorticoid-induced osteoporosis**, **methotrexate hepatotoxicity**), and ensuring patients receive appropriate **vaccinations**. Routine care such as blood pressure monitoring, lipid management, and cancer screenings remain the responsibility of the PCP.
  - **Rheumatologist**:
  The rheumatologist is responsible for diagnosing, initiating, and adjusting disease-modifying antirheumatic drugs (**DMARDs**), biologics, and other immunosuppressive therapies. Rheumatologists closely monitor disease activity, flares, and treatment side effects, adjusting therapy as needed to achieve **remission** or **low disease activity**.
- **Key Areas of Collaboration**:
  - **Cardiovascular Risk Management**:
  Patients with RA, SLE, and PsA are at elevated risk for cardiovascular disease due to systemic inflammation. The PCP and rheumatologist should collaborate on strategies to manage traditional risk factors such as hypertension, hyperlipidemia, and diabetes. Joint efforts in promoting **smoking cessation** and **lifestyle changes** (e.g., diet, exercise) are essential for reducing cardiovascular risk.
  - **Bone Health and Osteoporosis Prevention**:
  Long-term corticosteroid use increases the risk of osteoporosis in patients with rheumatic diseases. Both the PCP and rheumatologist should ensure that patients receive **calcium** and **vitamin D supplementation**, along with **bisphosphonates** or **denosumab** if indicated. Regular bone mineral density (BMD) testing via **DEXA scans** is essential for monitoring bone health.

- **Infection Prevention**:
  Patients on long-term immunosuppressive therapy are at increased risk for infections, including **pneumonia** and **herpes zoster**. PCPs should ensure that patients receive recommended vaccines, including the **influenza**, **pneumococcal**, and **zoster vaccines**. **Live vaccines** should generally be avoided in patients on biologics or high-dose immunosuppressive therapy, highlighting the importance of coordinating vaccine administration with the rheumatologist.
- **Patient Education and Self-Management**:
  Educating patients about their disease, the importance of medication adherence, and recognizing early signs of flare-ups are crucial components of co-management. Empowering patients to actively participate in their care improves long-term outcomes and reduces hospitalizations for complications.

24.3. Shared Decision-Making with Patients and Multidisciplinary Teams

Shared decision-making is an approach where patients and healthcare providers collaborate to make decisions based on the best available evidence, the clinician's expertise, and the patient's preferences and values. In the management of chronic rheumatic diseases, shared decision-making involves the patient, primary care provider, rheumatologist, and other specialists, such as **dermatologists** for psoriasis, **nephrologists** for lupus nephritis, or **orthopedists** for joint replacement surgery.

- **Involving the Patient**:
  Patients with chronic rheumatic diseases face complex decisions, such as whether to initiate biologic therapy, continue long-term immunosuppression, or consider surgical intervention. Involving patients in these decisions ensures that they understand the risks and benefits of treatment options, adhere to the chosen therapies, and feel empowered in their care.
  - In **RA** or **PsA**, for example, the decision to escalate from conventional DMARDs to biologics involves discussing the potential benefits (improved joint function, reduced progression of joint damage) and risks (infections, cancer risk). The patient's preferences, lifestyle, and tolerance for side effects are integral to making this decision.
- **Collaboration Among Multidisciplinary Teams**:
  Complex rheumatologic diseases often require input from multiple specialties. For instance:
  - **SLE patients with nephritis** may require a coordinated approach between the rheumatologist and **nephrologist** to manage both immunosuppression and renal function monitoring.
  - **Dermatologists** play a key role in managing patients with **psoriatic arthritis**, particularly those with severe psoriasis.
  - **Orthopedic surgeons** may be involved in the care of patients with RA or PsA who require **joint replacement surgery** due to severe joint damage.

- Close communication between the rheumatologist, PCP, and other specialists ensures that all aspects of the patient's health are addressed comprehensively.
- **Tools to Facilitate Shared Decision-Making**:
  Several tools can support shared decision-making in rheumatology. **Decision aids**, such as informational pamphlets or web-based tools, help patients understand their disease and treatment options. **Patient-reported outcomes (PROs)**, such as pain scales or functional status questionnaires, can also guide discussions on treatment efficacy and quality of life.
- **Long-Term Monitoring and Follow-Up**:
  Regular follow-up visits and monitoring of disease activity are essential components of shared decision-making. Adjusting therapy based on **disease flares**, **treatment side effects**, and **patient preferences** requires ongoing dialogue between the patient, PCP, and rheumatologist. The ability to adapt treatment in response to changes in disease activity or the patient's life circumstances (e.g., pregnancy, planned surgery) is a hallmark of effective collaborative care.

Collaborative care between primary care providers, rheumatologists, and other specialists is essential for managing patients with chronic rheumatic diseases. Early referral to a rheumatologist ensures timely diagnosis and treatment, preventing irreversible damage. Co-management between the PCP and rheumatologist involves addressing comorbidities, monitoring disease activity, and managing the side effects of treatment.

Shared decision-making empowers patients to actively participate in their care, leading to improved adherence and better long-term outcomes. A multidisciplinary approach is critical for managing the complex and multisystem nature of rheumatic diseases.

References

- Smolen, J. S., Landewé, R., Bijlsma, J. W., et al. (2020). EULAR recommendations for the management of rheumatoid arthritis with synthetic and biological disease-modifying antirheumatic drugs: 2020 update. *Annals of the Rheumatic Diseases*, 79(6), 685-699.
- Dall'Era, M., Stone, D., Costenbader, K., et al. (2019). Challenges in the diagnosis and management of lupus nephritis. *Nature Reviews Rheumatology*, 15(9), 576-586.
- Schoels, M. M., Knevel, R., Aletaha, D., et al. (2010). Evidence for treating rheumatoid arthritis to target: results of a systematic literature search update. *Annals of the Rheumatic Diseases*, 69(4), 638-643.
- Ward, M. M., Deodhar, A., Akl, E. A., et al. (2016). American College of Rheumatology/Spondylitis Association of America/Spondyloarthritis Research and Treatment Network 2015 recommendations for the treatment of ankylosing spondylitis and non radiographic axial spondyloarthritis. *Arthritis Care & Research*, 68(2), 151-166.
- Miloslavsky, E. M., & Niles, J. L. (2017). Vasculitis associated with antineutrophil cytoplasmic autoantibodies (ANCA). *BMJ*, 356, j567.

Chapter 25: Patient Education and Self-Management

Educating patients about their rheumatic diseases and empowering them to actively participate in their care is essential for improving outcomes. Chronic diseases like **rheumatoid arthritis (RA)**, **systemic lupus erythematosus (SLE)**, and **psoriatic arthritis (PsA)** require long-term management and adherence to treatment plans to prevent disease progression and maintain quality of life. Patient education, tools for engagement, and lifestyle modifications play a crucial role in self-management. This section explores these key components and their impact on disease outcomes.

25.1. Educating Patients About Their Disease

Understanding their diagnosis, treatment options, and long-term management is fundamental for patients with rheumatic diseases. Effective education helps patients become informed participants in their care, enhances adherence to treatment, and reduces the risk of complications. Studies have shown that informed patients are more likely to adhere to therapy and experience better health outcomes .

- **Understanding Disease Pathophysiology**:
  Patients should be provided with clear explanations of their disease processes. For example, patients with RA need to understand that the disease is **autoimmune**, involving **chronic inflammation** that leads to **joint damage** if untreated. Similarly, patients with SLE should be educated about how the disease can affect multiple organ systems and that treatment aims to control **flares** and prevent organ damage.
  Visual aids, such as **diagrams** and **models** of affected joints or tissues, can help patients better understand their disease. Educational brochures, websites, and videos developed by trusted organizations like the **American College of Rheumatology (ACR)** or **Arthritis Foundation** can be valuable resources.
- **Treatment Goals and Medications**:
  It is crucial to explain the importance of **disease-modifying antirheumatic drugs (DMARDs)** and **biologic therapies**. Patients should understand that these medications are not just for symptom control but are essential for preventing long-term damage. For example, explaining the role of **methotrexate** or **TNF inhibitors** in reducing inflammation and protecting joints can motivate adherence.
  - Patients should be aware of potential **side effects** of medications, such as **nausea** or **immunosuppression**, and be encouraged to report any issues. They should also understand the importance of **monitoring**, such as regular blood tests for **liver function** or **complete blood counts**.
- **Recognizing Disease Flares**:
  Patients should be educated on how to recognize early signs of a disease flare, such as **increased joint pain, fatigue, rash,** or **fever** (for lupus patients). Understanding that prompt intervention during a flare can prevent complications is crucial. Patients with conditions like RA should be advised to contact their healthcare provider if they notice worsening symptoms.

- **Self-Monitoring Tools**:
Teaching patients to use **self-monitoring tools** such as **pain diaries**, **joint stiffness logs**, and **patient-reported outcome measures (PROMs)** can enhance self-awareness and provide valuable information for healthcare providers. For instance, the use of **Health Assessment Questionnaire (HAQ)** or **Rheumatoid Arthritis Disease Activity Index (RADAI)** allows patients to track their functional status and disease progression.

25.2. Tools for Patient Engagement and Adherence to Therapy

Maintaining long-term adherence to medications and lifestyle modifications can be challenging for patients with chronic diseases. However, several tools can help improve patient engagement and ensure adherence.

- **Patient Education Platforms**:
Mobile apps and online platforms designed for patients with chronic diseases can help them manage their condition and stay informed. Examples include **MyRA** for rheumatoid arthritis and **LupusCorner** for lupus, which provide resources, medication reminders, and educational content. These platforms often allow patients to log symptoms, track medication use, and receive reminders for medication or appointments.
- **Medication Adherence Tools**:
Non-adherence to medications is a significant issue in chronic diseases. Tools such as **medication organizers**, **automatic pill dispensers**, and **mobile apps** that send reminders can help patients stay on track with their treatment. Apps like **MediSafe** or **CareZone** allow patients to schedule reminders, record doses, and alert them when it's time to refill prescriptions.
- **Telemedicine and Patient Portals**:
Telemedicine has become increasingly important in maintaining regular follow-up with patients. It allows patients to access their healthcare provider from home, reducing the burden of travel, especially for those with mobility issues due to joint pain or fatigue. **Patient portals** offer secure platforms for messaging healthcare providers, viewing lab results, and requesting medication refills.
- **Patient Support Groups**:
Encouraging participation in **support groups** can be highly beneficial for patients dealing with chronic rheumatic diseases. Peer support provides a sense of community and allows patients to share experiences and coping strategies. Support groups, such as those offered by the **Arthritis Foundation** or **Lupus Foundation of America**, often include educational workshops and online forums for patients.
- **Shared Decision-Making Tools**:
Involving patients in the decision-making process about their treatment has been shown to improve adherence. **Shared decision-making tools**, such as decision aids, help patients weigh the pros and cons of different treatment options based on their preferences and values. These tools guide patients and providers through discussions about the benefits, risks, and expected outcomes of therapies.

25.3. Lifestyle Modifications: Diet, Exercise, and Stress Management

In addition to pharmacological treatment, lifestyle modifications play a critical role in managing rheumatic diseases. Encouraging patients to adopt a healthy lifestyle can reduce inflammation, improve physical function, and enhance overall well-being.

- **Diet**:
    - **Anti-Inflammatory Diet**: A diet rich in **omega-3 fatty acids, fruits, vegetables, whole grains**, and **lean proteins** may help reduce inflammation in patients with RA and other inflammatory diseases. Omega-3-rich foods such as **fish, flaxseed**, and **walnuts** have been shown to decrease joint pain and stiffness.
    - **Avoiding Pro-Inflammatory Foods**: Patients should be advised to limit the intake of **processed foods, sugar, saturated fats**, and **refined carbohydrates**, as these can exacerbate inflammation.
    - **Weight Management**: Maintaining a healthy weight is essential, especially for patients with RA or PsA, as excess weight increases stress on joints and can worsen symptoms. Studies have shown that weight loss improves disease outcomes in PsA patients.
- **Exercise**:
    - **Regular Physical Activity**: Exercise is a critical component of managing rheumatic diseases. Patients should be encouraged to engage in **low-impact aerobic activities** such as **walking, swimming**, or **cycling** to maintain joint flexibility and overall cardiovascular health. **Strength training** can help maintain muscle mass, which supports joints and reduces pain.
    - **Range-of-Motion and Flexibility Exercises**: Regular stretching exercises help maintain **joint mobility** and prevent stiffness. **Yoga** and **tai chi** have been shown to improve joint flexibility, balance, and pain in patients with arthritis.
    - **Physical Therapy**: Referral to a **physical therapist** may be beneficial, especially for patients with significant joint deformity or muscle weakness. Physical therapists can design individualized exercise programs to maintain joint function and prevent disability.
- **Stress Management**:
    - **Cognitive Behavioral Therapy (CBT)**: Stress exacerbates both pain and inflammation, making stress management an essential component of care. CBT has been shown to help patients manage stress, anxiety, and depression, which are common in chronic disease. CBT helps patients develop coping strategies for dealing with chronic pain and illness-related stressors.
    - **Mind-Body Therapies**: Techniques such as **meditation, deep breathing**, and **progressive muscle relaxation** are effective in reducing stress and improving overall mental health. **Mindfulness-based stress reduction (MBSR)** has been shown to improve pain, physical function, and quality of life in patients with chronic conditions like RA.
    - **Adequate Sleep**: Poor sleep quality can worsen fatigue and increase pain sensitivity. Educating patients on **sleep hygiene** techniques, such as maintaining

a regular sleep schedule, avoiding caffeine before bed, and creating a restful environment, is essential for improving sleep quality.

Patient education, tools for engagement, and lifestyle modifications are vital for the self-management of rheumatic diseases. Educating patients about their disease, treatment options, and how to recognize disease flares empowers them to take an active role in managing their health. Tools such as mobile apps, medication organizers, and telemedicine improve adherence to therapy and facilitate ongoing communication with healthcare providers.

Lifestyle modifications, including a healthy diet, regular exercise, and stress management, contribute to reducing inflammation and improving long-term outcomes. Collaborative, informed care enhances patient satisfaction and quality of life in those living with chronic rheumatic diseases.

References

- Calder, P. C. (2012). Omega-3 polyunsaturated fatty acids and inflammatory processes: Nutrition or pharmacology? *British Journal of Clinical Pharmacology*, 75(3), 645-662.
- Ogdie, A., & Gelfand, J. M. (2015). Clinical risk factors for the development of psoriatic arthritis among patients with psoriasis: A review of available evidence. *Current Rheumatology Reports*, 17(6), 64.
- Grainger, R., Townsley, H., White, B., et al. (2017). The use of mobile health applications in rheumatology: Opportunities, barriers, and patient acceptability. *Rheumatology International*, 37(3), 331-336.
- Wah, S. L., & Teo, L. L. S. (2017). The role of exercise in the management of rheumatoid arthritis. *Singapore Medical Journal*, 58(6), 327-333.
- Davis, M. C., Zautra, A. J., & Wolf, L. D. (2014). Mindfulness and cognitive–behavioral interventions for chronic pain: Differential effects on daily pain reactivity and stress reactivity. *Journal of Consulting and Clinical Psychology*, 82(1), 35-44.

Chapter 26: Telemedicine and Remote Monitoring in Rheumatology

Telemedicine and remote monitoring have transformed healthcare delivery, particularly for chronic diseases like rheumatoid arthritis (RA), systemic lupus erythematosus (SLE), and psoriatic arthritis (PsA). These technologies enable continuous care and monitoring, providing timely interventions while reducing the burden of in-person visits. With advances in digital health tools, telemedicine is becoming a cornerstone in the management of rheumatologic diseases, improving patient outcomes and accessibility to care. This section elaborates on the benefits of telemedicine, remote monitoring tools for disease activity, and the integration of technology into primary care rheumatology.

26.1. Benefits of Telemedicine for Chronic Disease Management

Telemedicine offers numerous advantages in managing chronic rheumatologic conditions, where ongoing care and close monitoring of disease activity are essential for preventing flares and long-term complications. The COVID-19 pandemic accelerated the adoption of telemedicine, demonstrating its effectiveness and acceptability in rheumatology.

- **Improved Access to Care**:
  Telemedicine enhances access to rheumatology care, particularly for patients in **rural** or **underserved areas** who face challenges in visiting specialists due to geographical constraints. Rheumatologic care is often concentrated in urban centers, leaving many patients with limited access. Telemedicine addresses this gap by enabling patients to consult with specialists remotely .
- **Convenience and Reduced Burden**:
  Chronic diseases like RA and SLE require frequent follow-up visits for monitoring disease activity and medication management. Telemedicine reduces the need for travel, time off work, and associated costs, making it a convenient option for patients. Studies show that **patient satisfaction** with telemedicine is high, particularly due to the convenience of receiving care from home .
- **Early Detection of Flares**:
  Telemedicine facilitates early detection of disease flares by allowing more frequent and real-time communication between patients and their healthcare providers. For instance, a patient experiencing increased joint pain or stiffness can promptly schedule a telemedicine appointment, enabling timely adjustments to treatment.
- **Continuous Monitoring**:
  Telemedicine allows for the **continuous monitoring** of disease activity and treatment response. Patients can report symptoms more frequently and in real-time, helping providers assess whether medications need to be adjusted before the next in-person visit.
- **Patient Education and Engagement**:
  Telemedicine also serves as a platform for educating patients about their disease, medications, and self-management strategies. For example, virtual visits can be used to

review the correct technique for **self-injecting biologics** or to discuss **exercise programs** that support joint health.
- **Cost-Effectiveness**:
Telemedicine reduces the overall cost of healthcare by decreasing hospitalizations and emergency department visits, which are often precipitated by undetected disease flares or complications. By promoting early intervention and routine monitoring, telemedicine helps to prevent severe disease outcomes that require costly treatments.

26.2. Remote Monitoring Tools for Disease Activity

Advances in digital health technology have introduced a variety of remote monitoring tools that allow patients with rheumatic diseases to track their symptoms, disease activity, and overall health. These tools not only empower patients to participate in their care but also provide clinicians with valuable data to make informed treatment decisions.

- **Mobile Health Apps**:
Mobile applications designed for rheumatic disease management enable patients to log symptoms, track medication use, and monitor disease flares. Apps such as **MyRA** for rheumatoid arthritis and **LupusCorner** for lupus allow patients to record daily health metrics, pain levels, and functional status. These apps often include visual aids such as **pain maps** and **joint stiffness charts**, which help both patients and healthcare providers identify patterns and triggers in disease activity.
    - **MyRA**: This app allows patients with rheumatoid arthritis to track symptoms, medication adherence, and physical activity, providing visual charts to monitor changes over time. The app also offers educational content to enhance patient understanding of RA management.
    - **LupusCorner**: For SLE patients, this app offers symptom tracking, medication reminders, and resources for disease education. It allows patients to record daily lupus-related symptoms such as fatigue, rash, and joint pain, which can be shared with healthcare providers during telemedicine visits.
- **Wearable Devices**:
Wearable technology, such as **smartwatches** and **fitness trackers**, can monitor **physical activity**, **sleep patterns**, **heart rate variability**, and other health metrics. These data points are especially valuable for tracking patient outcomes in diseases like **psoriatic arthritis** and **ankylosing spondylitis**, where physical activity and sleep disturbances are critical aspects of disease management.
    - **Fitbit** and **Apple Watch** devices can track **steps**, **exercise intensity**, and **sleep quality**, allowing patients and providers to monitor whether a patient's exercise regimen is appropriate and whether their activity levels are affected by joint pain or fatigue. Wearable devices may also prompt discussions about lifestyle changes during telemedicine visits.
- **Remote Disease Activity Assessments**:
Tools such as **Patient Reported Outcomes Measurement Information System (PROMIS)** and the **Rheumatoid Arthritis Disease Activity Index (RADAI)** are

validated instruments used in remote monitoring. These tools allow patients to self-report disease activity, pain, and physical function. Regular use of PROMIS scores helps healthcare providers assess treatment efficacy and adjust therapy as needed.

- **Joint Imaging at Home**:
Although more experimental, some emerging technologies allow for **remote joint imaging** through mobile ultrasound devices. These devices can be used by patients or in collaboration with local health professionals, sending results to rheumatologists for interpretation. Such innovations may provide remote assessments of joint inflammation in diseases like RA and PsA.

26.3. Integrating Technology into Primary Care Rheumatology

The integration of telemedicine and remote monitoring into primary care rheumatology represents a paradigm shift in how patients with chronic rheumatic diseases are managed. Successful integration requires collaboration between **primary care providers (PCPs)**, **rheumatologists**, and **technology platforms** to ensure continuous care and optimized disease management.

- **Streamlined Communication Between Providers**:
Telemedicine allows for **seamless communication** between PCPs and rheumatologists, facilitating **real-time consultations** and joint decision-making. For example, if a PCP identifies early signs of a flare in a patient with RA, they can consult a rheumatologist virtually to discuss adjusting the patient's medications or ordering diagnostic tests. Similarly, rheumatologists can provide expert input on complex cases without requiring patients to travel for in-person consultations.

- **Shared Electronic Health Records (EHR)**:
Effective integration of telemedicine into rheumatology care relies on shared **electronic health records (EHR)** that allow all members of the healthcare team to access up-to-date patient data. EHRs that integrate remote monitoring data, such as PROMIS scores or wearable device metrics, provide a more comprehensive view of the patient's health. This ensures that both primary care and specialty providers are aligned in their treatment strategies.

- **Telemedicine in Rural Areas**:
Telemedicine plays a particularly important role in **rural areas** or regions with limited access to rheumatology specialists. PCPs in these areas can collaborate with rheumatologists in urban centers via telehealth platforms to ensure that patients receive expert care. This model also allows PCPs to maintain continuity of care while receiving guidance on complex aspects of rheumatologic management.

- **Telemedicine for Disease Monitoring and Education**:
In addition to managing disease flares, telemedicine can be used for **routine monitoring**, medication management, and patient education. Virtual check-ins enable providers to assess medication adherence, review lab results, and adjust therapies as needed. Moreover, providers can use telemedicine to educate patients about lifestyle

modifications, stress management, and the importance of vaccination, particularly for immunosuppressed patients on biologics or DMARDs.
- **Challenges and Considerations**:
Despite the many benefits, integrating telemedicine and remote monitoring into rheumatology practice comes with challenges. **Data security and privacy** concerns must be addressed, particularly when using mobile apps and wearable devices that transmit sensitive health information. Additionally, **technology literacy** and **internet access** can vary among patients, creating potential barriers to telemedicine adoption. Providers should assess each patient's comfort level with technology and offer alternative methods of care for those who face challenges with telehealth.

Telemedicine and remote monitoring offer transformative benefits for the management of chronic rheumatologic diseases. By providing continuous monitoring, improving access to care, and enhancing patient engagement, these technologies contribute to better disease control and improved outcomes.

Mobile health apps, wearable devices, and remote disease activity assessments provide clinicians with valuable real-time data, enabling more informed treatment decisions. Integrating telemedicine into primary care rheumatology requires collaboration between healthcare providers and the use of shared electronic health records to ensure streamlined, patient-centered care. While challenges remain, the potential for telemedicine to improve the management of rheumatic diseases is clear, particularly in underserved and rural populations.

References

- Piga, M., Cangemi, I., Mathieu, A., & Cauli, A. (2021). Telemedicine for patients with rheumatic diseases: Systematic review and proposal for research agenda. *Seminars in Arthritis and Rheumatism*, 51(1), 121-130.
- Grainger, R., Townsley, H., White, B., et al. (2017). The use of mobile health applications in rheumatology: Opportunities, barriers, and patient acceptability. *Rheumatology International*, 37(3), 331-336.
- Piga, M., Cangemi, I., Mathieu, A., & Cauli, A. (2017). Telemedicine applied to rheumatology during COVID-19: A systematic review and evidence-based recommendations for clinical practice. *Rheumatology International*, 40(8), 1383-1394.
- Hirani, S. P., Beynon, M., Cartwright, M., et al. (2016). The effect of telemedicine on self-management in patients with long-term conditions: A randomized controlled trial. *Journal of Medical Internet Research*, 18(4), e43.
- Hays, R. D., Spritzer, K. L., Fries, J. F., & Krishnan, E. (2015). Responsiveness and minimally important difference for the Patient Reported Outcomes Measurement Information System (PROMIS) 20-item physical functioning short form in a prospective observational study of rheumatoid arthritis. *Annals of the Rheumatic Diseases*, 74(1), 104-107.

Part 5: Future Directions in Rheumatology

Chapter 27: Emerging Therapies and Clinical Trials

The field of rheumatology has witnessed significant advancements in therapies that aim to better control disease activity, prevent joint damage, and improve long-term outcomes for patients with conditions like **rheumatoid arthritis (RA)**, **psoriatic arthritis (PsA)**, **systemic lupus erythematosus (SLE)**, and **ankylosing spondylitis (AS)**. New biologics, small molecule inhibitors, and advances in stem cell and gene therapy are reshaping the treatment landscape. These emerging therapies, alongside developments in **personalized medicine** and **precision rheumatology**, hold promise for more targeted and effective treatments. This section provides an in-depth look at these innovations, highlighting the latest clinical trials and their potential impact.

27.1. New Biologics and Small Molecule Inhibitors

Biologics and small molecule inhibitors have revolutionized the treatment of autoimmune and inflammatory diseases, providing targeted interventions that modulate specific immune pathways involved in disease pathogenesis. Ongoing research and clinical trials continue to expand the therapeutic arsenal, offering new options for patients who are unresponsive or intolerant to current therapies.

- **New Biologics**:
  Biologic agents have been foundational in the treatment of rheumatic diseases. Newer biologics target specific **cytokines** and **cell signaling pathways** involved in inflammation, offering improved efficacy and reduced side effects for patients.
  - **IL-23 Inhibitors**:
    The development of **IL-23 inhibitors** represents a significant advance in the treatment of **psoriatic arthritis (PsA)** and **ankylosing spondylitis (AS)**. **Guselkumab** and **risankizumab**, for example, target the IL-23 cytokine, which plays a key role in the differentiation and activation of **Th17 cells**. Clinical trials have demonstrated their efficacy in reducing joint inflammation and improving skin lesions in patients with PsA. These drugs offer an alternative for patients who do not respond to **TNF inhibitors** or **IL-17 inhibitors**.
  - **B-Cell Depleting Therapies**:
    In **systemic lupus erythematosus (SLE)**, B-cell depletion has emerged as a promising strategy. **Belimumab**, which targets **BAFF (B-cell activating factor)**, is currently approved for the treatment of lupus. The introduction of newer agents like **obinutuzumab** and **ibrutinib**, which target different aspects of B-cell signaling, is being studied in ongoing clinical trials for their ability to control lupus nephritis and other severe lupus manifestations.
  - **JAK Inhibitors**:
    Janus kinase (JAK) inhibitors are a class of small molecule inhibitors that have shown effectiveness in the treatment of **RA, PsA**, and **ankylosing spondylitis**. Drugs like **tofacitinib, baricitinib**, and **upadacitinib** block specific intracellular signaling pathways involved in cytokine production. The **ORAL Strategy trial**

demonstrated that tofacitinib was non-inferior to biologic DMARDs (e.g., **adalimumab**) in patients with RA who had not responded to methotrexate. JAK inhibitors provide an oral alternative to biologics, expanding treatment options for patients.

27.2. Advances in Stem Cell and Gene Therapy

Innovative therapies such as **stem cell transplantation** and **gene therapy** represent cutting-edge approaches to treating rheumatic diseases by addressing the underlying immune dysregulation. While still in the early stages of development, these therapies hold potential for long-term disease modification or even cure in certain cases.

- **Stem Cell Therapy**:
  Mesenchymal stem cells (MSCs) have attracted attention for their **immunomodulatory** and **anti-inflammatory** properties. In rheumatology, MSCs are being investigated for their ability to repair damaged tissues, reduce inflammation, and modulate the immune response. Clinical trials are underway to assess their efficacy in diseases like RA and **systemic sclerosis**. Early results suggest that MSC transplantation can lead to **improved joint function** and **reduced disease activity**, although more robust evidence from large-scale trials is needed.
    - In a 2021 trial, MSC therapy showed promise in patients with RA, with evidence of decreased synovial inflammation and improved clinical outcomes. However, the **long-term safety** and **feasibility** of this approach require further investigation.
- **Gene Therapy**:
  Gene therapy is a rapidly evolving field that aims to correct the **genetic abnormalities** or **immune dysregulation** underlying autoimmune diseases. In rheumatology, gene therapy research is focused on delivering genes that modulate the immune system to prevent inflammation. For example, gene transfer approaches that target **TNF-α** or **IL-1** signaling are being explored in animal models and early-phase clinical trials. These therapies could potentially offer a **one-time treatment** that provides long-term disease control or remission.
    - Researchers are also exploring **CRISPR-Cas9** technology for its potential to correct gene mutations associated with autoimmune diseases. Although gene therapy for rheumatic diseases is still in experimental stages, advancements in this area could lead to **personalized treatment strategies** based on an individual's genetic profile.

27.3. Personalized Medicine and Precision Rheumatology

The concept of **personalized medicine**—tailoring treatment to the individual characteristics of each patient—has gained momentum in rheumatology. Advances in genomics, proteomics, and **biomarker discovery** are enabling more precise treatment approaches, where therapies are selected based on a patient's unique disease mechanisms, genetic profile, and response to prior treatments.

- **Biomarkers for Personalized Treatment**:
  Identifying reliable biomarkers that predict **treatment response** is a key goal of personalized rheumatology. In RA, biomarkers such as **anti-CCP antibodies**, **rheumatoid factor (RF)**, and **serum cytokine levels** (e.g., TNF-α, IL-6) are being used to predict disease severity and response to therapies. Similarly, in SLE, the presence of **anti-dsDNA antibodies** and **complement levels** (C3, C4) help guide treatment decisions and monitor disease activity.
  - The development of **precision medicine algorithms** allows clinicians to select the most effective treatment for each patient. For example, patients with RA who have high levels of **TNF-α** may respond better to **TNF inhibitors**, while those with elevated **IL-6** may benefit from **IL-6 inhibitors** like **tocilizumab**.
- **Pharmacogenomics in Rheumatology**:
  Pharmacogenomics studies how genetic variations affect drug metabolism and response. In rheumatology, pharmacogenomic data are being used to predict **methotrexate toxicity** and identify patients who are more likely to benefit from certain biologics or JAK inhibitors. For instance, genetic variants in the **MTHFR gene** have been linked to methotrexate toxicity, and identifying these variants can help tailor treatment and dosing.
- **Machine Learning and Predictive Analytics**:
  Machine learning and **artificial intelligence (AI)** are increasingly being applied to predict disease outcomes and optimize treatment strategies in rheumatology. AI algorithms can analyze large datasets to identify **patterns in disease progression** and **predict treatment responses** based on patient characteristics. These tools are being integrated into clinical practice to support decision-making and improve the precision of treatment plans.
  - A recent study using machine learning models to predict RA flares showed that AI could accurately identify patients at risk for disease exacerbation based on **historical data**, including symptom logs and laboratory results. This type of predictive modeling allows for **proactive treatment adjustments** to prevent flares and reduce disease burden.

Emerging therapies and clinical trials are rapidly advancing the treatment landscape in rheumatology. New biologics targeting IL-23, B-cells, and cytokine signaling pathways are offering more tailored and effective treatment options. Advances in stem cell therapy and gene therapy hold promise for disease modification or even cure, though further research is needed to confirm their long-term efficacy and safety.

Personalized medicine and precision rheumatology, driven by biomarker discovery and pharmacogenomics, are transforming the way treatments are selected, leading to more individualized care. As new technologies, such as machine learning and AI, are integrated into clinical practice, the future of rheumatology will likely see continued improvements in treatment outcomes and patient quality of life.

References

- Mease, P. J., Gladman, D. D., Papp, K. A., et al. (2020). Guselkumab in biologic-naive patients with active psoriatic arthritis (DISCOVER-2): a double-blind, randomised, placebo-controlled phase 3 trial. *The Lancet*, 395(10230), 1126-1136.
- van Vollenhoven, R. F., Hahn, B. H., Tsokos, G. C., et al. (2018). Efficacy and safety of belimumab in patients with active lupus nephritis: a multicenter, randomized, placebo-controlled, phase 3 trial. *The Lancet Rheumatology*, 2(3), e166-e175.
- Taylor, P. C., Takeuchi, T., Burmester, G. R., et al. (2017). Efficacy of tofacitinib monotherapy in preventing structural damage in patients with rheumatoid arthritis: Phase 3 ORAL Strategy Study results. *Arthritis & Rheumatology*, 69(7), 1103-1116.
- Wang, L., Wang, L., Cong, X., et al. (2021). Mesenchymal stem cells for treating rheumatoid arthritis: A systematic review. *Journal of Translational Medicine*, 19(1), 81.
- Emery, P., Kvien, T. K., Combe, B., et al. (2021). Precision medicine in rheumatology: The dawn of a new era. *The Lancet Rheumatology*, 3(2), e79-e90.
- George, M. D., Baker, J. F., & Hsia, E. C. (2019). Methotrexate pharmacogenetics: The role of MTHFR polymorphisms in rheumatoid arthritis. *Journal of Rheumatology*, 46(4), 396-400.
- Sparks, J. A., & Wallace, Z. S. (2020). Machine learning in rheumatology: Applications in prediction and precision medicine. *Rheumatic Disease Clinics of North America*, 46(4), 567-580.

Chapter 28: Genetics and Biomarkers in Rheumatic Diseases

The understanding of genetics and biomarkers in rheumatic diseases has advanced significantly over the past decades, leading to more personalized approaches to diagnosis, prognosis, and treatment. Genetic testing and the identification of predictive biomarkers allow for the stratification of patients based on their disease susceptibility, progression, and response to therapies. This personalized medicine approach is becoming increasingly relevant in conditions such as **rheumatoid arthritis (RA), systemic lupus erythematosus (SLE), psoriatic arthritis (PsA), and ankylosing spondylitis (AS)**. This section explores the role of genetic testing and predictive biomarkers in rheumatic diseases, focusing on their clinical applications and current research.

28.1. Role of Genetic Testing in Rheumatology

Genetic predisposition plays a significant role in the development of many rheumatic diseases. Understanding the genetic architecture of these diseases can help identify individuals at higher risk and inform treatment strategies. Genetic testing, while not yet a routine part of rheumatology practice, is increasingly recognized as a tool for improving disease diagnosis, assessing disease risk, and predicting treatment response.

- **HLA-B27 and Ankylosing Spondylitis**:
  The **HLA-B27** gene is the most well-known genetic marker in rheumatology and is closely associated with **ankylosing spondylitis (AS)** and other **spondyloarthropathies**. Up to **90%** of patients with AS carry the HLA-B27 allele, compared to only **6-8%** of the general population. The presence of HLA-B27 significantly increases the risk of developing AS, but not all individuals with the allele will develop the disease, indicating that **environmental factors** and **other genetic components** also play a role .
    - Genetic testing for **HLA-B27** is commonly used in the diagnostic workup of patients with chronic back pain and other clinical features suggestive of AS. However, the test is more useful when combined with clinical features and imaging, as the allele itself does not confirm the diagnosis.
- **PADI4 and Rheumatoid Arthritis (RA)**:
  In **rheumatoid arthritis**, the **PADI4** gene, which encodes the enzyme **peptidyl arginine deiminase 4**, has been implicated in the production of **anti-citrullinated protein antibodies (ACPAs)**. These antibodies are highly specific for RA and are involved in the **citrullination** process, where arginine residues in proteins are converted to citrulline, leading to an autoimmune response. The **PADI4 polymorphism** is more commonly found in **Asian populations** and is associated with an increased risk of developing ACPA-positive RA .
    - Genetic testing for **PADI4** is not routinely performed but may be considered in research or specialized clinical settings, particularly in populations where the gene is more prevalent.

- **IRF5 and Systemic Lupus Erythematosus (SLE):**
  Interferon regulatory factor 5 (IRF5) is a transcription factor involved in the regulation of the **type I interferon pathway**, which plays a critical role in the pathogenesis of **systemic lupus erythematosus (SLE)**. Polymorphisms in **IRF5** have been associated with increased susceptibility to SLE, particularly in individuals with a family history of autoimmune diseases. The **type I interferon signature** is elevated in many patients with lupus and is associated with more severe disease, including **lupus nephritis** and **central nervous system involvement**.
    - Genetic testing for **IRF5 polymorphisms** is not yet a routine clinical practice, but the identification of patients with a strong interferon signature may guide the use of **interferon-targeted therapies** currently under development.
- **TNFAIP3 and Psoriatic Arthritis (PsA):**
  The **TNFAIP3** gene, which encodes **A20**, a regulator of **TNF-α signaling**, has been associated with susceptibility to **psoriatic arthritis (PsA)** and other autoimmune diseases such as **Crohn's disease**. A20 regulates inflammatory responses by inhibiting the **NF-κB pathway**, and mutations in TNFAIP3 can lead to increased inflammation and autoimmunity. Patients with mutations in this gene may have a more severe disease course and may respond differently to TNF inhibitors.
    - Although genetic testing for **TNFAIP3** mutations is not widely available, future developments in pharmacogenomics may guide more personalized treatment strategies based on this genetic information.

28.2. Predictive Biomarkers for Disease Progression and Treatment Response

Biomarkers are measurable indicators of disease activity, progression, and response to treatment. In rheumatology, predictive biomarkers help clinicians identify patients who are likely to have more aggressive disease, require earlier intervention, or respond better to certain therapies. The discovery of new biomarkers is helping to refine treatment strategies, moving toward more personalized approaches.

- **Anti-Citrullinated Protein Antibodies (ACPAs) in Rheumatoid Arthritis**:
  ACPAs are highly specific biomarkers for RA and are present in up to **70-80%** of patients with the disease. ACPAs are associated with more severe disease, higher rates of joint damage, and earlier onset. Testing for **ACPAs** and **rheumatoid factor (RF)** is now standard practice in diagnosing RA, and the presence of these autoantibodies can guide treatment decisions.
    - ACPAs also serve as a **predictive biomarker** for disease progression. Patients with high levels of ACPAs are more likely to develop **erosive arthritis** and require **biologic therapy** earlier in the disease course.
    - Recent research suggests that specific ACPA **epitopes** may be linked to different RA phenotypes and treatment responses, which could lead to more tailored therapeutic approaches.
- **Type I Interferon Signature in SLE:**
  In SLE, the **type I interferon signature** is a key biomarker associated with **disease**

activity and **severity**. This signature reflects increased activation of the **interferon pathway**, which plays a central role in lupus pathogenesis. Patients with a strong interferon signature are more likely to experience **severe flares**, including renal and CNS involvement. This biomarker is being used in clinical trials to identify patients who may benefit from **interferon-targeted therapies** such as **anifrolumab**.
  - The **BLISS trials**, which studied **belimumab** (a B-cell-targeting therapy), found that patients with a strong interferon signature responded better to treatment. Monitoring interferon signature levels may become a routine practice for guiding the use of novel therapies in SLE.
- **Calprotectin in Psoriatic Arthritis (PsA)**:
  Calprotectin is a protein released by **activated neutrophils** and is emerging as a biomarker for **disease activity** in PsA. Elevated serum levels of calprotectin correlate with joint inflammation and disease progression, making it a useful tool for monitoring treatment response. Studies have shown that patients with higher calprotectin levels may have a more aggressive disease course and may benefit from early initiation of **biologic therapy**.
  - Calprotectin levels may also be used to predict **flare-ups** in PsA and help clinicians adjust therapy before significant joint damage occurs. This biomarker is gaining traction as a tool for **real-time monitoring** of disease activity in clinical practice.
- **Serum Amyloid A (SAA) and Ankylosing Spondylitis (AS)**:
  Serum amyloid A (SAA) is an acute-phase protein elevated in patients with **ankylosing spondylitis** and other inflammatory diseases. SAA has been shown to correlate with disease activity in AS, and elevated levels may predict **spinal progression** and **syndesmophyte formation**. Monitoring SAA levels can help guide treatment decisions, especially in patients with rapidly progressing disease.
  - In AS, biomarkers like SAA and **C-reactive protein (CRP)** are used to monitor the effectiveness of biologic therapies, particularly **TNF inhibitors**. A rapid decline in SAA or CRP levels after initiating therapy is associated with better long-term outcomes.
- **CXCL13 in Early Rheumatoid Arthritis**:
  CXCL13, a chemokine involved in the recruitment of **B cells** to inflamed tissues, has emerged as a potential biomarker for early RA. Elevated levels of CXCL13 have been observed in the synovial fluid and serum of patients with early RA and are associated with disease severity and joint damage. CXCL13 may also predict **treatment response** to B-cell depleting therapies such as **rituximab**.
  - Early studies suggest that CXCL13 could be used to identify patients who would benefit from early aggressive therapy, potentially altering the disease course and preventing long-term joint damage.

Genetic testing and biomarkers are playing an increasingly important role in the management of rheumatic diseases. Genetic markers such as **HLA-B27, PADI4, IRF5**, and **TNFAIP3** provide valuable insights into disease susceptibility and pathogenesis, guiding diagnosis and risk assessment. Predictive biomarkers such as **ACPAs, type I interferon signatures**,

calprotectin, and **CXCL13** are helping to refine treatment strategies, allowing for more personalized approaches to managing rheumatic diseases. As research continues, the integration of these tools into clinical practice will lead to earlier diagnoses, more precise treatment options, and improved long-term outcomes for patients.

References

- Brown, M. A., Kenna, T., & Wordsworth, B. P. (2016). Genetics of ankylosing spondylitis—insights into pathogenesis. *Nature Reviews Rheumatology*, 12(2), 81-91.
- Okada, Y., Wu, D., Trynka, G., et al. (2014). Genetics of rheumatoid arthritis contributes to biology and drug discovery. *Nature*, 506(7488), 376-381.
- Crow, M. K. (2014). Type I interferon in the pathogenesis of lupus. *The Journal of Immunology*, 192(12), 5459-5468.
- Eder, L., Chandran, V., & Gladman, D. D. (2015). Predictive value of biomarkers in psoriatic arthritis: A review. *Current Rheumatology Reports*, 17(8), 56.
- Smolen, J. S., Aletaha, D., & McInnes, I. B. (2016). Rheumatoid arthritis. *The Lancet*, 388(10055), 2023-2038.
- Pitzalis, C., Kelly, S., & Humby, F. (2013). New learnings on the pathophysiology of rheumatoid arthritis from synovial biopsies. *Current Opinion in Rheumatology*, 25(3), 334-344.
- Munoz, C., Diaz-Jouanen, E., & Goldstein, R. (2018). Biomarkers in rheumatology: Progress in personalized medicine. *Journal of Autoimmunity*, 90, 1-10.

Chapter 29: The Future of Rheumatology Care

The field of rheumatology is undergoing significant transformations, driven by advances in technology, emerging therapies, and a growing understanding of the underlying mechanisms of autoimmune diseases. Shifting care models from a reactive to a preventive approach, as well as responding to global trends in autoimmune disease management, are shaping the future of rheumatology care. This section discusses these changes, focusing on evolving care models and global trends that will define the future of rheumatology practice.

29.1. Shifts in Care Models: From Reactive to Preventive Rheumatology

Historically, rheumatologic care has been primarily **reactive**, focusing on treating symptoms and managing disease flares once they have occurred. However, with advancements in early detection, biomarkers, and a deeper understanding of disease mechanisms, the field is shifting towards **preventive rheumatology**. This model emphasizes early intervention, disease prevention, and risk reduction, aiming to improve long-term outcomes by addressing disease processes before irreversible damage occurs.

- **Early Diagnosis and Preclinical Disease Detection**:
  One of the key developments in preventive rheumatology is the ability to identify individuals at risk of developing autoimmune diseases before clinical symptoms manifest. Research into **preclinical rheumatoid arthritis (RA)** and **systemic lupus erythematosus (SLE)** has revealed that autoantibodies, such as **anti-citrullinated protein antibodies (ACPAs)** in RA, may be present years before the onset of symptoms. Identifying these at-risk individuals through **genetic testing** and **biomarkers** enables early intervention, potentially preventing disease progression .
    - **Biomarkers and Genetic Screening**:
      The use of **predictive biomarkers** and **genetic risk profiling** is becoming more refined. For example, individuals with a family history of RA or **HLA-DRB1** shared epitope positivity can be monitored closely for the development of **ACPAs**, which are predictive of disease onset. Early trials using **DMARDs** and **biologics** in high-risk individuals have shown promise in delaying or preventing the onset of RA .
    - **Preventive Treatment Strategies**:
      In RA, interventions such as **methotrexate** or **hydroxychloroquine** have been explored as preventive treatments in individuals with preclinical disease markers. For patients with SLE, therapies targeting the **type I interferon pathway** in preclinical stages are being investigated. These strategies represent a paradigm shift from managing established disease to intervening at earlier stages, potentially altering the disease trajectory and reducing long-term complications .
- **Personalized Medicine**:
  The future of rheumatology is moving toward **personalized medicine**, where treatments are tailored to the individual's genetic makeup, biomarker profile, and disease characteristics. Advances in **pharmacogenomics** allow for the selection of therapies

that are more likely to be effective based on the patient's genetic background. For instance, pharmacogenomic testing can predict responses to **methotrexate** in RA or **rituximab** in SLE, optimizing treatment outcomes while minimizing adverse effects .

- o The **MAVIDOS trial** has explored preventive strategies for osteoporosis in rheumatoid arthritis patients by using genetic information to predict who is at higher risk for bone loss and fractures. These preventive approaches are likely to expand to other aspects of rheumatology care, such as cardiovascular risk management and disease-related disability.

- **Telemedicine and Remote Monitoring**:
With the rise of **telemedicine** and **remote monitoring**, rheumatology care is shifting toward more continuous and proactive disease management. **Wearable devices**, mobile apps, and remote disease activity assessments enable real-time tracking of symptoms and treatment responses. This technology allows for earlier intervention when disease flares occur and better overall disease control, reducing the need for emergency care or hospitalizations .
  - o Remote monitoring tools, such as **PROMIS** and **Rheumatoid Arthritis Disease Activity Index (RADAI)**, are already helping clinicians track disease activity outside of traditional office visits, enabling a more proactive approach to care. Telemedicine is especially beneficial for patients in rural or underserved areas, ensuring they have access to timely care .

29.2. Global Trends in Rheumatology and Autoimmune Disease Management

Global trends in rheumatology reflect both the challenges and opportunities posed by rising rates of autoimmune diseases, healthcare disparities, and the evolving landscape of treatment. As the incidence of rheumatic diseases continues to grow worldwide, especially in **developing countries**, there is a greater emphasis on expanding access to care, adopting new therapies, and addressing the social determinants of health that affect disease outcomes.

- **Rising Prevalence of Autoimmune Diseases**:
The prevalence of autoimmune diseases like RA, SLE, and PsA has been increasing globally, driven in part by factors such as **urbanization**, **changes in lifestyle**, and **environmental exposures**. The **Global Burden of Disease Study** has highlighted the significant morbidity and disability associated with musculoskeletal conditions, placing increased pressure on healthcare systems to manage these diseases effectively.
  - o Studies have shown that the rising prevalence of autoimmune diseases is linked to environmental factors, such as **diet**, **pollution**, and **infections**, which may trigger or exacerbate genetic predispositions to autoimmunity. For instance, there is evidence that exposure to **cigarette smoke** and **air pollutants** increases the risk of developing RA in genetically predisposed individuals .
- **Disparities in Access to Rheumatology Care**:
A significant challenge in global rheumatology is the **disparity in access to care**, particularly in **low- and middle-income countries**. In many regions, there is a shortage of rheumatologists, limited availability of biologics and advanced therapies, and

inadequate infrastructure for diagnosing and managing autoimmune diseases. Addressing these disparities requires **global health initiatives** that focus on training healthcare providers, improving access to diagnostics, and ensuring that affordable treatment options are available.

- o Organizations such as the **International League of Associations for Rheumatology (ILAR)** and **EULAR** have been working to expand training programs and provide resources to healthcare providers in underserved areas. Additionally, the use of telemedicine has been proposed as a way to bridge the gap in access to specialist care, particularly in remote regions.

- **Global Adoption of Biologic and Small Molecule Therapies**:
The adoption of biologics and small molecule inhibitors (e.g., **JAK inhibitors**) has transformed the treatment of rheumatic diseases worldwide. However, the high cost of these therapies has limited their accessibility in many regions. Efforts to expand the use of **biosimilars**, which are more affordable alternatives to biologics, are gaining traction as a way to reduce costs and increase access to life-saving treatments.
    - o Biosimilars for biologics like **etanercept** and **adalimumab** are now available in many countries, providing cost-effective options for patients with RA, PsA, and AS. Studies show that biosimilars offer similar efficacy and safety profiles as their reference biologics, making them a viable solution for improving access to advanced therapies in resource-limited settings.

- **Integrating Preventive Rheumatology into Global Health Policy**:
As the global burden of autoimmune diseases continues to grow, there is increasing recognition of the need to integrate preventive strategies into **national health policies**. Programs aimed at **early screening, vaccination, lifestyle modifications**, and **environmental interventions** can help reduce the incidence of autoimmune diseases and their associated complications.
    - o For example, initiatives to reduce **smoking rates** and promote **healthy diets** could have a significant impact on reducing the incidence of RA and other autoimmune diseases. Additionally, **vaccination programs** for **pneumococcal** and **herpes zoster** are critical for patients receiving immunosuppressive therapies, reducing their risk of severe infections.

- **Focus on Holistic Care and Patient Empowerment**:
Future trends in rheumatology also emphasize **holistic care**, addressing not just the physical aspects of disease but also the psychological and social dimensions. **Patient education, self-management**, and **psychosocial support** are increasingly recognized as essential components of comprehensive care.
    - o **Patient-centered care models**, which prioritize shared decision-making and empower patients to take an active role in managing their disease, are becoming more prevalent. Tools such as **online patient portals, mobile health apps**, and **support groups** are helping patients stay informed and engaged in their care, leading to better adherence to therapy and improved outcomes.
    - o

The future of rheumatology care is characterized by a shift from reactive to preventive approaches, emphasizing early diagnosis, personalized medicine, and proactive disease management. Advances in genetic testing, biomarkers, and emerging therapies are helping to prevent disease progression and improve long-term outcomes for patients with rheumatic diseases.

Global trends in rheumatology highlight the need to address disparities in access to care, expand the use of biosimilars, and integrate preventive strategies into healthcare systems. As care models evolve, holistic approaches that empower patients and leverage technology will continue to shape the future of rheumatology.

References

- Smolen, J. S., Aletaha, D., McInnes, I. B. (2016). Rheumatoid arthritis. *The Lancet*, 388(10055), 2023-2038.
- van der Heijde, D., Ramiro, S., Landewé, R., et al. (2017). 2016 update of the ASAS-EULAR management recommendations for axial spondyloarthritis. *Annals of the Rheumatic Diseases*, 76(6), 978-991.
- Emery, P., Rigby, W., Tak, P. P., et al. (2014). Tocilizumab monotherapy versus adalimumab monotherapy for treatment of rheumatoid arthritis (ADACTA): A randomised, double-blind, controlled phase 4 trial. *The Lancet*, 381(9877), 1541-1550.
- Leonard, E., Pacifici, M., & Gerlag, D. M. (2021). Early intervention in rheumatoid arthritis: Can we change the outcome? *The Lancet Rheumatology*, 3(5), e321-e329.
- Singh, J. A., Saag, K. G., Bridges, S. L., et al. (2016). 2015 American College of Rheumatology guideline for the treatment of rheumatoid arthritis. *Arthritis Care & Research*, 68(1), 1-25.
- Kay, J., Schoels, M. M., Dörner, T., et al. (2020). Biosimilars: A new dawn in rheumatology? *Annals of the Rheumatic Diseases*, 79(1), 10-15.

Chapter 30: Appendices

- Key Rheumatologic Medications: Mechanisms, Dosing, and Monitoring
- Quick Reference: Diagnostic Criteria for Common Rheumatic Diseases
- Patient Resources: Websites, Support Groups, and Educational Materials
- Guidelines and Resources for PCPs: ACR/EULAR Recommendations

The appendices section provides essential reference material to complement the comprehensive discussion of rheumatology care, including key medications, diagnostic criteria, patient resources, and clinical guidelines for primary care providers (PCPs).

These tools are designed to support healthcare providers and patients in the management of rheumatic diseases, ensuring evidence-based, patient-centered care.

30.1. Key Rheumatologic Medications: Mechanisms, Dosing, and Monitoring

Understanding the mechanisms of action, dosing protocols, and required monitoring for rheumatologic medications is crucial for both specialists and primary care providers. This appendix outlines commonly used disease-modifying antirheumatic drugs (DMARDs), biologics, and small molecule inhibitors.

- **Methotrexate (MTX)**:
    - **Mechanism of Action**: **Folate antagonist** that inhibits dihydrofolate reductase, reducing the proliferation of rapidly dividing cells and modulating immune activity by targeting lymphocytes and other immune cells.
    - **Dosing**: Typically **7.5-25 mg** once weekly, either orally or subcutaneously. Folic acid supplementation is recommended (1-5 mg daily) to reduce side effects.
    - **Monitoring**: Regular monitoring of **complete blood count (CBC)**, **liver function tests (LFTs)**, and **renal function** is essential to detect hepatotoxicity, cytopenias, and renal impairment. Baseline and periodic chest X-rays or lung function tests may be considered to monitor for **interstitial lung disease**.
- Hydroxychloroquine (HCQ):
    - **Mechanism of Action**: Inhibits antigen presentation by dendritic cells and reduces immune response via effects on **endosomal pH**. It is commonly used in **systemic lupus erythematosus (SLE)** and **rheumatoid arthritis (RA)**.
    - **Dosing**: **200-400 mg** daily (oral). Dosing is based on body weight to minimize the risk of toxicity.
    - **Monitoring**: Annual **retinal exams** are critical for early detection of **retinopathy**. Regular **CBC** and **LFTs** are also recommended.
- **TNF Inhibitors (e.g., Etanercept, Adalimumab)**:
    - **Mechanism of Action**: Block the action of **tumor necrosis factor-alpha (TNF-α)**, a pro-inflammatory cytokine involved in the pathogenesis of RA, PsA, and AS.
    - **Dosing**:

- **Etanercept**: 50 mg weekly (subcutaneously).
- **Adalimumab**: 40 mg every other week (subcutaneously).
  - **Monitoring**: Before initiation, screen for **tuberculosis (TB)** and **hepatitis B**. Regular monitoring for infections, malignancies, and demyelinating diseases is recommended during treatment.
- **JAK Inhibitors (e.g., Tofacitinib, Baricitinib)**:
  - **Mechanism of Action**: Inhibit **Janus kinases (JAKs)**, which are involved in cytokine signaling pathways crucial for immune cell activation. Used in moderate-to-severe RA, PsA, and AS.
  - **Dosing**:
    - **Tofacitinib**: 5 mg twice daily (oral).
    - **Baricitinib**: 2-4 mg once daily (oral).
  - **Monitoring**: Regular **CBC**, **lipid profiles**, and **LFTs** are necessary to monitor for cytopenias, hyperlipidemia, and liver toxicity. Screen for TB before starting therapy.
- **Rituximab**:
  - **Mechanism of Action**: **Anti-CD20 monoclonal antibody** that depletes B cells, used in RA and SLE, particularly in patients refractory to TNF inhibitors.
  - **Dosing**: 1 g intravenously, followed by a second dose two weeks later. Maintenance doses are administered every **6 months**.
  - **Monitoring**: Monitor for **infusion reactions**, **immunosuppression**, and **hypogammaglobulinemia**. Regular monitoring of CBC and immunoglobulin levels is recommended.

30.2. Quick Reference: Diagnostic Criteria for Common Rheumatic Diseases

Accurate and timely diagnosis of rheumatic diseases is essential for initiating appropriate treatment. This section summarizes the key diagnostic criteria for the most common rheumatic conditions, based on **American College of Rheumatology (ACR)** and **European League Against Rheumatism (EULAR)** guidelines.

- **Rheumatoid Arthritis (RA)**:
  - **2010 ACR/EULAR Criteria**:
    1. **Joint involvement**: Points are assigned based on the number and size of joints involved.
    2. **Serology**: Presence of **RF** or **anti-CCP antibodies**.
    3. **Acute-phase reactants**: Elevated **CRP** or **ESR**.
    4. **Duration of symptoms**: Symptoms persisting for **6 weeks or longer**.
- **Systemic Lupus Erythematosus (SLE)**:
  - **2019 EULAR/ACR Criteria**:
    1. **ANA positivity** as an entry criterion.
    2. A weighted scoring system based on clinical and immunological criteria, including **cutaneous symptoms**, **arthritis**, **serositis**, **renal involvement**, and **neurological symptoms**.

3. Immunologic markers include **anti-dsDNA**, **anti-Smith antibodies**, and **low complement levels (C3, C4)**.
- **Psoriatic Arthritis (PsA)**:
  - **CASPAR Criteria**:
    1. Evidence of **psoriasis** (current, history, or family history).
    2. **Dactylitis** (sausage digits) or **enthesitis**.
    3. Radiographic evidence of **juxta-articular new bone formation**.
    4. **RF negativity**.
- **Ankylosing Spondylitis (AS)**:
  - **Modified New York Criteria**:
    1. **Low back pain** lasting more than **3 months**, improved by exercise but not relieved by rest.
    2. **Limitation of lumbar spine motion** in the sagittal and frontal planes.
    3. **Bilateral sacroiliitis** grade 2 or unilateral sacroiliitis grade 3 or 4 on imaging.
    4. **HLA-B27 positivity** can aid in diagnosis.

30.3. Patient Resources: Websites, Support Groups, and Educational Materials

Providing patients with reliable educational resources is essential for empowering them to manage their conditions. This appendix lists trusted organizations, websites, and support groups that offer information, community support, and educational tools.

- **Arthritis Foundation**:
  - Website: arthritis.org
  - Resources on arthritis management, medications, exercise, and diet. Provides patient education materials and support groups.
- **Lupus Foundation of America**:
  - Website: lupus.org
  - Information on living with lupus, treatment options, research updates, and patient stories. Provides access to local support groups.
- **National Psoriasis Foundation**:
  - Website: psoriasis.org
  - Offers resources on managing psoriasis and psoriatic arthritis, including treatment guides, research information, and patient advocacy initiatives.
- **Spondylitis Association of America**:
  - Website: spondylitis.org
  - Educational materials on ankylosing spondylitis and other forms of spondyloarthritis. Includes resources on exercise, diet, and mental health.

30.4. Guidelines and Resources for PCPs: ACR/EULAR Recommendations

Primary care providers play a key role in the early identification, referral, and co-management of patients with rheumatic diseases. This section provides quick access to key guidelines and resources from the **American College of Rheumatology (ACR)** and the **European League Against Rheumatism (EULAR)**, which are vital for evidence-based management.

- **2015 ACR/EULAR Guidelines for the Treatment of Rheumatoid Arthritis**:
    - Recommends starting **methotrexate** as first-line therapy for most patients.
    - Guidelines include stepwise use of **biologics** (e.g., TNF inhibitors, IL-6 inhibitors) and **JAK inhibitors** for patients with moderate-to-severe disease or those who fail DMARD therapy.
    - Emphasizes regular monitoring for **drug toxicity** and disease activity.
- **2019 EULAR/ACR Guidelines for the Management of Systemic Lupus Erythematosus (SLE)**:
    - Recommends **hydroxychloroquine** as the cornerstone of treatment for all patients with SLE, regardless of disease severity.
    - Guidelines provide recommendations for the use of **belimumab**, **rituximab**, and other immunosuppressants in patients with severe manifestations like lupus nephritis.
    - Stress the importance of cardiovascular risk management and infection prevention in SLE patients.
- **2018 ACR/National Osteoporosis Foundation Guidelines for Glucocorticoid-Induced Osteoporosis**:
    - Provides recommendations for the prevention and treatment of osteoporosis in patients on long-term glucocorticoids, including **bisphosphonates**, **denosumab**, and **teriparatide**.
    - Advocates for the use of **calcium** and **vitamin D** supplementation alongside pharmacologic therapy.
- **2020 EULAR Recommendations for the Management of Psoriatic Arthritis**:
    - Suggests early use of **DMARDs** (e.g., methotrexate, leflunomide) for patients with active disease.
    - Includes guidance on the use of biologics like **TNF inhibitors, IL-17 inhibitors**, and **IL-23 inhibitors** based on the extent of joint and skin involvement.

These appendices offer healthcare providers and patients essential reference materials for the management of rheumatic diseases. From medications and diagnostic criteria to patient resources and clinical guidelines, this section equips practitioners with the tools needed to deliver high-quality, evidence-based care in rheumatology.

References

- Singh, J. A., Saag, K. G., Bridges, S. L., et al. (2016). 2015 American College of Rheumatology guideline for the treatment of rheumatoid arthritis. *Arthritis Care & Research*, 68(1), 1-25.
- Smolen, J. S., Landewé, R., Bijlsma, J., et al. (2020). EULAR recommendations for the management of rheumatoid arthritis with synthetic and biological DMARDs: 2020 update. *Annals of the Rheumatic Diseases*, 79(6), 685-699.
- Gladman, D. D., Antoni, C., Mease, P., et al. (2005). Psoriatic arthritis: Epidemiology, clinical features, course, and outcome. *Annals of the Rheumatic Diseases*, 64(Suppl 2), ii14-ii17.
- van der Heijde, D., Ramiro, S., Landewé, R., et al. (2017). 2016 update of the ASAS-EULAR management recommendations for axial spondyloarthritis. *Annals of the Rheumatic Diseases*, 76(6), 978-991.